D0204592

Controversies
in
Food and Nutrition

The Greenwood Press **Contemporary Controversies series** is designed to provide high school and college students with one-volume reference sources that each explore controversies in seven specific areas important to contemporary life: sports, music, entertainment, medicine, education, business, and law. Students will discover that difficult problems occur across disciplines, that they manifest themselves in many different ways, and that not all of these problems have easy answers. The series' unique focus on those in high-profile professions is designed to help readers consider the importance of ethics in all sectors of society. Students will be encouraged to develop their critical thinking by examining the history of these topics, exploring various solutions and drawing their own conclusions.

Other Titles in Contemporary Controversies

Controversies of the Sports World
Douglas Putnam

Controversies in the Practice of Medicine
Myrna Chandler Goldstein and Mark A. Goldstein, M.D.

Controversies of the Music Industry
Richard D. Barnet and Larry L. Burriss

Controversies
in
Food and Nutrition

Myrna Chandler Goldstein
and Mark A. Goldstein, M.D.

Contemporary Controversies

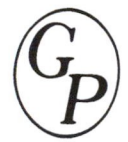

GREENWOOD PRESS
Westport, Connecticut • London

Library of Congress Cataloging-in-Publication Data

Goldstein, Myrna Chandler, 1948–
    Controversies in food and nutrition / Myrna Chandler Goldstein and Mark
  A. Goldstein, M.D.
        p.   cm.—(Contemporary controversies, ISSN 1522–2047)
    ISBN 0–313–31787–9 (alk. paper)
    1. Food.   2. Nutrition.   I. Goldstein, Mark A. (Mark Allan), 1947–
  II. Title.   III. Series.
  TX355.5.G65   2002
  641.3—dc21   2002069605

British Library Cataloguing in Publication Data is available.

Library of Congress Catalog Card Number: 2002069605
ISBN: 0–313–31787–9
ISSN: 1522–2047

First published in 2002

Greenwood Press, 88 Post Road West, Westport, CT 06881
An imprint of Greenwood Publishing Group, Inc.
www.greenwood.com

Printed in the United States of America

The paper used in this book complies with the
Permanent Paper Standard issued by the National
Information Standards Organization (Z39.48–1984).

10 9 8 7 6 5 4 3 2 1

In Loving Memory

Craig Abraham Chandler
March 18, 1920–December 22, 1994

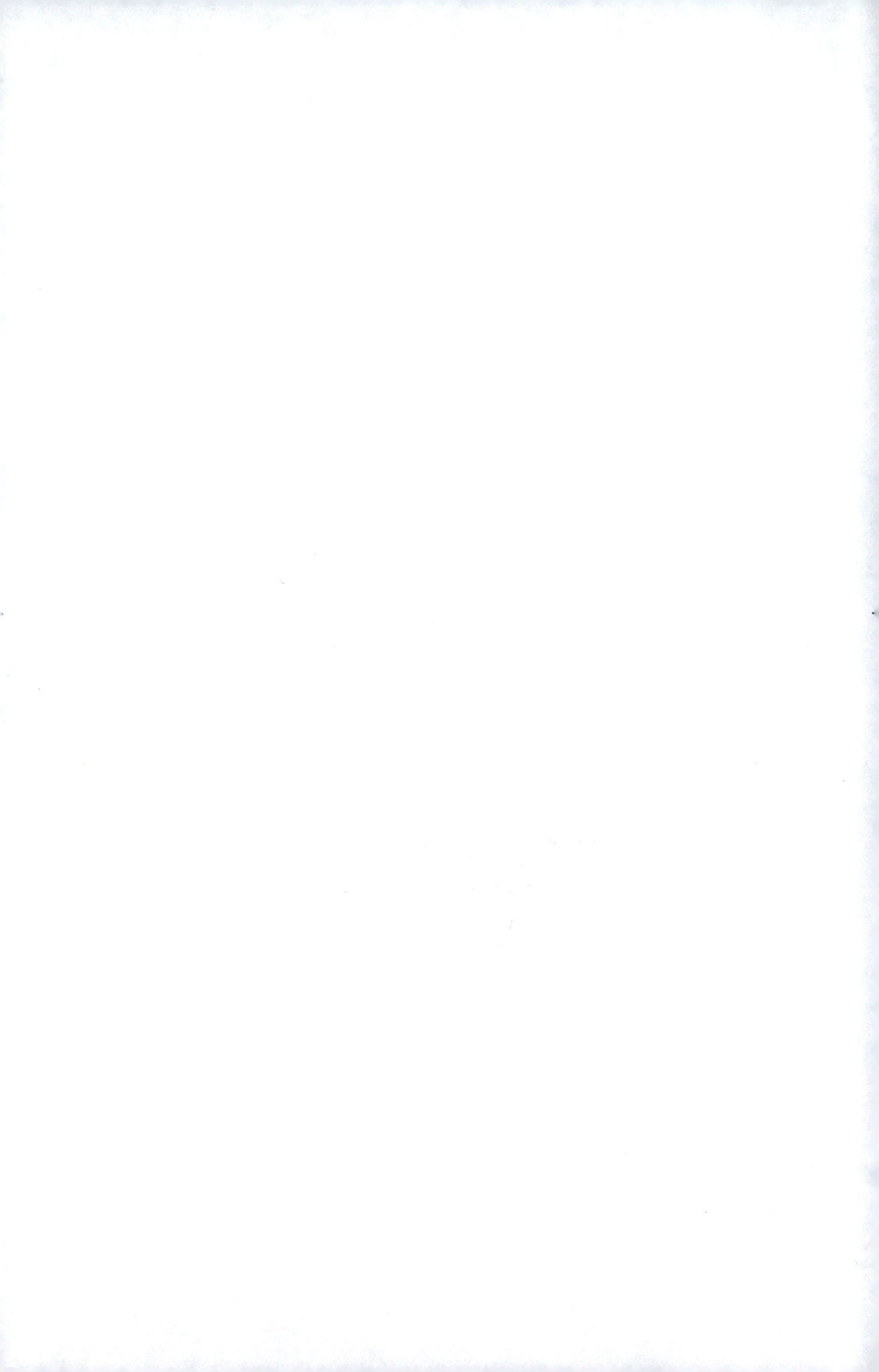

Contents

Acknowledgments

First and foremost, I would like to thank Mark A. Goldstein, M.D., my husband and coauthor. Researching and writing a scholarly book is a monumental task. It is extraordinarily helpful to have someone to share ideas and provide continuous input. Of course, like many other physicians, Mark is a superb editor whose editorial skills proved invaluable on a number of occasions.

I must also thank Emily Birch, our former editor. It was pure joy to work with Emily. When we signed the contract to write this book, Mark and I had already written two other books with Emily. Not surprisingly, in view of her many talents, about midway through this book, Greenwood asked Emily to direct a new division of the company. It could not have been easy for Debby Adams, her successor, to step into Emily's shoes, but she has carefully and conscientiously reviewed all the remaining chapters and offered important insights. Since our first exchange, it has always been evident how strongly Debby is committed and dedicated to her work.

Finally, I need to thank the librarians at our local library in Lincoln, Massachusetts. They connected the library's database to my home office. That enabled me to conduct a large portion of my research from my home. Thanks to the interlibrary loan system, the librarians obtained the countless numbers of books that I required. I truly appreciate how graciously the librarians have fulfilled my seemingly endless number of requests.

I have dedicated this book to my father, Craig Abraham Chandler. Though he died before my first book was published in 1996, he always felt enormous pride in my writings and other accomplishments. I am quite certain that he could be thrilled to know that this work is written in his memory.

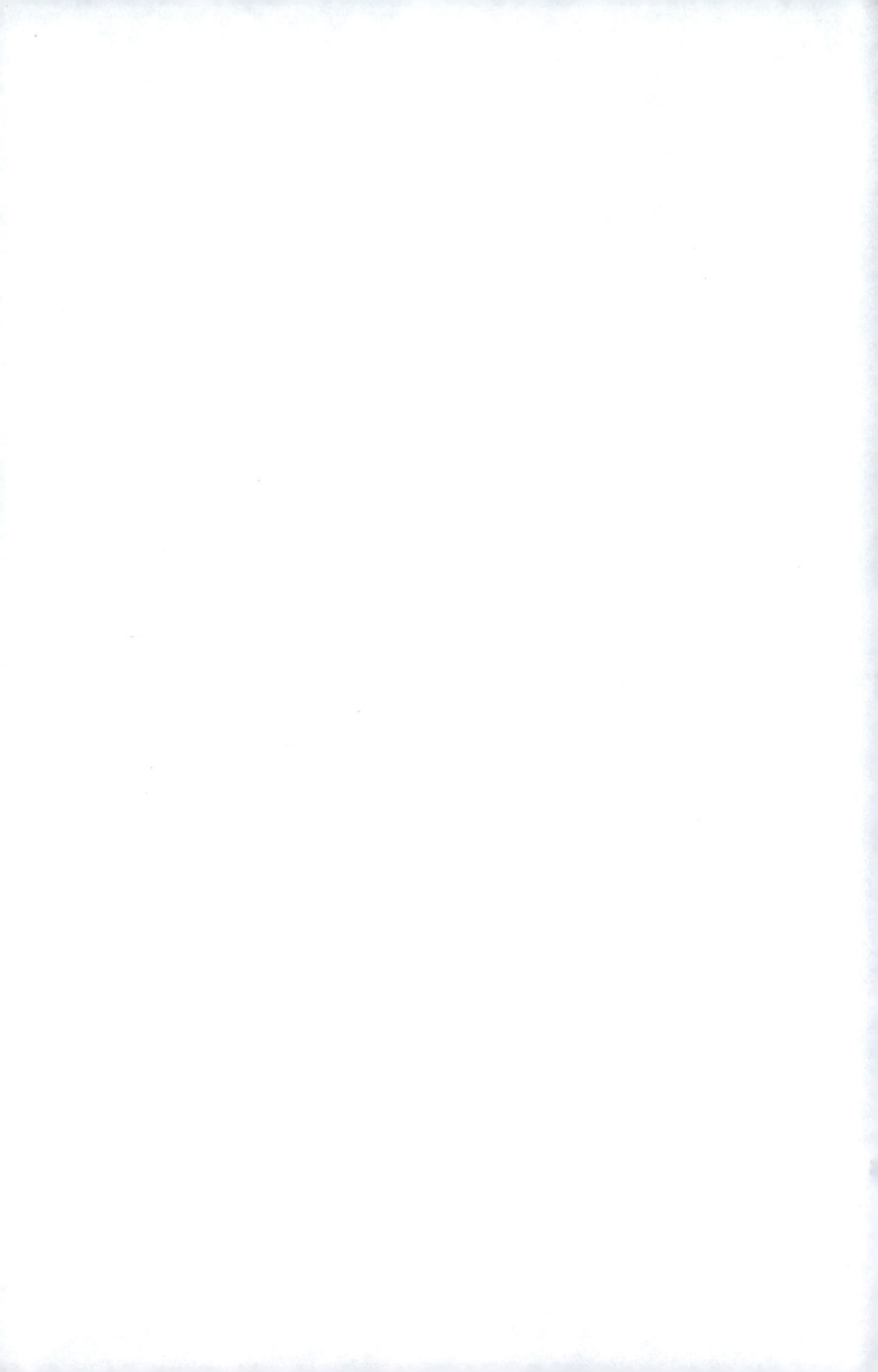

Introduction

Society is bombarded with messages about food and nutrition. These messages often conflict with one another. One expert may tell us that food irradiation is perfectly safe and should be used far more often to preserve the safety and integrity of our foods. Another expert may question whether exposing food to radiation places people who eat the food at risk for certain illnesses. In a country that is dealing with record rates of obesity, none of the experts agree on the best way to lose weight. Should one eat a diet that is high in protein and low in carbohydrates or one high in carbohydrates and low in protein? Should one eat foods only in certain combinations, or cut out meat entirely? The average consumer is at a clear disadvantage. It is not easy to sort through the options and opinions.

While there are a seemingly endless number of food and nutrition controversies, this book has focused on just fifteen. We attempted to select those concerns that were most commonly discussed in the media and that would be of interest to most people. The chapters are designed to serve as introductions, presenting the various sides of the controversies. Each of the topics has been studied extensively by researchers and continues to be. Many of them have been the subjects of books. If your interest is sparked, you may easily find more resources to review, such as the numerous references listed at the end of each chapter. All the chapters close with listings of Web sites.

1

Food Additives

Foods often contain a host of different additives. Some are considered safe. Others are believed to trigger undesirable reactions in some people. Open your kitchen cabinets. Most of the items inside probably contain some food additives. For example, look at the list of ingredients on the label of a can of chicken noodle soup:

> Chicken broth, enriched penne pasta (semolina, egg whites, niacin, ferrous sulfate, thiamin mononitrate, riboflavin, folic acid), carrots, celery, salt, monosodium glutamate, hydrolyzed corn and soy protein, chicken fat, onion powder, autolyzed yeast extract, parsley, natural flavor.

All these products are contained in one 19-ounce can. Some of them—such as chicken broth, carrots, celery, chicken fat, onion powder, and parsley—are straightforward, but why add monosodium glutamate or hydrolyzed corn and soy protein?

According to the Center for Food Safety and Applied Nutrition of the U.S. Food and Drug Administration, food additives—substances that are usually not eaten alone but are added to other foods—play an important role in enhancing the quality of our food supply. Additives can help keep food wholesome and appealing while it is being transported to markets thousands of miles from where it was grown or manufactured. And, additives that enhance taste, texture, consistency or color can also improve the nutritional value and physical appeal of foods.

Legally, a food additive is "any substance the intended use which results or may reasonably be expected to result—directly or indirectly—in its becoming a component or otherwise affecting the characteristics of any food." As such, the term "includes any substance used in the production, processing, treatment, packaging, transportation or storage of food" (Center for Food Safety and Nutrition Web site).

The Center for Food Safety and Applied Nutrition lists five main reasons for using food additives:

1. To maintain product consistency. Emulsifiers give products a consistent texture and prevent them from separating. Stabilizers and thickeners give smooth uniform texture. Anti-caking agents help substances such as salt to flow freely.

2. To improve or maintain nutritional value. Vitamins and minerals are added to many common foods, such as milk, flour, cereal and margarine to make up for those likely to be lacking in a person's diet or lost in processing. Such fortification and enrichment has helped reduce malnutrition among the U.S. population. All products containing added nutrients must be appropriately labeled.

3. To maintain palatability and wholesomeness. Preservatives retard product spoilage caused by mold, air, bacteria, fungi or yeast. Bacterial contamination can cause foodborne illness, including life-threatening botulism. Antioxidants are preservatives that prevent fats and oils in baked goods and other foods from becoming rancid or developing an off-flavor. They also prevent cut fresh fruits such as apples from turning brown when exposed to air.

4. To prevent leavening or control acidity/alkalinity. Leavening agents that release acids when heated can react with baking soda to help cakes, biscuits and other baked goods to rise during baking. Other additives help modify the acidity and alkalinity of foods for proper flavor, taste and color.

5. To enhance flavor or impart desired color. Many spices and natural synthetic flavors enhance the taste of foods. Colors, likewise, enhance the appearance of certain foods to meet consumer expectations. (Center for Food Safety and Applied Nutrition Web site)

In their book *The Food Jungle*, Nancy and Eduardo Balingasa, professional writers with a special interest in nutrition, health, and fitness, describe two main types of additives. Direct additives are added to food for a definite purpose. Indirect additives are unintentionally added through packaging, storage, or handling. Further, food additives are categorized according to their source. Natural additives are derived from plants and other living sources, and synthetic additives are produced in a laboratory.

Food additives have a long history. The Center for Food Safety and Applied Nutrition says that "our ancestors used salt to preserve meats and fish; added herbs and spices to improve the flavor of foods; preserved fruit with sugar; and pickled cucumbers in a vinegar solution" (Center for Food Safety and Applied Nutrition Web site). In *Additives*, Rhoda Nottridge, a professional writer, comments that "in the 1700s, so many people wanted white bread that bakers added dried, ground-up bones, chalk, and even poisonous white lead. These additives helped make brown bread look whiter" (Nottridge: 5).

Additives are now more regulated. The Federal Food, Drug, and Cosmetic (FD&C) Act of 1938 gave the Food and Drug Administration (FDA) authority over food and food ingredients and defined requirements for truthful labeling of ingredients. "The Food Additives Amendment to the FD&C Act, passed in 1958, requires FDA approval for the use of an additive prior to its inclusion in food. It also requires the manufacturer to prove an additive's safety for the way it will be used" (Center for Food Safety and Applied Nutrition Web site).

There are exemptions. "All substances that FDA or the U.S. Department of Agriculture (USDA) had determined were safe for use in specific food prior to the 1958 amendment were designated as prior-sanctioned substances. Examples of prior-sanctioned substances are sodium nitrite and potassium nitrite used to preserve luncheon meats." Also excluded were foods that were generally recognized as safe (GRAS) "based on their extensive history of use in food before 1958 or based on published scientific evidence" (Center for Food Safety and Applied Nutrition Web site). Hundreds of additives are classified as GRAS. These include products such as salt, sugar, spices, vitamins, and monosodium glutamate.

In 1960, legislation governing color additives was passed. These laws "require dyes used in foods, drugs, cosmetics and certain medical devices to be approved by FDA prior to their marketing. In contrast to food additives, colors in use before the legislation were allowed continued use only if they underwent further testing to confirm their safety. Of the original 200 provisionally listed color additives, 90 have been listed as safe and the remainder have either been removed from use by the FDA or withdrawn by industry" (Center for Food Safety and Applied Nutrition Web site).

Every year, the FDA receives about 100 requests for the approval of food additives. Of these, the vast majority are for indirect additives such as packaging materials. The approval process is comprehensive. A petition for a food or color additive must provide persuasive proof that the proposed additive functions as it is intended. Frequently, animal studies with large doses of the additive have been conducted. There may also have been studies on humans. The FDA reviews a number of factors about the additive, such as the amount that is likely to be consumed and any long-term effects. "Absolute safety of any substance can never be proven. Therefore, [the] FDA must determine if the additive is safe under the proposed conditions of use, based on the best scientific knowledge available. If an additive is approved, FDA issues regulations that may include the types of foods in which it can be used, the maximum amounts to be used, and how it should be identified on food labels" (Center for Food Safety and Applied Nutrition Web site).

Even after a food additive is approved, scrutiny continues by the FDA's Adverse Reaction Monitoring System (ARMS), a program that "monitors and investigates all complaints by individuals or their physicians that are believed to be related to specific foods; food and color additives; or vitamin and mineral supplements. The ARMS computerized database helps officials decide whether reported adverse reactions represent a real public health hazard associated with food, so that appropriate action can be taken" (Center for Food Safety and Applied Nutrition Web site). For example, a small percentage of the population is sensitive to sulfites, which may be added to a variety of foods. When these people consume sulfites, they may experience reactions such as hives, nausea, diarrhea, shortness of breath, or perhaps fatal shock. The FDA has estimated that "one out of 100 people may suffer asthma attacks due to sulfites" (Rowlands and Bregman: 16–18). As a result, in 1986 FDA banned the use of sulfites on fresh fruits and vegetables that are sold or served raw to consumers. When added to packaged and processed foods, sulfites must be noted on the product label (Center for Food Safety and Applied Nutrition Web site). People who are sensitive to sulfites may still be at risk because sulfites may be in unlabeled products, such as bulk foods, or in alcoholic beverages from other countries that do not require labeling (Sussman and Yang: 2834). Similarly, as a result of reports that FD&C Yellow No. 5 or tartrazine, a color additive, caused hives in fewer than 1 out of 10,000 people, whenever it is added to foods or taken internally, it must be listed on the label so that people who may be sensitive can be aware of its presence (Center for Food Safety and Applied Nutrition Web site).

In the early 1970s, studies conducted in the former Soviet Union questioned the safety of Red Dye No. 2, but further tests found no hazards. Although the FDA's tests were inconclusive, interest in Red Dye No. 2 grew when the consumer-oriented Health Research Group petitioned the FDA to ban the color. The FDA's Toxicology Advisory Committee studied numerous reports and concluded that there was no reason for concern but still advised follow-up analysis. After further evaluation, agency scientists decided that there was some evidence that feeding Red Dye No. 2 to female rats increased their incidence of tumors. "There still was no positive proof of either potential danger or safety. FDA ultimately decided to ban the color because it had not been shown to be safe" (Center for Food Safety and Applied Nutrition Web site.).

It should also be mentioned that there are individual differences in responses to additives. Nancy and Eduardo Balingasa write that some

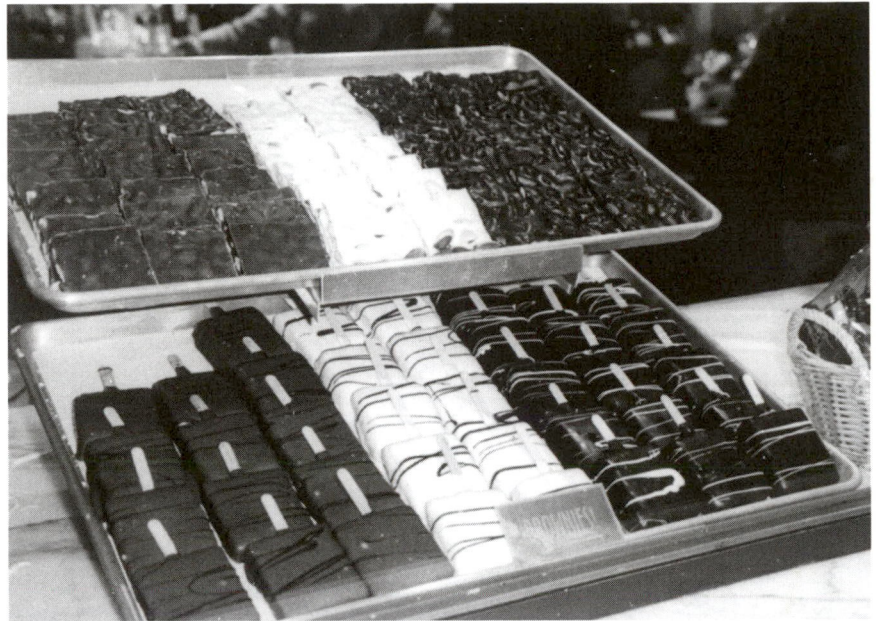

Common foods may have artificial colors and flavors. Photo by Mark A. Goldstein.

products are approved even though they may harm a small number of people. "To protect the consumer, a margin of safety at the level of 1/100th of the harmful amount is set as the limit. Because of myriad differences in our physiological make up, one man's food may be another man's poison" (Balingasa and Balingasa: 23).

In a story that appeared in 2000 in *Insight on the News*, Linda Joyce Forristal described how she ended a day of sightseeing by enjoying a salmon dinner. Within several hours, she was "itching inside and out, as if every blood vessel were dilated." Three days later, she had an even worse reaction when she ate salmon again. After that, she learned that the red coloring of farmed salmon comes from the two food dyes that it is fed—canthaxanthin and astaxanthin. The process is called "color finishing." While Forristal said that there have been no reports of documented allergic reactions, she is clearly sensitive to the additives. In the future, Forristal will eat only wild salmon. These salmon obtain their color naturally from "feeding on colorful crustaceans, plankton and algae" (Forristal: 26–27).

On the average, Americans eat 150 pounds of additives each year (Nottridge: 22), and the vast majority of the almost 3,000 approved food additives appear to generate little or no controversy. Food additives play a pivotal role in improving the taste, safety, and appearance of foods. Generally viewed as safe, additives sometimes serve a positive public health function. For example, the addition of folic acid in cereal grain products caused the level of folic acid found in women of childbearing age to nearly triple in only five years (Charatan: 1176). Women with low levels of folic acid are at greater risk for giving birth to children with neural tube defects. The many vitamins added to bread—hence the term "enriched bread"—have certainly been of enormous benefit, especially to growing children, teens, and the elderly. Likewise, large numbers of products, such as orange juice, that may contain added calcium are helping to prevent future cases of osteoporosis.

Some people have a negative opinion about all additives. "Consumer-protection groups voice concern over some chemical additives' potential health hazards. And a renewed interest in healthy foods had led many food makers to trumpet 'No Additives or Preservatives' on their packages" (Rowlands and Bregman: 16–18). Many people believe that there is a strong relationship between food additives and hyperactivity in children, which may appear in a syndrome known as attention deficit hyperactivity disorder (ADHD). "Children with this disorder are hard to manage, disruptive at home and in the classroom, and they often fail in school. The main symptoms are difficulty concentrating, short attention spans, easy distractibility, excessive activity and impulsiveness." A report issued in 1999 reviewed 23 studies completed since the mid-1970s that examined the relationship between dietary factors and ADHD as well as statements from a number of influential organizations such as the American Academy of Pediatrics. The report found "that for some children, behavioral disorders are caused or aggravated by certain food additives, artificial food colors, the foods themselves or a combination" (Brody: Section F, page 8).

MSG

One of the most controversial additives is monosodium glutamate (MSG). "Monosodium glutamate is the most common form of glutamic acid, one of the building blocks of proteins. Glutamic acid is found in natural, unadulterated foods—and even in the human body—and is not harmful. It's also not a flavor enhancer. It's when glutamic acid is processed to create 'free glutamates' that it becomes a flavor enhancer—and potentially hazardous" (Boyle: Page 1/ZZ1).

The Center for Food Safety and Applied Nutrition states that MSG is a "flavor enhancer in a variety of foods prepared at home, in restaurants, and by food processors." MSG may be found in many different foods. Some of these include canned and dry soups, potato chips, prepared snacks, canned meats, prepared meals, international foods such as Chinese food, diet foods, weight-loss powders, cured and luncheon meats, sauces such as tomato and barbecue sauce, salad dressing, and mayonnaise (Diamond and Moore: 3132). In *The Feel Good Handbook*, Annie Costa, a researcher in the field of nutritional health, notes that "MSG is not like a spice such as salt, oregano or pepper. These lend their own taste to food." Instead, "Its strength is its ability to stimulate receptors in your brain, telling your senses, much like a drug, that what you are tasting is a larger, more robust taste than the food itself might portray on its own" (Costa: 31).

In *The Crazy Makers*, Carol Simontacchi, a certified clinical nutritionist, says that "MSG first appeared when the Japanese added a sea vegetable called kombu to foods to enhance the natural flavors of the food" (Simontacchi: 96). Early in the twentieth century, scientists determined that MSG gave kombu its intense flavors. In response, the Ajinomoto Company began producing MSG and hydrolyzed vegetable protein, which contains MSG, and started exporting it around the world. After World War II, American food-processing companies started adding millions of pounds of MSG to processed foods, including baby foods. The Ajinomoto Company is still the largest producer of MSG in the world.

Research on glutamate—a group of chemicals that includes MSG—has raised questions about its safety. Simontacchi says that "in 1957, two ophthalmologist . . . tested MSG on infant mice to learn if it could be used to treat retinal dystrophy. To their dismay, they found that MSG destroyed the nerve cells in the inner layers of the animal's retinas. Ten years later researcher John Olney, M.D., found that not only was MSG toxic to the retina [in animals] but that specialized cells in the hypothalamus were destroyed as well. . . . The hypothalamus is unprotected by the blood-brain barrier and is therefore susceptible to damage from the influx of toxic materials" (Simontacchi: 96–97).

In *Excitotoxins*, Russell L. Blaylock writes that Olney's "findings should have been earthshaking to say the least. Why? Because millions of babies all over the world were eating baby foods containing large amounts of MSG and hydrolyzed vegetable protein. . . . In fact, the concentrations of MSG found in baby foods was equal to that used to create brain lesions in experimental animals. And in all of these experiments, immature animals were found to be much more vulnerable to the toxic effects of MSG than were older animals" (Blaylock: xix).

According to the Center for Food Safety and Applied Nutrition, "The body uses glutamate, an amino acid, as a nerve impulse transmitter in the brain and . . . there are glutamate-responsive issues in other parts of the body, as well. Abnormal function of glutamate receptors has been linked with certain neurological diseases, such as Alzheimer's disease and Huntington's chorea. Injections of glutamate in laboratory animals have resulted in damage to nerve cells in the brain." The center contends that for most people this does not occur when food is consumed. Still, there are two groups of people who may experience a condition known as MSG symptom complex. One group consists of those who react to MSG when it is eaten in large quantities, and the other group includes people with "severe, poorly controlled asthma" (Center for Food Safety and Applied Nutrition Web site).

Though repeated scientific reviews have demonstrated the safety of MSG, the Adverse Reaction Monitoring System has received hundreds of complaints about the additive. The most common MSG-related symptom was headache. The Center for Food Safety and Applied Nutrition also notes that several books and a TV news show have reported numerous cases of adverse reactions to MSG, even when small amounts were ingested. However, these reports are unconfirmed and have failed to show a clear causal link between MSG and the reactions.

Nevertheless, a comprehensive study completed by the Federation of American Societies for Experimental Biology (FASEB) in the mid-1990s determined that an unknown percentage of the population does indeed react to the ingestion of MSG by developing MSG symptom complex. People with this medical problem may experience one or more of the following symptoms:

- Burning sensation in the back of the neck, forearms, and chest
- Numbness in the back of the neck, radiating to the arms and back
- Tingling, warmth, and weakness in the face, temples, upper back, neck, and arms
- Facial pressure or tightness
- Chest pain
- Headache
- Nausea
- Rapid heartbeat
- Bronchospasm (difficulty breathing) in MSG-intolerant people with asthma
- Drowsiness
- Weakness (Center for Food Safety and Applied Nutrition Web site)

In addition, the FASEB concluded the following:

- In otherwise healthy MSG-intolerant people, the MSG symptom complex tends to occur within one hour after eating 3 grams or more of MSG on an empty stomach or without other food. A typical serving of glutamate-treated food contains less than 0.5 grams of MSG. A reaction is most likely if the MSG is eaten in a large quantity or in a liquid, such as a clear soup.

- Severe, poorly controlled asthma may be a predisposing medical condition for MSG symptom complex.
- No evidence exists to suggest that dietary MSG or glutamate contributes to Alzheimer's disease, Huntington's chorea, amyotropic lateral sclerosis, AIDS dementia complex, or any other long-term or chronic disease.
- No evidence exists to suggest that dietary MSG causes brain lesions or damages nerve cells in humans.
- The level of vitamin B6 in a person's body plays a role in glutamate metabolism, and the possible impact of marginal B6 intake should be considered in future research.
- There is no scientific evidence that the levels of glutamate in hydrolyzed proteins causes adverse effects or that other manufactured glutamate had effects different from glutamate normally found in foods. (Center for Food Safety and Applied Nutrition Web site)

At present, FDA regulations require that MSG be listed in ingredient labels. "While technically MSG is only one of several forms of free glutamate used in foods, consumers frequently use the term MSG to mean all free glutamate. For this reason, FDA considers foods whose labels say 'No MSG' or 'No Added MSG' to be misleading if the food contains ingredients that are sources of free glutamates, such as hydrolyzed protein" (Center for Food Safety and Applied Nutrition Web site). This is a widespread practice. It is also not at all unusual for MSG to be "concealed in dozens of commonly used additives including hydrolyzed soy protein and yeast extract found in many processed foods" (Bonvie and Bonvie: 21). If MSG is added to an ingredient that is listed on the label, for example, hydrolyzed vegetable protein, the food manufacturer does not need to list MSG on the label, even if a large amount of MSG is used (Walsh: 50). A person who is sensitive to MSG may become horribly ill and have absolutely no ability to locate the offending food.

Nevertheless, the FDA has not taken action to require clear and precise labeling for all products that may contain MSG. "In 1994, FDA received a citizen's petition requesting changes in labeling requirements for foods that contain MSG or related substances. The petition asks for mandatory listing of MSG as an ingredient on labels of manufactured and processed foods that contain manufactured free glutamic acid. It further asks that the amount of free glutamic acid or MSG in such products be stated on the label, along with a warning that MSG may be harmful to certain groups of people" (Center for Food Safety and Applied Nutrition Web site). Thus far, there have been no changes in the FDA policy on this issue.

In a multicenter study published in 2000 in the *Journal of Allergy and Clinical Immunology*, researchers tested the response to MSG with or without the consumption of food. "The results suggest that large doses of MSG given without food may elicit more symptoms than a placebo in individuals who believe that they react adversely to MSG. However, neither persistent nor serious effects from MSG ingestion are observed, and the responses were not consistent on retesting" (Geha et al.: 973–980).

However, it is true that some people are extremely sensitive to MSG. A 1997 article in the *Journal of the American Dietetic Association* described a two-year-old boy with "signs and symptoms of uncontrollable seizures of multiple types mimicking that of Lennox-Gastaut syndrome" (Shovic, Bart, and Stalcup: 793–794). Lennox-Gastaut syndrome is a rare form of epilepsy that is unresponsive to antiseizure medications. Eventually, it was decided to place the boy on an MSG-free diet. The seizures ended. After several uneventful months, the boy's mother decided to test the veracity of the diagnosis, and he ate a commercial hot dog. Later in the same week, he ate a bag of chips with MSG. The boy had trouble sleeping and was clumsy in school. He also exhibited behavior problems and urinary incontinence. When the article was published, the boy was seven years old. Remaining on a MSG-free diet, he was healthy and no longer required seizure medication.

Adrienne and Jack Samuels, founders of the Truth in Labeling Campaign, a nonprofit organization in Illinois, also claim that monosodium glutamate is far more insidious than the federal government acknowledges. Years ago, Jack experienced a number of Alzheimer's disease–like symptoms. After reading *In Bad Taste: The MSG Syndrome*, by George R. Schwartz, Adrienne eliminated all processed free glutamic acid from Jack's diet. He improved dramatically. Adrienne also reviewed the literature on the topic. She wrote that she found two kinds of studies. Those sponsored by the glutamate industry invariably concluded that MSG was safe. Those by independent neuroscientists and other researchers found that MSG kills brain cells and causes neuroendocrine disorders, learning disabilities, and various disorders such as tachycardia (rapid heart rate) and seizures (Truth in Labeling Campaign Web site).

The Truth in Labeling Campaign asserts that monosodium glutamate is far more harmful than most people realize and that it is a neurotoxin that is potentially toxic to everyone, even those who do not have obvious adverse reactions. The Truth in Labeling Campaign has compiled the following list of adverse reactions to the ingestion of MSG (this list does not prove cause and effect):

Cardiac
Arrhythmia
Atrial fibrillation
Tachycardia
Rapid heartbeat
Palpitations
Slow heartbeat
Angina
Extreme rise or drop in blood pressure
Circulatory
Swelling
Gastrointestinal
Diarrhea
Nausea/vomiting
Stomach cramps
Irritable bowel
Swelling of hemorrhoids and/or anus area
Rectal bleeding
Bloating
Muscular
Flu-like achiness
Joint pain
Stiffness
Neurological
Depression
Mood swings
Rage reactions
Migraine headaches
Dizziness
Light-headedness
Loss of balance
Mental confusion
Anxiety
Panic attacks
Hyperactivity

Behavioral problems in children

Attention deficit disorders

Lethargy

Sleepiness

Insomnia

Numbness or paralysis

Seizures

Sciatica

Slurred speech

Chills and shakes

Visual

Blurred vision

Difficulty focusing

Pressure around eyes

Respiratory

Asthma

Shortness of breath

Chest pain

Tightness in the chest

Runny nose

Sneezing

Urological/Genital

Swelling of the prostate

Swelling of the vagina

Vaginal spotting

Frequent urination

Nocturia

Skin

Hives (may be both internal and external)

Rash

Mouth lesions

Temporary tightness or partial paralysis (numbness or tingling) of the skin

Flushing

Extreme drying of the mouth

Face swelling

Tongue swelling

Bags under eyes

The Truth in Labeling Campaign notes that these reactions are no more diverse than the side effects of certain neurological drugs. It is not known why some people experience reactions while others do not. It is also not known whether MSG causes the reaction or aggravates some underlying condition. However, all forms of MSG cause these reactions in MSG-sensitive people.

Since MSG is contained in most processed foods, it is not easy to avoid. It is also found in a plant "growth enhancer" called AuxiGro and other fertilizers and fungicides that are sprayed on growing crops. "Processed free glutamic acid (MSG) is hidden in food, drugs, cosmetics, and pesticides.... The glutamate industry must certainly understand ... that if the MSG in food, drugs, and cosmetics was disclosed on the product labels, people who reacted adversely to those products might realize that it was the MSG they were reacting to, and might, therefore, refrain from buying any products that contain MSG" (Truth in Labeling Campaign Web site).

The Truth in Labeling Campaign notes many hidden sources of MSG. The following additives and foods always contain MSG: glutamate, monosodium glutamate, monopotassium glutamate, yeast extract, hydrolyzed protein, glutamic acid, calcium caseinate, sodium caseinate, sodium caseinate, yeast food, gelatin, textured protein, yeast nutrient, and autolyzed yeast. The following items often have MSG or create MSG during processing: carrageenan, natural pork flavoring, bouillon, natural beef flavoring, stock, whey protein concentrate, whey protein, whey protein isolate, flavors, flavorings, natural flavors, natural flavorings, maltodextrin, broth, natural chicken flavoring, anything ultrapasteurized, barley malt, pectin, protease, protease enzymes, anything enzyme modified, enzymes, malt extract, malt flavoring, soy protein isolate, soy protein, soy protein concentrate, anything protein fortified, anything fermented, and seasonings (Truth in Labeling Campaign Web site).

A 1997 article in *JAMA: The Journal of the American Medical Association* suggested that elderly persons who have diminished capacities for taste might benefit from food prepared with flavor enhancers such as MSG. While some express fear of MSG, others advise using it to improve the taste of the food the elderly, even the frail elderly, eat (Schiffman: 1357–1362).

ASPARTAME

Aspartame, a low-calorie sweetener that is sold under the brand names of NutraSweet or Equal, is another controversial food additive. About 200 times sweeter than sugar, it does not cause tooth decay. According to the International Food Information Council, "Aspartame is made by joining two protein components, aspartic acid and phenylalanine, and a small amount of methanol. Aspartic acid and phenylalanine are building blocks of protein and are found naturally in all protein-containing foods, including meats, grains and dairy products. Methanol is found naturally in the body and in many foods such as fruit and vegetable juices. Aspartame is digested just like any other protein. Upon digestion, aspartame breaks down into its basic components and is absorbed into the blood. Neither aspartame nor its components accumulate in the body over time" (International Food Information Council Web site).

Aspartame is used to sweeten a wide variety of foods. Because it does not have the higher calories of sugar, some people prefer it. It is found in "instant breakfasts, breath mints, cereals, sugar-free chewing gum, cocoa mixes, beverages, frozen desserts, gelatin desserts, juice beverages, laxatives, multivitamins, milk drinks, pharmaceuticals and supplements, shake mixes, soft drinks, tabletop sweeteners, tea beverages, instant teas and coffees, topping mixes, wine coolers, and yogurt" (Simontacchi: 183–184). However, when heated, the components separate. As a result, it is not recommended for foods that require longer heating or baking times, though it may be added near the end of the cooking or baking.

The FDA contends that aspartame is safe. Only a few cautions are noted. "Persons with a rare hereditary disease known as phenylketonuria (PKU) must control their phenylalanine intake from all sources, including aspartame. These persons are diagnosed at birth by a blood test performed on all babies. Products sweetened with aspartame carry a statement on the label that they contain phenylalanine" (International Food Information Council Web site). Additionally, the FDA recommends that the Acceptable Daily Intake (ADI) levels of aspartame be 50 milligrams per kilogram (mg/kg) of body weight. The FDA believes that most people consume far less than that limit.

The following list (from the International Food Information Council Web site) outlines the number of servings an individual would need to ingest to reach the ADI of aspartame:

50-lb. Child	150-lb. Adult	
7	20	12-ounce containers of carbonated soft drink
11	34	8-ounce servings of powdered soft drink
14	42	4-ounce servings of gelatin dessert
32	97	Packets of tabletop sweetener

The International Food Information Council states that aspartame is one of the most thoroughly studied food additives. It was widely tested in animals and humans, including normal adults and children, lactating women, and persons with diabetes, obesity and special genetic conditions, in amounts many times higher than an individual would consume, before the FDA approved it in 1981. Aspartame is approved for use in more than 90 nations throughout the world. It has been deemed safe by the Joint Expert Committee on Food Additives (JECFA) of the United Nations Food and Agricultural Organization and World Health Organization.

The American Diabetes Association considers aspartame an appropriate sugar substitute, and the Epilepsy Institute, an organization concerned with seizure-related problems, has concluded that aspartame is not linked to epileptic seizures (International Food Information Council Web site).

The International Food Information Council Web site claims that aspartame is unable to become a carcinogen. When consumed, aspartame is broken down into dietary components such as amino acids, aspartic acid, and phenylalanine that are eaten in other foods such as milk, meat, fruits, and vegetables. Aspartame components are digested in the same way as those from other food sources. Tests of large doses of aspartame in rats and mice have shown no evidence of any kind of tumors (International Food Information Council Web site).

Aspartame also has no effect on vision. Large quantities of methanol can effect vision, but the small amount of methanol in aspartame is safe and indeed less than that found in many fruits and vegetable juices (International Food Information Council Web site).

Does aspartame trigger adverse reactions in people with no special medical condition? The International Food Information Council claims that there is no scientific evidence linking aspartame to adverse reactions in people. The FDA has investigated all complaints since 1980 and has reported a declining trend of complaints of adverse reactions to aspartame since a peak in 1985 (International Food Information Council Web site).

A study published in 1998 in the *American Journal of Clinical Nutrition* attempted to learn if aspartame could "disrupt cognitive, neurophysiologic or behavioral functioning in normal individuals" (Spiers et al.: 531–537). For one month, the 48 participants ate a diet that included no aspartame. "Subjects then consumed sodas and capsules with placebo, aspartame, or sucrose for 20 days each." Researchers found that on the days participants consumed aspartame, the amounts of phenylalanine in the blood increased notably. Nevertheless, "large daily doses of aspartame had no effect on neuropsychologic, neurophysiologic or behavioral functioning in healthy young adults" (Spiers et al.: 531–537).

One of the best-known studies, which was published in 1997 in the *Journal of the National Cancer Institute*, appears to have been a response to allegations made in 1996 by John Olney. At the time, Olney noted that the rate of brain tumors has been rising since the mid-1980s, a few years after the 1981 approval of aspartame. Could aspartame play a role in the development of brain cancer? The researchers analyzed the exposure to aspartame of 56 case patients and 94 control subjects. Additionally, they studied intake of aspartame by mothers during pregnancy and breast-feeding. The researchers found no relationship between aspartame consumption and the incidence of brain cancer in children (Gurney et al.: 1072–1074). Moreover, a 1999 article in *FDA Consumer* says that an "analysis of the National Cancer Institute's database on cancer incidence showed that cases of brain cancers began increasing in 1973—well before aspartame was approved—and continued to increase through 1985. In recent years, brain tumor frequency has actually decreased slightly" (Henkel: 12). Even a 1997 article in *Prevention* says that the original research was flawed. "Part of the observed increase in brain cancer is probably due to improved diagnosis" (McCord: 56).

A number of prominent organizations have issued statements supporting the safety of aspartame, including the American Cancer Society, the American Diabetes Association, the American Dietetic Association, and the American Heart Association. The National Multiple Sclerosis Society has refuted the occasionally theorized notion that aspartame causes multiple sclerosis and other neurological illnesses (Hinson-Smith: 8).

Not everyone agrees. In *The Crazy Makers*, Carol Simontacchi wrote, "Of the thousands of adverse reactions [to aspartame] reported to the FDA, most concerned abnormal brain functions, i.e. depression, fatigue, irritability, insomnia, vision problems, hearing loss, anxiety attacks, slurred speech, loss of the sense of taste, tinnitus, vertigo, and memory loss. Also included were a number of chronic illnesses, including brain tumors, multiple sclerosis, epilepsy, chronic fatigue syndrome, Parkinson's disease, Alzheimer's, mental retardation, lymphoma. birth defects, fibromyalgia, and diabetes" (Simontacchi: 186). These were self-reported reactions that people believed were from aspartame, but there was no proof.

In an article that appeared in June 2000 in the *Ecologist*, Ed Metcalfe, Betty Martini, and Mark Gold note that "in a recent survey of 166 studies on the effects of the sweetener aspartame on human health, 74 had industry-related funding and 92 were independently funded. Of the industry-sponsored articles, 100 percent attested to aspartame's safety. Of the non-industry-sponsored articles, 92 percent demonstrated some type of adverse reaction" (Metcalfe, Martini, and Gold: 16). The authors seem to suggest that the industry only published articles that supported the safety of aspartame, while independent surveys showed that this might not be true.

In *Sweet Poison*, Janet Starr Hull outlined her debilitating battle with illness. Formerly healthy, Hull, after increasing her intake of diet foods and drinks to lose weight, began experiencing severe headaches, nausea, splitting and tearing nails, racing heartbeat, abnormal breathing, moodiness, dry skin, hair loss, and vision irregularities. As her symptoms worsened, so did her marriage. Laboratory tests were inconclusive. In desperation, Hull checked herself into the hospital. There she was diagnosed with Graves' disease, a condition in which the thyroid gland produces too much hormone. Though the physician recommended the immediate destruction of the thyroid gland with radioactive iodine, Hull was hesitant. In Graves' disease, the patient generally loses weight. While trying to lose weight, she had gained 30 pounds. Hull rejected the physician's assessment and began her own search for a solution to her deteriorating health.

Hull located a specialist in nutrition. Under his guidance, she replaced her diet soda with water and monitored everything she and her family ingested. "I began to understand how people pollute their bodies the same way they pollute the environment. Chemicals aren't meant to be eaten and can accumulate in the body like toxic waster accumulates in a river" (Hull: 42). Her health improved. After three months, a laboratory test determined that her thyroid function was normal.

It did not take Hull long to focus her attention on aspartame. She learned that the manufacturing of aspartame was a huge business and that there were serious flaws in much of the pro-aspartame research. "As I looked into the general method that the FDA uses when approving a product, I learned that, basically, what the FDA does is review other scientists' studies—scientists usually paid by the company requesting the approval. . . . Unfortunately . . . reports can be biased, facts can be shaped, and objectivity blighted" (Hull: 163–164).

Since then, Hull has spent a great deal of time researching aspartame and writing her book. She also became a certified nutritionist. Today, with her health completely restored, she has a new attitude toward food. "After my horrific experience with aspartame, I have learned to avoid processed, artificial, counterfeit, sugar-free, fat-free, calorie-free, responsibility-free foods. I only eat *real* food" (Hull: 231).

In *Aspartame (NutraSweet*): Is It Safe?* H.J. Roberts writes that he was initially supportive of aspartame because he welcomed the availability of a safe sugar-free product that could satisfy the sweet tooth of patients with reactive hypoglycemia (attacks of low blood sugar). But one day, a 16-year-old patient named Tammy, who had initially been treated for convulsions, had a recurrent seizure in his office. Roberts could find no obvious cause for the problem. Tammy's mother explained that to prevent low blood sugar, her daughter ate a snack every afternoon, just as Roberts recommended. On that afternoon, she had eaten aspartame-sweetened chocolate pudding. Tammy's mother also mentioned that Tammy's grandmother had severe reactions to aspartame. She added that Tammy had been drinking more diet beverages during the preceding two weeks to avoid sugar, just as Roberts had prescribed (Roberts: 4).

To Roberts, the wisest course for Tammy appeared to be to eliminate all sources of aspartame. Three weeks later, Tammy felt much better, and there had been no further seizures. To test his thesis, Roberts arranged for Tammy to ingest the pudding in his laboratory. She soon began to show signs of a seizure. Feeding her milk and crackers prevented a full-blown convulsion (Roberts: 5).

As he investigated aspartame, Roberts said that he was alarmed by three issues. "First, not enough was known about this synthetic chemical. Second, aspartame had been approved *without any extensive pre-marketing trials on humans*. Third, it did not come under intense FDA scrutiny because of its classification as a food 'additive' rather than a drug" (Roberts: 6). Accepting no money from anyone connected with the sugar, sweetener, or drug industries, Roberts began to study aspartame reactions among his patients. In the end, he was able to evaluate 551 aspartame reactors. His book is filled with anecdotes of the huge numbers of negative physical and psychological responses to aspartame. Roberts concludes that aspartame poses a significant public health risk. "It is imperative that researchers who are not influenced by producer-corporations gather detailed data concerning the incidence of rates of epilepsy, visual problems, allergies, Parkinsonism, brain tumors and Alzheimer's disease, among aspartame consumers. The same applies to other disorders—including the frequency of birth defects, seizures, impaired intelligence and behavioral abnormalities among the children of women who ingested aspartame products at conception and during pregnancy" (Roberts: 213).

OLESTRA

Olestra, a nondigestible fat substitute developed by the Procter and Gamble Company, is marketed under the brand name Olean. After almost three decades of research and development, including 150 animal and human studies and 150,000 pages of data, olestra was approved by the FDA in 1996. This approval was confirmed more than two years later by the FDA's Food Advisory Committee. Olestra replaces fat used in such foods as potato chips. Thus potato chips processed with olestra "contain no fat and only 75 calories vs. 10 grams of fat and 150 calories in regular chips" (Winter: 304). When consumed, olestra, or sucrose polyester, is not digested or absorbed by the body. "In theory, substitution of olestra for natural fats could help people reduce their intake of calories, fat, saturated fat, and cholesterol and, therefore, reduce the risk of obesity and related diseases: coronary heart disease, certain cancers, and diabetes. The potential uses of olestra in commonly consumed foods—and the potential economic returns to P&G investors—are enormous" (Nestle: 508–520). By 1999, "Americans [had] consumed 1.5 billion servings of snacks containing Olean" (Billings: 132–135).

Some people who eat foods with olestra have complained of gastrointestinal reactions such as cramping and loose stools. "In addition, olestra affects the absorption of fat-soluble vitamins but does not affect the absorption of water-soluble vitamins." Thus, when products containing olestra are eaten "with foods containing vitamins A, D, E, or K [fat-soluble vitamins], the fat substitute could have an effect on the absorption of these nutrients." As a result, the FDA has required that these vitamins be added to foods containing olestra in the following amounts: "170 IU vitamin A per gram olestra, 12 IU vitamin D per gram olestra, 2.8 IU vitamin E per gram olestra, and 8 (micro)gram vitamin K per gram olestra" (Prince and Welschenbach: 565–569). But olestra also "lowers blood carotenoids such as beta-carotene that are associated with cancer prevention." Walter Willett, the chair of the Department of Nutrition at the Harvard School of Public Health, has found that eating "as few as 16 olestra chips a day can reduce blood carotenoids by more than 50." A higher level of beta-carotene in the blood has been shown to be a marker for reduced cancer risk (Billings: 132–135). Labeling of foods containing olestra must indicate the presence of added vitamins and the potential for triggering gastrointestinal symptoms. There is also unease about any potential lasting effects of olestra. "Many studies of the effects of olestra have been of short duration, and, therefore, unable to address the long-term risk of gastrointestinal problems or nutrient depletion" (Nestle: 508–520).

In a 1996 article in the *New England Journal of Medicine*, Henry Blackburn voiced this discomfort. He also expressed dismay that, as in the case of other products, the vast majority of the research that was used to support the approval of olestra was sponsored by Procter and Gamble. "There were no relevant reports from disinterested investigators and no independent studies sponsored by the FDA.... What appeared to me to be collusion with industry is not only legal but also deliberate FDA policy—supportive and collaborative rather than adversarial—in considering petitions from industry" (Blackburn: 984–986).

Since the approval of olestra, further studies have been published. A 1999 report that appeared in the *Annals of Internal Medicine* found that "the incidence of diarrhea and cramping was the same in the olestra group and the control group.... In fact, the frequency of cramping was greater in the control group than in the olestra group among men. Of note, participants who ate the highest amounts of control (regular) chips reported loose stools and more frequent bowel movements less often than participants who consumed lower amounts of control chips." The researchers speculate that the responses of some of the participants were influenced by the type of chip they thought they were eating. Those who believed that they were eating the chips with olestra were about 50% more likely to report gastrointestinal symptoms than those who assumed what they were eating regular chips. "Among participants who said that they did not know which product they were eating, the percentage of participants reporting gastrointestinal symptoms was intermediate between the percentages of participants who guessed that they were eating olestra chips and those who guessed that they were eating regular chips" (Sandler et al.: 253–261).

A study that appeared in 2000 in the *Archives of Internal Medicine* evaluated the role that olestra has played in improving the overall health of 335 participants. In particular, the researchers investigated how eating products containing olestra impacted the weight and serum-lipid levels of the participants. The researchers found "a statistically significant decrease in total serum cholesterol associated with olestra intake." Additionally, "although not statistically significant, there was some evidence that olestra intake was associated with weight loss. In the two highest olestra intake categories, there was a mean 0.55–kg weight loss, compared with no weight change in nonusers of olestra. Trends in changes in LDL cholesterol [bad cholesterol] paralleled those for total cholesterol but were not statistically significant. There were no associations of changes in HDL cholesterol [good cholesterol] or triglycerides with olestra consumption." The researchers concluded that they "found the first evidence from a population-based sample of adults that consumption of a fat-modified food (e.g., olestra-containing savory snack) is associated with decreases in fat intake and total serum cholesterol levels" (Patterson: 2600–2604).

An article published in 2000 in the *Annals of Internal Medicine* raised a cautionary note that people who eat olestra may be erroneously misdiagnosed with malabsorption syndrome. "Consumption of foods containing olestra may cause large amounts of fat to be excreted in fecal material. . . . Researchers measured the amount of fat in fecal material from 10 healthy volunteers after they ate regular potato chips or potato chips containing olestra. When participants ate 40 grams of olestra per day, they excreted as much fat as patients with malabsorption syndrome" (Balasekaran et al.: 279).

CONCLUSION

It is apparent that society is becoming increasingly aware of some of the potential problems associated certain additives. As this trend continues, there will probably be more pressure placed on members of the food industry to eliminate those that are not absolutely necessary.

TOPICS FOR DISCUSSION

1. Are you concerned about the large numbers of foods that contain additives? Why or why not?
2. Do you believe that the complaints about additives are legitimate? Why or why not?
3. Do you think the regulation of food additives is appropriate? Why or why not?
4. Why do you think that the FDA has not taken action to require clear and precise labeling for all products that may contain MSG?
5. Has sufficient testing been conducted on food additives, especially controversial ones? Why or why not?

REFERENCES AND RESOURCES

Books

Balingasa, Nancy, and Eduardo Balingasa. *The Food Jungle.* The Woodlands, Texas: (PM) Printed Matters, 1999.

Blaylock, Russell L. *Excitotoxins.* Santa Fe, New Mexico: Health Press, 1995.

Costa, Annie. *The Feel Good Handbook.* San Mateo, California: Lighthouse Press, 1998.

Dibb, Sue. *What the Label Doesn't Tell You.* London: Thorsons, 1997.

Haas, Elson M. *The Staying Healthy Shopper's Guide.* Berkeley, California: Celestial Arts, 1999.

Hull, Janet Starr. *Sweet Poison.* Far Hills, New Jersey: New Horizon Press, 1999.

Lacey, Richard W. *Hard to Swallow.* New York: Cambridge University Press, 1994.

Nottridge, Rhoda. *Additives.* Minneapolis: Carolrhoda Books, 1993.

Renders, Eileen. *Food Additives, Nutrients, and Supplements A-To-Z.* Sante Fe, New Mexico: Clear Light Publishers, 1999.

Roberts, H.J. *Aspartame (NutraSweet*): Is it Safe?* Philadelphia: Charles Press, 1990.

Simontacchi, Carol. *The Crazy Makers.* New York: Jeremy P. Tarcher/Putnam Books, 2000.

Walsh, William E. *Food Allergies.* New York: John Wiley and Sons, 2000.

Winter, Ruth. *A Consumer's Dictionary of Food Additives.* 5th ed. New York: Three Rivers Press, 1999.

Magazines, Journals, and Newspapers

Balasekaran, Ranga, Jack L. Porter, Carol A. Santa Ana, and John S. Fordtran. "Positive Results on Tests for Steatorrhea in Persons Consuming Olestra

Potato Chips." *Annals of Internal Medicine*, February 15, 2000, 132(4): 279–282.

Billings, Laura. "Food Fright." *Women's Sports and Fitness*, November 1999, 3(1): 132–135.

Blackburn, Henry. "Olestra and the FDA." *New England Journal of Medicine*, April 11, 1996, 334(15): 984–986.

Blakeslee, Sandra. "With MSG Sensitivity Still at Issue in Studies, Label Rules Tighten." *New York Times*, March 6, 1990: Section C, page 3.

Bonvie, Linda, and Bill Bonvie. "A Game of Hide and Seek." *Vegetarian Times*, September 1998, 253: 21.

Boyle, Caitlin. "Digesting MSG: How to Break It Down." *San Francisco Chronicle*, April 14, 1999: Page 1/ZZ1.

Brody, Jane E. "Diet Change May Avert Need for Ritalin." *New York Times*, November 2, 1999: Section F, page 8.

Bryant, Tim. "Lawsuit Blames Illnesses on MSG; Activists Demanding Labels for Additive." *St. Louis Post-Dispatch*, June 9, 1996: Page 1C.

Burros, Marian. "A Little Medicine with Your Food?" *New York Times*, December 30, 1998: Section F, page 5.

Charatan, Fred. "Fortification of Flour Raises Folate Levels in US Women, Says CDC." *British Medical Journal*, November 11, 2000, 321(7270): 1176.

Diamond, Seymour, and Kenneth L. Moore. "The Many Faces of MSG." *Consultant*, November 1999, 39(11): 3132.

Elash, Anita. "Also Containing—Watching Those Extras in Prepared Foods." *Maclean's*, October 27, 1997, 110(43): 59.

Forristal, Linda Joyce. "The Great Salmon Scam." *Insight on the News*, June 12, 2000, 16(22): 26–27.

Geha, Raif S., Alexa Beiser, Clement Ren, Roy Patterson, Paul A. Greenberger, Leslie C. Grammer, Anne M. Ditto, Kathleen E. Harris, Martha A. Shaughnessy, Paul R. Yarnold, Jonathan Corren, and Andrew Saxon. "Multicenter, Double-Blind, Placebo-Controlled, Multiple-Challenge Evaluation of Reported Reactions to Monosodium Glutamate." *Journal of Allergy and Clinical Immunology*, November 2000, part 1, 106(5): 973–980.

Gurney, James G., Janice M. Pogoda, Elizabeth A. Holly, Stephen S. Hecht, and Susan Preston-Martin. "Aspartame Consumption in Relation to Childhood Brain Tumor Risk: Results from a Case-Controlled Study." *Journal of the National Cancer Institute*, July 16, 1997, 89(14): 1072–1074.

Henkel, John. "Sugar Substitutes." *FDA Consumer*, November 1999, 33(6): 12.

Hinson-Smith, Vicki. "Not-So-Sweet Talk." *Real Life with Multiple Sclerosis*, October 1999, 6(10): 8.

Kleiner, Susan M. "Fake Sugars and Fats: Net Benefits or Real Risks?" *Physician and Sportsmedicine*, April 1997, 25(4): 133.

Kuntz, Lynn. "Attacks on Aspartame Are Falling Short." *Supermarket News*, January 13, 1997, 47(2): S27.

McCord, Holly. "To Aspartame or Not to Aspartame." *Prevention*, August 1997, 49(8): 56.

Metcalfe, Ed, Betty Martini, and Mark Gold. "Sweet Talking." *Ecologist*, June 2000, 30(4): 16.

Nestle, Marion. "The Selling of Olestra." *Public Health Reports*, November/December 1998, 113: 508–520.

Patterson, Ruth E., Alan R. Kristal, John C. Peters, Marian L. Neuhouser, Cheryl L. Rock, Lawrence J. Cheskin, Dianne Neumark-Sztainer, and Mark D. Thornquist. "Changes in Diet, Weight, and Serum Lipid Levels Associated with Olestra Consumption." *Archives of Internal Medicine*, September 25, 2000, 160(17): 2600–2604.

Prawirohardjono, Widharto, Iwan Dwiprahasto, Indwiani Astuti, Soeliadi Hadiwandowo, Erna Kristin, Mustofa Muhammad, and Michael Kelly. "The Administration to Indonesians of Monosodium L-Glutamate in Indonesian Foods: An Assessment of Adverse Reactions in a Randomized Double-Blind, Crossover, Placebo-Controlled Study." *Journal of Nutrition*, April 2000, 130(4S): 1074S–1076S.

Prince, Diane M., and Marilyn A. Welschenbach. "Olestra: A New Food Additive." *Journal of the American Dietetic Association*, May 1998, 98(5): 565–569.

Rowlands, Philippa, and Mark Bregman. "Food Additives." *Science World*, November 2, 1998, 55(5): 16–18.

Sandler, Robert S., Nora L. Zorich, Thomas G. Filloon, Heather B. Wiseman, Dennis J. Lietz, Michael H. Brock, Mary G. Royer, and Robert K. Miday. "Gastrointestinal Symptoms in 3181 Volunteers Ingesting Snack Foods Containing Olestra or Triglycerides." *Annals of Internal Medicine*, February 16, 1999, 130(4): 253–261.

Schiffman, Susan S. "Taste and Smell Losses in Normal Aging and Disease." *JAMA: The Journal of the American Medical Association*, October 22, 1997, 278(16): 1357–1362.

Shaywitz, Bennett A., Colleen M. Sullivan, George M. Anderson, Sheila M. Gillespie, Barbara Sullivan, and Sally E. Shaywitz. "Aspartame, Behavior, and Cognitive Function in Children with Attention Deficit Disorder." *Pediatrics*, January 1994, 93(1): 70–75.

Shovic, Anne, Robert D. Bart, and Apryll M. Stalcup. " 'We Think Your Son Has Lennox-Gastaut Syndrome'—A Case Study of Monosodium Glutamate's Effect on a Child." *Journal of the American Dietetic Association*, July 1997, 97(7): 793–794.

Simon, Ronald A. "Additive-Induced Urticaria: Experience with Monosodium Glutamate (MSG)." *Journal of Nutrition*, April 2000, 130(4S): 1063S–1066S.

Spiers, Paul A., LuAnn Sabounjian, Allison Reiner, Diane K. Myers, Judith Wurtman, and Donald L. Schomer. "Aspartame: Neuropsychologic and Neurophysiologic Evaluation of Acute and Chronic Effects." *American Journal of Clinical Nutrition*, September 1998, 68(3): 531–537.

Stevenson, Donald D. "Monosodium Glutamate and Asthma." *Journal of Nutrition*, April 2000, 130(4S): 1067S–1073S.

Sussman, Gordon L., and William Yang. "When Sulfites Pose a Hidden Danger." *Consultant*, December 1998, 38(12): 2834.

Woessner, Katharine M., Ronald A. Simon, and Donald D. Stevenson. "Monosodium Glutamate Sensitivity in Asthma." *Journal of Allergy and Clinical Immunology*, August 1999, part 1, 104(2): 305–310.

Organizations to Contact

Center for Food Safety and Applied Nutrition
Food and Drug Administration
5100 Paint Branch Parkway
College Park, MD 20740-3835
Phone: 1-888-SAFEFOOD
http://vm.cfsan.fda.gov/list.html (January 1, 2001)

Center for Science in the Public Interest
1875 Connecticut Ave. NW, Suite 300
Washington, DC 20009
Phone: 202-332-9110
http://www.cspinet.org/ (January 26, 2001)

International Food Information Council
1100 Connecticut Avenue NW, Suite 430
Washington, DC 20036
Phone: 202-296-6540
http://www.ific.org (January 14, 2001)

Olean
Procter & Gamble
P.O. Box 599
Cincinnati, OH 45201
Phone: 800-224-7665
http://olean.com (January 25, 2001)

Truth in Labeling Campaign
P.O. Box 2532
Darien, IL 60561
Phone: 858-481-9333
http://www.truthinlabeling.org (January 9, 2001)

2

Food Irradiation

Every year millions of people become ill from the food they eat. One way to improve the safety of food is to treat it with radiation. Many are opposed because they fear health risks. In 1993, two sisters, ages four and two, were eager to visit the newly built fast-food restaurant that had opened in their Seattle neighborhood. Early in January, their father treated them to cheeseburgers, fries, and milk. Six days later, the older child, who was suffering from cramps and bloody diarrhea, was rushed to the hospital. Soon her sister was also hospitalized. Both girls were horribly ill, and during the course of her sickness, the older child often teetered close to death.

Their illness was caused by food poisoning. The hamburger meat in the cheeseburgers was contaminated with *Escherichia coli* 0157:H7 (E. coli), a deadly bacterium. Fortunately, both sisters survived their ordeal, but others did not. During that West Coast outbreak, several children died.

Food is supposed to nourish and sustain us. On occasion, food is improperly handled. When that occurs, deadly bacteria are provided an ideal medium in which to flourish. Statistics from the Centers for Disease Control and Prevention (CDC) have estimated that every year between 6 and 33 million people in the United States experience a foodborne disease. Of these, about 9,000 die. That means that on the average, every week slightly fewer than 200 people in the United States die from something they have eaten. While anyone is vulnerable, the young and the old or those with impaired immune systems are most at risk for serious morbidity or death (Centers for Disease Control and Prevention Web site).

Salmonella and campylobacter are two of the most frequent pathogens that cause foodborne illness. "The Centers for Disease Control and Prevention estimates that Salmonella—commonly found in poultry, eggs, meat and milk—sickens as many as four million and kills 1,000 per year nationwide. Campylobacter, found mostly in poultry, is responsible for six million illnesses and 75 deaths per year in the United States," and "nationally, E. coli 0157:H7 causes about 20,000 illnesses and 500 deaths a year" (Henkel: 12–17).

The financial toll is also high. "In 1996, the estimated cost of direct medical care and lost productivity resulting from all intestinal and food-borne infectious disease was about $28 billion" (Prier and Solnick: 245). Companies lose money because they have to buy back contaminated products and pay huge settlements to affected families. Not factored into this equation is the senseless loss of human life.

The CDC contends that about 97% of all food-related illnesses are a direct result of improper handling. Of these, 79% occur in a commercial setting; 21% take place at home. Not everyone is aware of or understands the concept of improperly handled food. Food can be inappropriately handled in a number of ways. It may be inadequately cooked or may be allowed to remain too long at a temperature that fosters bacterial growth. Also, unless people preparing the food frequently wash their hands, most notably after using the restroom, they have the potential to spread germs, especially if they are ill. Further, there is the problem of cross-contamination. "Cross-contamination may occur when raw contaminated food comes in contact with other foods, especially cooked foods through direct contact or indirect contact on food preparation surfaces" (Shewmake and Dillon: 125–129). Ground beef is particularly risky "because the grinding process spreads any pathogens that may be present on the surface of the meat throughout the ground beef," and because "an individual hamburger patty may contain meat from many cattle" (Morrison, Buzby, and Lin: 33–37), thereby increasing the number of sources of contaminants.

Clearly, these figures could be lowered somewhat if people were more informed. Some believe that a far broader effort must be made. They call for the commercial irradiation of many types of food, a process that exposes food to radiation and is known to minimize the number of pathogens as well as extend the useful life of perishable foods. Irradiation is already used to reduce the bacteria in hospital supplies, medical instruments, wine-bottle corks, and cosmetics. Since 1972, American astronauts have eaten foods that have been irradiated (Henkel: 12–17). "Some hospitals and nursing homes serve irradiated food to people with compromised immune systems, including burn victims and those undergoing chemotherapy" ("Irradiation Back": 4).

Since radiation evokes images of atomic explosions and nuclear war, it is often thought of as being dangerous. As might be imagined, some people strongly support the irradiation of food, while others just as vehemently oppose it. The vast majority of people are poorly informed about irradiation. "In 1995, researchers at the University of Georgia reported that 87.5 percent of consumers had heard of irradiation but knew little about it" (Henkel: 12–17). A Food Marketing Institute telephone survey in 1996 found that 47% of the 1,007 respondents knew nothing about food irradiation (Morrison, Buzby, and Lin: 33–37). In *The Food That Would Last Forever*, Gary Gibbs wrote, "If you were to ask the average person on the street what he or she thinks of food irradiation, the most likely response would be a puzzled, 'What is that?' Few Americans know that the next time they bite into a slice of bread, they may be eating irradiated wheat, or that when they pour spaghetti sauce on their pasta, they may be eating irradiated herbs and spices" (Gibbs: 3).

HISTORY OF FOOD IRRADIATION

Irradiation has an interesting history. Shortly before the end of the nineteenth century, the French physicist Antoine-Henri Becquerel discovered radiation, or radiant energy. Soon thereafter, Samuel Prescott, a biology professor at the Massachusetts Institute of Technology in Cambridge, Massachusetts, demonstrated that bacteria in food could be killed with gamma rays from radium. He suggested that radiation be used to help preserve a variety of foods, including meat, fruits, vegetables, and grains (Skerrett: 28–36). "By 1930, patents had been granted for food irradiation in both the United States and France" (Gibbs: 11), but more extensive studies did not begin until the World War II era. In 1953, President Dwight D. Eisenhower's Atomic Energy Commission spearheaded the "Atoms for Peace" program designed to find nonviolent means to use atomic energy. Food irradiation, or the exposure of food to "very high-energy invisible lightwaves" (National Food Safety Database Web site), was one such use of atoms.

Other countries were also entering the field. "The Soviet Union led the way by permitting the irradiation of potatoes (to prevent sprouting) in 1958 and the irradiation of grain (for disinfestations) in 1959. West Germany, although the first to actually employ commercial food irradiation in 1957 for the sterilization of spices used in sausage, dropped back in the race in 1958, when it banned food irradiation for use on foods consumed within its own country" (Gibbs: 11).

The Food, Drug, and Cosmetic Act of 1958 defined food irradiation as an additive rather than a process, such as pasteurization. "In practical terms, this means that every single irradiated food, as well as most forms of packaging, must be approved by the FDA. (When animal products are involved, the operational details of a specific irradiation program must also be approved by USDA [U.S. Department of Agriculture])" (Demetrakakes: 20–26).

Soon the FDA was giving its approval to irradiation of various foods. In 1963, irradiation of wheat and flour was approved, followed by potatoes, dried spices and vegetable seasonings, pork, fruits and vegetables, and poultry during the next three decades. FDA approved irradiation of red meat on December 2, 1997, after three years of study and "a series of high-profile food poisonings and meat recalls" (Demetrakakes: 20–26). Irradiated foods must be labeled either "treated with radiation" or "treated by irradiation" and must contain a picture of the radura, the international symbol of irradiation. These rules only affect food products sold in stores. "When used as ingredients in other foods . . . the label of the other food does not need to describe these ingredients as irradiated" (Henkel: 12–17). Also, food need not be labeled if one of its minor ingredients, such as a spice, has been irradiated.

No one refutes the effectiveness of food irradiation, which is sometimes called cold pasteurization because it kills bacteria without heat. Radiation energy alters molecules and breaks chemical bonds. In so doing, it has the potential to retard spoilage, thus reducing the chance of human illness.

Not all foods are suitable candidates for irradiation. "Cucumbers, grapes and some tomatoes turn mushy when radiation breaks cell walls and release enzymes that digest the food and speed up rotting" (Skerrett: 28–36). Oysters and other raw shellfish may be irradiated, but the process damages or kills the live oyster, thus greatly diminishing its quality. Eggs are also not good candidates for irradiation. "Irradiation causes the egg whites to become milky and more liquid, which means it looks like an older egg, and may not serve as well in some recipes" (Centers for Disease Control and Prevention Web site).

TYPES OF FOOD IRRADIATION

At present there are several main types of food irradiation. The most common variety uses cobalt 60 as its radiation source. A cobalt-based irradiator requires space for a deep pool of shielding water and is thus impractical for most food plants. "Processors who wish to irradiate their food with cobalt must ship it to the facility, which represents an ongoing expense and logistical problem" (Demetrakakes: 20–26).

The first such facility was built in the early 1990s in Mulberry, Florida. "The heart of the plant . . . is a shiny rack of 400 gamma-ray-emitting cobalt-60 'pencils,' each 18 inches long and the diameter of a fat crayon, housed in a chamber surrounded by a concrete wall six feet thick. When not in use, the rack is submerged in a 15-foot-deep pool of cooled water that absorbs and neutralizes the gamma rays. At the push of a button, hydraulic arms slide into the irradiation chamber on an overhead monorail. The boxes follow a zig-zag pattern around the radioactive rack so gamma rays can reach all sides. Treatment times vary—fresh strawberries pass through in five to eight minutes, frozen chicken takes as long as 20 minutes" (Skerrett: 28–36).

Cesium irradiators require much less space—only an 8- to 10-foot area—and use fuel from decommissioned nuclear weapons, "which makes for a cheaper supply than cobalt (although not as stable)" (Demetrakakes: 20–26). Because there are only a small number of nuclear-weapons-reprocessing facilities throughout the world, there are only a few cesium irradiators.

Electron-beam irradiators are safer for workers and the environment because they may be turned off. It is also easier to change their elements. Although they deliver faster and higher doses of radiation than most other sources, they lack penetrating power. "Radioactive source irradiators emit gamma rays, which consist of photons. Because photons are units of electromagnetic energy with no mass, they penetrate relatively well, which allows the irradiator to process entire pallets at a time. The electrons in electron beams, on the other hand, have mass, which greatly reduces their penetrating power. In practical terms, the average electron-beam irradiator can penetrate only two to four inches, meaning that only relatively flat products (like hamburger patties) and/or packages are suitable" (Demetrakakes: 20–26).

X-ray irradiators—more powerful versions of the types of machines used in hospitals and dental offices—are still in development. "A beam of electrons is directed at a thin plate of gold or other metal, producing a stream of X-rays coming out the other side. Like cobalt gamma rays, X-rays can pass through thick foods, and require heavy shielding for safety. However, like e-beams [electron beams], the machine can be switched on and off, and no radioactive substances are involved" (Centers for Disease Control and Prevention Web site).

In all forms of food irradiation, the food is irradiated after it has been packaged and sealed. Food that may have been tainted during any portion of the production process is cleaned.

Food irradiation is administered in one of three "doses." A dose is the amount of radiation absorbed by the food and is determined by the intensity of the radiation and the length of time it is applied. The following are examples of usages of treatment doses approved by the Food and Drug Administration (FDA): Low doses are used to control insects in grains, inhibit sprouting in white potatoes, control trichinae in pork, and inhibit decay and control insects in fruits and vegetables. Medium doses control salmonella, shigella, campylobacter, yersinia, and other bacteria that can cause food poisoning in meat, poultry, and fish, and delay mold growth on strawberries and other fruits. High doses kill microorganisms and insects in spices and commercially sterilize food (National Food Safety Database Web site).

Doses of irradiation are measured in Gray (GY) units. "This is a measure of the amount of energy transferred to food, microbe or other substance being irradiated. . . . A single chest X-ray has a dose of roughly a half of a milliGray (a thousandth of a Gray). To kill *Salmonella*, fresh chicken can be irradiated at up to 4.5 kiloGrays, which is about seven million times more irradiation than a single chest X-ray. . . . The killing effect of irradiation on microbes is measured in D-values. One D-value is the amount of irradiation needed to kill 90% of that organism. For example, it takes 0.3 kiloGrays to kill 90% of *E. coli 0157*, so the D-value of *E. coli* is 0.3 kGy" (Centers for Disease Control and Prevention Web site).

THE CASE FOR IRRADIATION

Currently, almost 40 countries have approved food irradiation for more than 40 different foods—"from apples in China and frog legs in France to rice in Mexico, raw pork sausages in Thailand, and wheat in Canada" (Skerrett: 28–36). Throughout the world, there are about 160 irradiators. "The plants, which must be approved by governmental authorities before construction, are subject to regular inspections, audits and other reviews to ensure that they are safely and properly operated" (National Food Safety Database Web site). Further, food irradiation has been endorsed by a wide range of powerful and prestigious groups, including the World Health Organization, the United Nations, the International Atomic Energy Association, the U.S. Public Health Service, the Food and Drug Administration, the American Medical Association, the American Public Health Association, and the American Dietetic Association (see Wood and Bruhn: 246). Every year, "about a half million tons of food products and ingredients are irradiated worldwide" (National Food Safety Database Web site).

The International Food Information Council, a Washington, DC–based nonprofit group that was formed to communicate information on food safety and nutrition, contends that years of research have proven that food irradiation is safe. "The first patents for food irradiation were granted in the United States and United Kingdom in 1905. Since then, hundreds of studies on the effects of food irradiation have been reviewed by the U.S. government and other governments worldwide. It is the most extensively studied food processing technology available" (International Food Information Council Web site).

The International Food Information Council says that irradiated food does not become radioactive. "The food irradiation process moves food through a radiant energy field, but the food never touches the energy source. Think of the irradiation process as the way light passes through a window" (International Food Information Council Web site). A March 2000 article in *Good Housekeeping* noted that "food never comes into direct

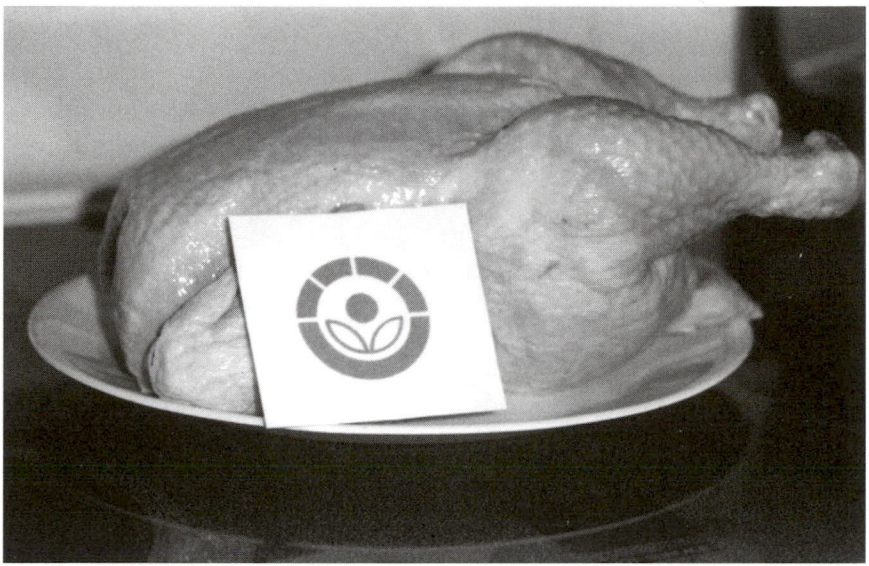

Irradiated foods are becoming more commonplace. Photo by Mark A. Goldstein.

contact with the radiation. . . . It's similar to what happens when you get an x-ray. The rays pass through your body, but don't leave YOU radioactive" (Holcomb: 75–76). Also, the environment in which we live contains trace amounts of radioactivity. In the course of everyday life, people are exposed to small amounts of radiation from sources such as their television sets.

How are the nutrients and flavors of food altered by irradiation? To these questions the International Food Information Council responds, "Irradiation produces virtually no heat within food and does not 'cook' foods. Foods processed with irradiation are just as nutritious and flavorful as other food in the marketplace. Changes in nutrient content or flavor from cooking, canning, or freezing are the same or lower with processing by irradiation." The council maintains that irradiation greatly improves the safety of food, but cautions that the food is still subject to spoilage or to contamination during food handling and preparation.

The process of irradiating food does affect its chemical composition. Could some of these changes be harmful? The National Food Safety Database, which is supported by the U.S. Department of Agriculture, comments that "in general, the irradiation process produces very little chemical change in food. None of the changes known to occur have been found to be harmful or dangerous" (National Food Safety Database Web site).

How about free radicals, which are known to be released during food irradiation? "Free radicals—which in scientific terms are atoms or molecules with an unpaired electron—can be formed during the irradiation process, as well as by certain other food treatments (toasting bread, frying and freeze-drying) and during normal oxidation processes in food." There is absolutely no proof that free radicals alter the safety of irradiated foods. "Free radicals disappear by reacting with each other in the presence of liquids such as saliva in the mouth. Consequently, their ingestion does not create any toxicological or other harmful effects." In a long-term laboratory study in which animals were fed dry milk powder irradiated by 45 kilogray, more than four times the maximum dose approved for food irradiation, "no mutagenic effects were noted and no tumors were formed. No toxic effects were apparent in the animals over nine successive generations. Similarly, toasted bread (unirradiated), which actually contains more free radicals than very dry foods that have been irradiated, can be expected to be harmless" (National Food Safety Database Web site).

Can food irradiation trigger genetic abnormalities? In the 1970s, studies conducted in India reported higher rates of multiple sets of chromosomes in rats, mice, monkeys, and malnourished children who had eaten wheat immediately after irradiation. No such results were found in subjects who had eaten wheat 12 weeks after irradiation. Since then, no other institution has replicated these results. Several years later, in the early 1980s, human volunteers in China were fed irradiated food, including irradiated wheat. In eight different studies, more than 400 people ate irradiated food for 7 to 15 weeks. "No significant difference between the number of chromosomal aberrations in the control and test groups could be discovered." Many subsequent studies have supported this finding. "Over the last 20 years millions of mice, rats and other laboratory animals have been bred and reared exclusively on an irradiated diet.... No transmittable genetic defects ... have been observed which could be attributed to the consumption of irradiated diets" (National Food Safety Database Web site).

There are other safety issues. Accidents have occurred at food-irradiation facilities, and people who work there are at risk from radiation-related accidents, but the National Food Safety Database believes that such problems are rare: "Over the past 25 years there have been a few major accidents at industrial irradiation facilities that caused injury or death to workers because of accidental exposure to a lethal dose of radiation. All of the accidents happened because safety systems had been deliberately bypassed and proper control procedures had not been followed. None of these accidents endangered public health and environmental safety." Accidents can also occur during the transportation of radioactive materials. According to the March 2000 issue of the *Tufts*

University Health and Nutrition Letter, these concerns should be "weighed against the fact that in all the decades medical equipment and various foods have undergone irradiation, there has never been a nuclear accident attributable to irradiation materials" ("Irradiation Back": 4). Moreover, "in the 50 or so years that medical supplies and various foods have undergone irradiation, there has not been a single nuclear accident in which a finger could be pointed at irradiation materials" (Lindner: Page Z11).

Some worry that food irradiation will dramatically raise the price of food. Building a food-irradiation plant costs between one and three million dollars. "This is within the range of plant costs for other food technologies. For example, a moderately-sized, ultra-high temperature plant for sterilizing milk, fruit juices and other liquids costs about US $2 million." There are also costs associated with running the plants and irradiating the food. "Broken down, irradiation costs range from US $10 to $15 per ton for a low-dose application (for example, to inhibit the growth of sprouts in potatoes and onions) to US $100 to $250 per ton for a high-does application (for example, to ensure hygienic quality of spices). These costs are competitive with alternative treatments. In some cases, irradiation can be considerably less expensive" (National Food Safety Database Web site).

A 1999 article in *Food Review* outlined the cost benefits of irradiating ground beef. It concluded, "If 25 percent of the seven billion pounds of ground beef consumed in the United States were irradiated, and this treatment successfully prevented 25 percent of foodborne illnesses . . . the net annual benefits would range from $57.5 million to $174.5 million in 1996 dollars" (Buzby and Morrison: 21–22). In spite of the positive reports, many retailers are reluctant to carry irradiated food. "This, experts say, is partially because many store owners and food producers fear consumers won't buy the products based on misgivings about radiation in general" (Henkel: 12–17).

Some stores and restaurants have taken the plunge. One of the first was Carrot Top, a grocery market in the Chicago area that started selling irradiated products in 1992. Jim Corrigan, the store's owner, has found that the food, which sells well, remains fresher for a far longer period of time. In 1998, an article in *Food Processing* reported that Church Street Station, an entertainment complex in Orlando, Florida, purchased 50,000 pounds of irradiated chicken in 1997. At the time, the executive chef of the complex noted that regular chicken had to be discarded after five days of refrigeration. The irradiated chicken remained fresh for three weeks (Demetrakakes: 20–26).

Many consumers seem willing to try such foods. A few years ago, the International Food Information Council paid for a series of focus groups to be conducted in four U.S. cities. "Participants from each group represented a diverse mix of consumers by age, gender, ethnic group, occupation, and education." The following were some of the findings:

- Most consumers do not fully understand and have not thought much about food irradiation as a processing or food-safety technology.
- After education, consumers were willing to try irradiated foods for themselves and their families, including children; however, for irradiated foods, taste was more important to consumers than price.
- Consumers embraced the food-safety benefits of food irradiation, but not as a substitute for safe food production, processing, and handling.
- When asked, unaided by text, about their understanding of the radura symbol that is used for identifying products treated with irradiation, most consumers thought the symbol was "cute," pleasant, or appealing.
- The FDA currently requires irradiated foods to include the radura on the label accompanied by the statement "treated with irradiation." Consumers wanted food products to identify the process, tell what the process does, and describe public health benefits.
- Consumers felt that terms such as "cold pasteurized (irradiated) to eliminate harmful bacteria" provided the most beneficial information.
- Consumers appreciated the safety benefit of irradiation "to eliminate harmful bacteria" more than extended shelf-life. Consumers did not want produce that would "last for several months." (International Food Information Council Web site)

The Centers for Disease Control and Prevention contends that if consumers were better informed about the health benefits of food irradiation, they would be supportive. "Consumers are interested in a process that eliminates harmful microbes from the food and reduces the risk of foodborne disease. In test marketing of specific irradiated foods, consumers have shown that they are willing to buy them. Typically at least half will buy the irradiated food, if given a choice between irradiated product and the same product non-irradiated. If consumers are first educated about what irradiation is and why it is done, approximately 80% will buy the product in these marketing tests" (Centers for Disease Control and Prevention Web site).

David A. Kessler, dean of the Yale University School of Medicine and a former FDA commissioner, has compared the past debate over the pasteurization of milk to the current dispute around food irradiation.

Although many people became sick from drinking milk, they remained skeptical about pasteurization. In 1889, Dr. Henry Koplik of New York City began an effort to make pasteurization a universally accepted practice. "The true point, however, in the public awareness and acceptance of pasteurization was when Nathan Straus, head of R.H. Macy's in New York City, launched a campaign to change the public's idea that pasteurized milk was a medicated product. Although Mr. Straus commended Dr. Koplik's work, he wanted a wider appeal for pasteurization and opened his first milk depot in 1893" (Grocery Manufacturers of America Web site).

Straus's effort kept growing. Soon he was writing the mayors of the country's largest cities, and milk depots were established in many cities, including Boston, Chicago, Cleveland, Philadelphia, and Pittsburgh. "In 1895, Nathan Straus predicted that 'the day is not far distant when it will be regarded as a piece of criminal neglect to feed young children with milk that has not been sterilized (pasteurized).' " Kessler concludes that "though the ideas of men would have to be altered and the industry would have to develop to handle large-scale commercial pasteurization before that prophecy could come true, it would come true. Today we recognize milk pasteurization as a necessary safety measure" (Grocery Manufacturers of America Web site).

THE OPPOSITION TO FOOD IRRADIATION

Despite widespread support, food irradiation is opposed by many. One of the more vocal opponents is Public Citizen, a watchdog organization founded in 1971 by consumer advocate Ralph Nader. Public Citizen says that there is really little evidence that food irradiation is safe. "Irradiation . . . changes the molecular structure of food. Irradiation creates new and potentially dangerous compounds, called radiolytic products, by smashing apart the chemical bonds in food and sending electrons flying." Public Citizen states that there have been no long-term studies proving that food irradiation is safe. "In fact, almost all research on toxicity was done before 1980 and did not use modern toxicological methods of research" (Public Citizen Web site).

Public Citizen maintains that food radiation reduces the nutritional value of food by destroying vitamins, essential amino acids, and polyunsaturated fatty acids. The longer shelf life of irradiated food can lead to even more loss of nutrients.

Public Citizen says that the FDA has chosen to ignore studies indicating that food irradiation may be dangerous and that it has caused health problems in laboratory animals such as shorter life spans, low birth weight, kidney damage, immune and reproductive problems, chromosomal abnormalities, and tumors. Unfortunately, since the FDA claims that much of this research was poorly done, the results were ignored. "Without exception, FDA officials have chosen to ignore any evidence that suggests irradiation may be dangerous" (Public Citizen Web site).

To Public Citizen, there is little value in comparing the radiation from televisions and microwaves to the amount of radiation used on food. "It would take 1.4 *billion* TVs to generate the amount of radiation generated when meat is 'treated' by an e-beam accelerator. In the case of microwave ovens, the devices use *non*-ionizing radiation, meaning that the radiation is not powerful enough to obliterate the chemical bonds that hold atoms and molecules together (which is also the case with visible and ultraviolet light)." Although food-irradiation advocates claim that the food never becomes radioactive, Public Citizen says that it may, at least for a brief period of time.

Moreover, according to Public Citizen, any comparison between food irradiation and pasteurization is absurd. "There is nothing proper about comparing a process by which milk is quickly heated and cooled to a process by which food is exposed to the equivalent of tens of millions of X-rays—more than enough to turn nutritious, good-tasting food into vitamin-depleted, chemically altered mush that can smell like a wet dog" (Public Citizen Web site).

The Organic Consumers Association has also taken a strong stand against food irradiation. At its Web site, the organization notes that there is no definitive long-term evidence that irradiated food is safe:

- The longest human feeding study was 15 weeks. No one knows the long-term effects of a lifelong diet that includes foods that are frequently irradiated, such as meat, chicken, vegetables, fruits, salads, sprouts, and juices.

- There are no studies on the effects of feeding babies or children diets containing irradiated foods, except a small study from India.

- Studies on animals fed irradiated foods have shown increased tumors, reproductive failures, and kidney damage. Some possible causes are irradiation-induced vitamin deficiencies, the inactivity of enzymes in the food, DNA damage, and toxic radiolytic products in the food.

- The FDA based its approval of irradiation on only 5 of 441 animal-feeding studies. Marcia van Gemert, the toxicologist who chaired the FDA committee that approved irradiation, later said, "These studies reviewed in the 1982 literature from the FDA were not adequate by 1982 standards, and are even less accurate by 1993 standards to evaluate the safety of any product, especially a food product such as irradiated food." The 5 studies were conducted using lower energies of irradiation than those approved for foods for human consumption.

- The science of today is totally inadequate to prove the long-term safety of food irradiation. (Organic Consumers Association Web site)

The Organic Consumers Association believes that food irradiation is an environmental hazard. If food irradiation grows in popularity, then the likelihood of accidents—whether in transport, operation, or disposal of nuclear wastes—will increase. There have already been problems. "In Georgia in 1988, radioactive water escaped from an irradiation facility. The taxpayers were stuck with $47 million in cleanup costs. Radioactivity was tracked into cars and homes. In Hawaii in 1967 and New Jersey in 1982, radioactive water was flushed into the public sewer system." "Numerous worker exposures have occurred in food irradiation facilities worldwide" (Organic Consumers Association Web site).

Further, while food irradiation does reduce the amount of bacteria in food, the Organic Consumers Association emphasizes that it does not ensure clean food. Consider the following:

- Bacteria that survive irradiation are by definition radiation-resistant. These bacteria will multiply and eventually work their way back to the slaughterhouses, perhaps through a slaughterhouse worker who ate irradiated meat for dinner. The bacteria that contaminate the meat will no longer be killed by currently approved doses of radiation, and stronger bacteria will contaminate our food supply.

- People may become more careless about sanitation if irradiation is widely used. In a few hours at room temperature, the bacteria remaining in meat or poultry after irradiation can multiply to the level existing before irradiation. Some bacteria (like the one that causes botulism), viruses, and prions (which are believed to cause mad cow disease) are not killed by current doses of irradiation.

- Irradiation encourages food producers to cut corners on sanitation, because they can irradiate the food just before it is shipped. (Organic Consumers Association Web site)

A third leader in the anti-food-irradiation movement is Food and Water, a national nonprofit food-safety and environmental organization based in Walden, Vermont. Food and Water states that the government is approaching the problem of foodborne illness from the wrong direction and is failing to address the primary reasons for the U.S. food-safety crisis. Instead of advocating the irradiation of meat, the government should implement immediate steps to clean up the current system of meat production (*Food Irradiation: An Activist Primer*: 4). Food and Water identifies the following causes of dirty meat:

- *Factory farms*: Factory farms and feed lots are the initial breeding ground of pathogens that contaminate the food supply. Cattle are frequently confined to inhumane pens, open and unprotected from weather, often in groups of 500 or more. Before even entering the slaughterhouse, cattle can be contaminated by feed, water, feces, and other animals.

- *Slaughtering facilities*: Industrial slaughtering facilities are fast, filthy, and dangerous. Many large slaughtering facilities operate at rates that exceed 300 cows per hour. These breakneck speeds are the reason that jobs in these facilities are now among the most dangerous in the country. At these high rates, filth and the spread of pathogen-containing fecal matter to consumable meat become commonplace.

- *Industrial food*: The nation's love affair with cheap, industrial, "fast," and processed food creates the demand that eventually leads to factory farming, an emphasis on consumption and devaluation of production, and a disconnection between citizens and their food sources. Until we come to grips with the fact that cheap industrial food is inherently unsafe (irradiated or not), we can only expect things to get worse.

- *Meat monopolies*: A mere three corporations control 77% of the meat market, giving them a monopoly-like control over beef production, slaughtering, and distribution. This kind of concentration translates to contamination as long as speed and profit, rather than health and public safety, remain the priorities of the meat industry. (*Food Irradiation*: 8)

In *Food Irradiation: An Activist Primer*, Food and Water includes quotes opposing food irradiation from such scientists as George L. Tritsch of the Roswell Park Cancer Institute in Buffalo, New York, John W. Gofman of the University of California at Berkeley, and Geraldine Dettman, radiation safety officer and biosafety officer at Brown University. These scientists raise concerns about carcinogens, chemicals, and mutated organisms produced by irradiation.

CONCLUSION

In a 1999 *Technology Review* article, Daniel Akst compared those who fear food irradiation to the Luddites, the "disaffected craftsmen who destroyed newfangled textile machinery in England in the early 19th century." Akst suggests that most people do not comprehend how food irradiation actually works. This lack of understanding leads to fear. In many ways this concern about food irradiation resembles a fear of flying. "You are probably safer on a major U.S. airline than in your bathtub, yet my mother-in-law (who smokes cigarettes) is still somewhat afraid to fly. Who understands, after all, what keeps airplanes aloft?" (81–83).

On the other hand, in an article in *Bulletin of the Atomic Scientists*, Linda Rothstein says that food irradiation seems to be a concept that has come and gone. "Apart from a very occasional piece of fruit—usually a papaya—irradiated foods are not in demand and rarely appear in the marketplace." Of course, that could always change. "The hearts of irradiation boosters must leap with each report of food contamination or news of yet another recall." New technologies are coming down the pipeline that may provide more alternatives to food irradiation. If that happens, "claiming that irradiation is the only way to assure the safety of the American food supply . . . [may become] yesterday's news" (Rothstein: 7–11).

TOPICS FOR DISCUSSION

1. Every year millions of people suffer from food poisoning. Have you ever become sick from something you ate? How do you think this could have been prevented?

2. Before reading this chapter, had you heard of food irradiation? If you had, did you think that it was a good idea?

3. Since reading this chapter, have your opinions changed? How and why?

4. Have you ever eaten irradiated food? Did you like it? Did you notice any difference between it and nonirradiated food? If so, how was it different?

5. Do you think that food irradiation will become more popular? Why or why not?

REFERENCES AND RESOURCES

Book

Gibbs, Gary. *The Food That Would Last Forever*. Garden City Park, New York: Avery Publishing Group, 1993.

Booklet

Food Irradiation: An Activist Primer. Walden, Vermont: Food and Water, 2000.

Magazines, Journals, and Newspapers

Akst, Daniel. "Ludd's Choosy Children." *Technology Review*, January 1, 1999, 102(1): 81–83.

Buzby, Jean C., and Rosanna Mentzer Morrison. "Food Irradiation." *Food Review*, May–August 1999, 22(2): 21–22.

Demetrakakes, Pan. "Zap!" *Food Processing*, February 1998, 59(2): 20–26.

Gormley, James J. "Food Irradiation—'Protecting' Us?" *Better Nutrition*, February 1998, 60(2): 10.

Grogan, David. "Rare and Deadly." *People Weekly*, February 15, 1993, 39(6): 48–50.

Henkel, John. "Irradiation: A Safe Measure for Safer Food." *FDA Consumer*, May–June 1998, 32(3): 12–17.

Holcomb, Betty. "How Safe Is Your Dinner?" *Good Housekeeping*, March 2000, 230(3): 75–76.

"Irradiation Back on the Front Burner." *Tufts University Health and Nutrition Letter*, March 2000, 18(1): 4.

Lindner, Lawrence. "Eating Right: In Harmony with Nature? Organic Food Purists May Blanch, But Irradiation Is Safe, Widespread, and Time-Tested." *Washington Post*, March 28, 2000: Page Z11.

Lingle, Rick. "Food Irradiation Accelerations." *Packaging Digest*, July 1999, 36(7): 44–48.

Linstedt, Sharon. "Irradiated Meat Seen as Tough Sell; At Least One Local Meat Seller Has Sized Up His Customers and Has Concluded They Won't Buy It." *Buffalo News*, March 5, 2000: Page 15B.

Lore, David. "Food Irradiation Grows, But Public Remains Wary." *Columbus Dispatch*, February 27, 2000: Page 7B.

Marandino, Cristin. "Is Zapping Food the Answer?" *Vegetarian Times*, December 1997, 244: 12–13.

Morrison, Rosanna Mentzer, Jean C. Buzby, and C.-T. Jordan Lin. "Irradiating Ground Beef to Enhance Food Safety." *Food Review*, January–April 1997, 20(1): 33–37.

Prier, Richard, and Jay V. Solnick. "Foodborne and Waterborne Infectious Diseases." *Post-Graduate Medicine*, April 2000, 107(4): 245–252, 255.

Rothstein, Linda. "An Idea Whose Time Has Come—and Gone?" *Bulletin of the Atomic Scientists*, July–August 1998, 54(4): 7–11.

Shewmake, Roger A., and Bonnie Dillon. "Food Poisoning." *Post-Graduate Medicine*, June 1998, 103(6): 125–129, 134, 136.

Skerett, P.J. "Food Irradiation: Will It Keep the Doctor Away?" *Technology Review*, November–December 1997, 100(8): 28–36.

Wood, Olivia Bennett, and Christine M. Bruhn. "Position of the American Dietetic Association: Food Irradiation." *Journal of the American Dietetic Association*, February 2000, 100(2): 246.

Organizations to Contact

Agricultural Research Service
James L. Whitten Building
United States Department of Agriculture
14th and Independence Ave. SW
Washington, DC 20250
Phone: 202-720-2791
http://www.ars.usda.gov (June 24, 2000)

Centers for Disease Control and Prevention
1600 Clifton Rd.
Atlanta, GA 30333
Phone: 800-311-3435, 404-639-3534, 404-639-3311
http://www.cdc.gov (June 24, 2000)

Foundation for Food Irradiation Education
Operated as a public service by Brookhaven Technology Group, Inc.
12–12 Technology Drive
Setauket, NY 11733
No phone number available
www.food-irradiation.com (June 24, 2000)

Grocery Manufacturers of America
1010 Wisconsin Ave. NW, Ninth Floor
Washington, DC 20007
Phone: 202-337-9400
http://www.gmabrands.com (July 13, 2000)

International Food Information Council
1100 Connecticut Avenue NW, Suite 430
Washington, DC 20036
Phone: 202-296-6540
http://www.ific.org (June 24, 2000)

The National Food Safety Database
University of Florida
Florida Energy Extension Service
P.O. Box 110940, Building 242
2610 SW 23rd Terrace
Gainesville, FL 32611
Phone: 352-392-7126
http://www.foodsafety.org (May 22, 2002)

Organic Consumers Association
6101 Cliff Estate Road
Little Marais, MN 55614

Phone: 218-226-4164
http://www.purefood.org (July 12, 2000)

Public Citizen
1600 20th St. NW
Washington, DC 20009
Phone: 202-588-1000
http://www.citizen.org (June 24, 2000)

3

Vegetarian/Vegan Diets

Is a vegetarian diet healthier than a diet that includes meat? Many believe that it is, but others contend that a vegetarian diet lacks sufficient vitamins and nutrients. A number of people also advocate a vegetarian diet for other reasons such as the environment and animal rights.

For the vast majority of Americans, eating some form of meat is an essential part of the daily diet. Breakfast would not be breakfast without eggs and sausage or bacon. Lunch would be incomplete without a cheeseburger and fries or a turkey club. Dinner is most enjoyable when it includes a medium-rare steak grilled to perfection. To these Americans, it would be unimaginable to have a Thanksgiving without turkey or an Easter celebration without a ham or a leg of lamb. In fact, the American Meat Institute Foundation notes that the use of meat, poultry and fish is higher than ever. "In 1997, meat, poultry and fish consumption was 223.6 pounds per person. Compare that to 214.6 pounds in 1987, 207.9 pounds in 1977 and 198 pounds in 1976" (American Meat Institute Foundation Web site).

Clearly, people may obtain valuable nutrients from meat. According to the National Cattlemen's Beef Association, beef is an excellent source of heme (animal-based) iron. The following chart from the National Cattlemen's Beef Association Web site, http://www.beefnutrition.org, shows that beef has more iron than other foods:

	Total Iron (mg)	Available Iron (mg)
Beef eye round, roasted, three ounces, lean only	1.7	.22
Chicken breast meat, roasted, three ounces	.90	.12

Baked beans, canned, plain, ½ cup	.40	.02
Egg, large, whole, hard-boiled	.60	.03
Brown rice, cooked, ½ cup	.50	.02
Apple, 1 medium	.20	.01
Spinach, raw, ½ cup	.80	.04

Beef is also rich in zinc. The National Cattlemen's Beef Association states that the zinc in meat, liver, eggs, and seafoods (especially oysters) more is available to the body than that in whole-grain products. Beef in the diet also improves the absorption of zinc from other foods. Moreover, a study commissioned by the National Cattlemen's Beef Association found that people who eat higher amounts of beef are more likely to meet 100% of the daily value for protein, iron, zinc, and B vitamins than people who eat lower amounts of beef or no beef (National Cattlemen's Beef Association Web site, http://www.beefnutrition.org).

In the past, some people stayed away from pork, a source of protein, because of its high fat content. That is no longer true. The National Pork Producers Council notes that pork today is leaner and lower in fat, calories, and cholesterol than it was 20 years ago. All of the loin cuts of pork—such as tenderloin and loin chops—"provide less than 180 calories and nine grams of fat per three-ounce serving." The council says that pork contains about a third less cholesterol than chicken and that there is only a slight difference in the amount of fat between pork and chicken. (National Pork Producers Council Web site).

The National Chicken Council states that fat content breast meat is the part of the chicken lowest in fat, but leg meat is very competitive with other types of meat and poultry. "According to the American Dietetic Association, three ounces of baked chicken drumstick with the skin removed has less total fat than the same amount of sirloin steak, beef tenderloin, pork chop, or salmon" The following table, from the National Chicken Council Web site, shows how the calories and fat content of chicken compare to other animal protein sources per three-ounce boneless, cooked portion:

Type of Meat	Calories	Total Fat (g)	Saturated Fat (g)	Cholesterol (mg)	Protein (g)
Filet of sole, baked	100	1.5	0.3	60	20
Chicken breast, no skin, baked	120	1.5	0.5	70	24

Chicken drumstick, no skin, baked	130	4.0	1.0	80	23
Salmon, baked	150	7.0	1.5	55	21
Chicken breast, with skin, baked	170	7.0	2.0	70	25
Beef sirloin steak, trimmed of visible fat, broiled	170	6.0	2.0	75	26
Chicken drumstick, with skin, baked	180	9.0	3.0	75	23
Beef tenderloin, trimmed of visible fat, broiled	180	9.0	3.0	70	24

Nevertheless, a growing number of Americans are deciding to eliminate animal products from their diets. According to a study conducted for the Vegetarian Resource Group, 2.5% of Americans may be considered vegetarians; they never eat meat, poultry, or fish. A higher proportion, 4.5%, said that they never eat meat. A similar statistic was obtained for poultry, and 9% said that they never eat fish or seafood. For dairy products, eggs, and honey, those statistics were 3.7%, 6.7%, and 15.4%, respectively (Vegetarian Resource Group Web site). That means that millions of Americans follow some form of vegetarian diet.

There are several types of vegetarians. Lacto-ovo vegetarians eat dairy and egg products in addition to fruits and vegetables; ovo vegetarians eat egg products; lacto vegetarians eat dairy products; and vegans (pronounced VEE-gn) refrain from all animal products including dairy, eggs, and honey (Vegetarian Resource Group Web site). "Beyond modifying their diet, many vegans refuse to consume any animal products. That means they do not wear leather or consume anything else derived from animal source" (Weiss: 7).

People give many reasons to eliminate animal products from the diet. These include "health, ecological and religious concerns, dislike of meat, compassion for animals, belief in non-violence, and economics. People often become vegetarian for one reason, be it health, religion, or animal rights, and later adopt some of the other reasons as well" (Vegetarian Resource Group Web site). An April 1999 article in *Vegetarian Times* lists 22 reasons for becoming a vegetarian. In essence, the article contends that vegetarians are healthier than nonvegetarians and have longer lives. "Vegetarians live about seven years longer, and vegans ... about 15 years longer than meat eaters." Vegetarians save money. "Replacing meat, chicken and fish with vegetables and fruits is estimated to cut food bills by an average of $4,000 a year." They also spare the lives of untold numbers of animals. "Each day, 22 million animals are slaughtered to support the American appetite for meat" (Dworkin: 90–93).

In *Vegan Nutrition: Pure and Simple*, Michael Klaper outlines some of the reasons that people may chose to follow a vegetarian diet. "We now live in a world of Salmonella-tainted chickens, Listeria-covered cheese, and beefburgers laced with estrogenic hormones and residues of potent antibiotics. These are very good reasons why people would want to obtain their daily nourishment without pouring fatty and contaminated meat and dairy products through their bloodstream every few hours. Many people are concerned about the high incidence of health threats that are linked to improper diet, like heart attacks, strokes, birth defects, breast, prostate and other cancers, high blood pressure, diabetes and other diseases. They are seeking more wholesome food alternatives for themselves and their families." He adds that eating meat products supports the violence that is part of killing animals for food, and it negatively impacts the environment. Humans have no nutritional requirement to eat any form of animal food or milk from cows (Klaper, 1998: 3).

According to the Physicians Committee for Responsible Medicine, the following are some of the long-term health reasons for eating a plant-based diet:

- A vegetarian diet lowers blood pressure in those people who are prone to high blood pressure.
- Vegetarians tend to have lower cholesterol levels.
- After controlling for socioeconomic status, body-mass index, and smoking, vegetarians have cancer rates that are 20 to 50% below population averages.
- When compared to the general population, vegetarians are far less likely to be obese.
- Plant-based diets tend to support later menarche. That finding has been correlated with a reduced risk for breast cancer. (Physicians Committee for Responsible Medicine Web site)

Vegetarians consume a plant-based diet. What does that mean? "Vegetarians eat a wide range of foods that come from the soil, including fruits, vegetables, grains and grain products, nuts, seeds and legumes, and dried beans and peas" (Havala: 4). Does such a diet have sufficient protein? Havala writes, "as long as you are eating enough wholesome foods to meet your calories needs and are getting a reasonable mix of vegetables, grains, and legumes over the course of the day, you should not have any problems getting enough protein or the appropriate mix of amino acids. At the same time, you will probably avoid the excessive amounts of protein that can be typical of the traditional Western-style diet" (Havala: 17).

HISTORY OF VEGETARIANISM

Vegetarianism is not a new concept. It has existed throughout history in cultures around the world. "Many of the world's greatest philosophers and intellects refused meat in times when such a choice was contrary to the dictates of the ruling class. In the west, the first of these was the Greek philosopher Pythagoras, who lived 2,500 years ago and is often considered 'the father of vegetarianism.' Until the late 19th century, when the word 'vegetarian' was coined, people who lived on a meatless diet were referred to as 'Pythagoreans' " (Melina, Davis, and Harrison: 7).

Born around 580 B.C., Pythagoras was multitalented. In addition to discoveries in mathematics and geometry and beliefs in planetary motion and the rotation of the Earth around the sun, "he also founded a society that pursued wisdom, believed in the transmigration of souls and practiced meditation. Among the Pythagoreans, materialism and meat-eating were taboo" (Melina, Davis, and Harrison: 7–8). Since Pythagoras, there have been a countless number of vegetarians, including Plato, Socrates, Newton, Leonardo de Vinci, Mahatma Gandhi, Albert Schweitzer, Albert Einstein, Paul and Linda McCartney, Richard Gere, *Spider-man* star Tobey Maguire, and Kim Basinger.

It should be noted that until the twentieth century, only the rich had the wherewithal to eat meat on a regular basis. "Even in the 18th and 19th centuries, well-to-do families of many European countries such as France and Holland could seldom afford to eat meat more than once a week. The truth is that the vast majority of the world's population has existed on a near-vegetarian diet and still does, though not necessarily by choice" (Melina, Davis, and Harrison: 9).

Donald Watson founded the vegan segment of the vegetarian movement in England in 1944. It "called for the abolition not only of all foods of animal origin but of all animal-based commodities as well. Furthermore, it emphasized the moral, spiritual, social, health, and economic advantages of living by humane principles" (Stepaniak: 5).

During the late 1960s and early 1970s, the vegetarian movement gained momentum, especially among counterculture groups that advocated ecology and natural living (Melina, Davis, and Harrison: 9). In 1971, *Diet for a Small Planet*, by Frances Moore Lappé, was published. Her arguments for the environment and fighting world hunger attracted many people to vegetarianism. Two more books, *Diet for a New America* (1987) and *May All Be Fed* (1992), both written by John Robbins, galvanized still more support with his arguments about the environment, world hunger, and the "degenerative diseases of affluence." He also took a strong stand in favor of animal rights (Melina, Davis, and Harrison: 9–10).

EFFECTS OF VEGETARIAN DIETS

During the 1990s, increasing numbers of health professionals saw the value of vegetarian diets. Shortly before his death in 1998 at the age of 94, Benjamin Spock, probably the best-known pediatrician in the United States, advocated vegetarian diets for children. Apparently Spock had become a vegetarian in 1991. According to his wife, that change of diet "greatly improved his health and enabled him to complete the revision of his world-famous book" (Brody: Section F, page 7, column 4). In the seventh edition of *Dr. Spock's Baby and Child Care*, Spock and Steven J. Parker wrote, "A vegetarian-based diet for children is generally more healthful than a diet containing the cholesterol, saturated fat, and excessive protein found in meat and dairy products." But this type of diet—derived from many leafy green vegetables, fruits, whole grains, and bean products—should not necessarily be low in calories. "Studies have shown that a well-balanced vegetarian diet had many advantages and does not interfere with a child's growth and development. A reliable vitamin B12 source such as a children's vitamin or cereal or soy milk fortified with B12 is recommended for vegetarians" (Spock and Parker: 342).

In *Pregnancy, Children, and the Vegan Diet*, Michael Klaper recommends a vegan diet for children. He claims that animal fats have been linked to clogged arteries in children as young as 9 months old. Fat in children's unbalanced diets is the basis for heart attacks and strokes when they are adults and sometimes in childhood. "A high-fat diet also promotes higher levels of sex and growth hormones that circulate in the body. The effects of these higher hormone levels are of great concern, as growth and maturation are crowded into disturbingly early years" (Klaper, 1997: 37).

Are vegetarian diets always beneficial? Do they provide all the essential vitamins and nutrients that people require? First, it should be noted that not all vegetarian diets are low in fat. Whole dairy products, such as cheese, milk, cream, and butter, are high in saturated fat, which is unhealthful. When consumed frequently, they may negate any of the advantages of a vegetarian diet. Though nuts, seeds, mono-unsaturated oils, avocados, and tofu—foods often eaten on a vegetarian diet—are also higher in fat and calories, they contain healthier fats.

Numerous studies indicate that a low-fat vegetarian diet may be helpful for people with a number of medical conditions. A short-term examination of 500 men and women published in the *American Journal of Clinical Nutrition* found that "a strict, very-low-fat vegetarian diet free from all animal products combined with lifestyle changes that include exercise and weight loss is an effective way to lower serum cholesterol and blood pressure" (McDougall, Saunders, and Spiller: 625S). Women with menstrual cramps and premenstrual syndrome (PMS) have obtained relief from a low-fat, vegetarian diet. Researchers at Georgetown University in Washington, D.C., followed 33 women with moderate to severe symptoms. "The women shunned meat, fish, dairy, and eggs, as well as butter, oils, and even, peanut butter." Their diets had only about 10% of the calories from fat, "the lowest healthy limit" (Walsh: 42). For many of the women, the results were quite dramatic. "They experienced less intense and less frequent menstrual pain and also noted increased energy, decreased water retention and fewer concentration problems. Some even lost weight and reduced their cholesterol levels" (Chipley: 14). "Researchers suspect that this eating style works by increasing sex hormone–binding globulin, which binds to and inhibits the effect of estrogen, which is a primary culprit in menstrual pain and discomfort" (Walsh: 42).

A vegetarian diet may be useful for those suffering from rheumatoid arthritis. Research conducted at the University of Kuopio in Finland showed that people with rheumatoid arthritis who ate an uncooked vegan diet that was rich in lactobacilli experienced a relief of symptoms. After three months, when they returned to their meat-eating diets, the symptoms returned (La Puma: 52). In another study, researchers examined how people with rheumatoid arthritis responded to 7 to 10 days of fasting, which was followed by 3½ months of a gluten-free, vegan diet, which was, in turn, followed by 9 months of a lacto-vegetarian diet. "For all clinical variables and most laboratory variables measured, the 27 patients in the fasting and vegetarian diet groups improved significantly compared with the 26 patients in the control group who followed their usual omnivorous diet throughout the study period" (Kjeldsen-Kragh: 5945–6005).

While most cancer patients are told to eat whatever they wish, Keith Block, medical director of the Block Medical Center in Evanston, Illinois, believes that this is a terrible mistake. He contends that fatty foods sanctioned by the National Cancer Institute support the cancer while starving the patient. In a cancer patient's body, "Metabolism speeds up as the immune system marshals its forces to fight the disease. Rapidly growing tumors become sinkholes for nutrients and calories. The body churns through protein, calories, vitamins and minerals, impairing immunity and leaving the patient increasingly susceptible to infection and unable to tolerate chemotherapy, radiation or drugs. Eventually, the cancerous tumors prevail, and severe malnutrition often leads to death" (O'Connor: 56–63).

Block contends that dietary recommendations should be part of cancer treatment, and he advises his patients to adhere to a strictly low-fat, vegetarian diet. More than half of all calories should come from complex carbohydrates; less than 15% of calories should come from fat. "Plant foods inhibit cancer. Phytochemicals in broccoli, cauliflower and other cruciferous vegetables help cancer-fighting enzymes purge carcinogens in cells. Garlic strengthens the immune system. Soyfoods contain genistein, a chemical that counteracts hormonal cancers and shrinks tumors. Carotenoids in orange-colored fruits and vegetables as well as leafy greens shield cells from careening free-radicals that can cause cancer" (O'Connor: 56–63).

There is research supporting Block's beliefs. One study conducted in Sweden found that breast cancer was more likely to reoccur two to four years after surgery in patients whose diets were higher in fat. A review of men with prostate cancer determined that men with advanced prostate cancer ate more saturated fat than a control population, indicating that animal fat could promote the growth of malignant tumors. Likewise, "Several epidemiological studies show a strong correlation between per capita fat intake and mortality from breast and other hormonal cancers, particularly for post-menopausal women. Other studies show that Italian and Asian women, who eat lower on the food chain and consume relatively little animal fat or protein, live longer with advanced breast cancer than American women" (O'Connor: 56–63).

While chemotherapy and radiation have been known to take a devastating toll on patients, Block has found that his patients manage the treatments with fewer ill effects. He is convinced that the phytochemicals in cruciferous vegetables detoxify the blood and flush poisonous residues of drugs and chemotherapy from the body (O'Connor: 56–63).

Not everyone agrees that vegetarian diets are beneficial. Some people maintain that a vegetarian diet has limitations. A May 2000 article in the *Journal of the American Dietetic Association* described a study of overweight to moderately obese men between the ages of 51 and 69 and resistance training. For 12 weeks, 9 of the men ate their usual meat-based diet. During the same time period, 10 men followed a lacto-ovo-vegetarian diet. The men who ate meat "experienced greater gains in fat-free mass and skeletal muscle in response to resistance training than those who ate a lacto-ovo-vegetarian (LOV) diet" ("Omnivorous vs. Vegetarian Diet": 596). Women who want to give birth to a son may need to think twice about vegetarianism. "Researchers at Nottingham University in England have found that mothers who don't eat meat or fish are more likely than carnivores to give birth to daughters. In the general British population, boys outnumber girls at birth 106 to 100, but girls outnumbered boys

100 to 81 among babies born to vegetarian moms in the study" (McLaughlin: 82).

The prime concern appears to be that vegetarian diets may fail to supply sufficient amounts of certain vitamins. A study of elderly Chinese vegetarians, with a mean age of 81, found that the vegetarian diet appeared to be useful in preventing chronic illness. However, the diet was deficient in several B vitamins as well as "lower in total energy, fat and protein calories" (Woo et al.: 455–461). Similarly, research published in the *American Journal of Clinical Nutrition* compared the nutritional intake and iron status of 50 vegetarian women between the ages of 18 and 45 to 24 age-matched meat-eating women. The vegetarians were found to have a relatively low intake of hemoglobin iron (Ball and Bartlett: 353). Another article, also published in the *American Journal of Clinical Nutrition*, compared the rates of anemia in vegetarian pregnant women to the rates in meat-eating women. Lacto-ovo-vegetarians "more frequently reported anemia during pregnancy, but this was not associated with any adverse pregnancy outcomes" (Drake, Reddy, and Davies: 628S).

The USDA Grand Forks Human Nutrition Research Center in North Dakota compared the zinc content in the diets of healthy young women who followed a lacto-ovo-vegetarian diet to women of a similar age who ate meat. "The lactoovovegetarian diet was associated with a 21% reduction in absorptive efficiency that, together with a 14% reduction in dietary zinc, reduced the amount of zinc absorbed by 35% (2.4 compared with 3.7 mg/d) and reduced plasma zinc by 5% within the normal range. Zinc balance was maintained with both diets." The researchers concluded that "although there is a greater risk of zinc deficiency in persons consuming lactoovovegetarian compared with omnivorous diets, with inclusion of whole grains and legumes zinc requirements can be met and zinc balanced maintained" (Hunt, Matthys, and Johnson: 421–430).

Whether vegetarians, especially vegans, consume adequate amounts of calcium is not clear. Some studies imply that the intake may be too low (Stepaniak: 215). Nevertheless, a March 1998 article in *Vegetarian Times* noted that calcium is found not only in dairy products. On the contrary, many plants have high amounts of calcium. "One cup of turnip or collard greens or one-half cup of sea vegetables, such as hijiki, nori or kelp, contains about as much calcium as a cup of milk. In addition, calcium fortified rice and soy milks, tofu, dried fruits and sesame seeds are valuable nondairy sources of calcium" (Turner: 48–53). The article said that the concern is not only about calcium intake, but also about how much is excreted. Some foods have the potential to increase the excretion of calcium. "For instance, it's believed that high-protein consumption interferes with calcium absorption, which means that dairy products can actually leach calcium even as they provide it. And dietary fiber will bind to calcium, effectively blocking its absorption—so it's best to eat high-fiber foods, such as enriched cereals, at separate meals from calcium-dense foods" (Turner: 48–53). Moreover, to maintain calcium levels in the blood, the body requires levels of certain nutrients. "Vitamin D helps regulate calcium absorption from the digestive tract, slowing the excretion of calcium and channeling it back into the blood and bones. Phosphorous plays a delicate balancing act: When its levels are too high, calcium is excreted, a good reason to avoid high-phosphorous products, such as soda. And other minerals, such as potassium and magnesium, are equally important in regulating calcium levels in blood and bones" (Turner: 48–53).

A number of studies have found that people who eat a plant-based diet are more at risk for vitamin B12 deficiency (Melina, Davis, and Harrison: 33–34). The consequences of such a deficiency "include a host of neurological problems that range from subtle tingling of extremities, to actual loss of sensation or paralysis, to changes in memory. In fact, some of the symptoms commonly attributed to senility in old age are actually believed to be the result of B12 deficiency" (Stepaniak: 217). According to Joanne Stepaniak, an educator and counselor who is the author of *The Vegan Sourcebook*, vegans risk deficiency unless they supplement their diet with vitamin B12 (Stepaniak: 216).

Is a vegetarian diet safe for children? Spock supported the diet for children, but others disagree. In an article that appeared in 1998, noted *New York Times* nutritional columnist Jane Brody wrote, "Placing children on a vegan diet is a recommendation that few experts in childhood nutrition endorse. Concerns center on the ability of small children to consume enough bulky plant foods to take in all the calories and nutrients they need to sustain normal growth. Particularly worrisome are the calcium and iron that are best absorbed from milk and meats, respectively." Brody added that most experts recommend "a less radical approach to children's diets" (Brody: Section F, page 7, column 4). Perhaps red meat and poultry may be eliminated, but fish, eggs, and diary products should be included.

In contrast, a March 15, 2000, article in *Patient Care* said that recent studies have found that vegetarian and nonvegetarian children grow at about the same rate. "Researchers typically concluded that a vegan or broader vegetarian diet did not impair a child's growth and development if known pitfalls were avoided. . . . Pitfalls referred to potential inadequacies in calories, protein, vitamins . . . , calcium, iron and zinc—problems usually confined to the vegan diet" (Labson et al.: 111–128).

How may problems be avoided? First, extra attention must be devoted to food planning. Without such care, "Food intake may be haphazard, or lack variety, be higher in fat than is desirable, or be short on nutrients or calories." Also, it may be advisable to ask your medical provider to screen for iron-deficiency anemia. Vitamin C intake should be encouraged. "Foods that contain vitamin C, such as citrus fruits, improve the absorption of nonheme iron [the type of iron in plant foods]. Vegetarians should be advised also to limit intake of foods that are high in substances such as phytates (whole grain, bran, and soy products) and oxalic acid (spinach). These substances decrease the absorption of iron" (Labson et al.: 111–128).

If dairy products have been eliminated, calcium and vitamin D should be taken in supplemental form. Parents should also be certain that their children consume adequate amounts of vitamin B12 and zinc. The consequences of a B12 deficiency have already been noted. As for zinc, inadequate amounts may cause "delays in cognitive development." Further, "poor appetite and slowing of growth are the most evident clinical signs of zinc deficiency in children, particularly during infancy and adolescence" (Labson et al.: 111–128).

The American Academy of Pediatrics maintains that some forms of vegetarian diets should be off limits for children. In the *Pediatric Nutrition Handbook*, fourth edition, the Academy provides guidelines for infants, toddlers, and older children. Infants are potentially at greatest risk from inappropriate restrictions of diet. They are particularly vulnerable during weaning if they are fed a macrobiotic diet. Providing calorically dense foods at the time of wearing is important so that the increased bulk of vegetarian diets does not interfere with adequate consumption of energy, protein, and other nutrients. Toddlers are also unable to tolerate bulky diets. Meal plans must include foods of high caloric density, such as nuts, olives, dates, and avocados. Older children and adolescents on vegetarian diets are at less risk for growth failure than younger children. However, adolescents must understand basic principles of food selection. Without adequate nutrition knowledge, adolescents who combine vegetarian eating habits with weight-loss schemes are vulnerable to malnutrition and growth failure (Kleinman: 581–582).

Adolescents who consider themselves vegetarians also have higher rates of eating disorders. In a study published in the August 1997 issue of the *Archives of Pediatrics and Adolescent Medicine*, researchers reported that "vegetarians were more likely to engage in all of the disordered eating behaviors examined in this study, which included frequent dieting, binge eating, self-induced vomiting and laxative use.... Vegetarianism may be serving as a marker for potentially harmful weight control behaviors.... It is possible that the adolescent is using vegetarianism as a socially acceptable way to avoid fat intake and to reduce energy intake" (Neumark-Sztainer et al.: 833–838).

Ann Louise Gittleman, an award-winning nationally recognized nutritionist, does not think that a vegetarian diet is appropriate for everyone. "Some people, because of their genetic inheritance and ancestry, are better designed biologically than others for a vegetarian or near-vegetarian diet. However, I believe everyone would be more healthy physically if they ate some meat."

During her college years, Gittleman went on a vegetarian diet. Her response was far from ideal. "By about the middle of my senior year, my hair started falling out and I couldn't stand the noise in the dorm. My nerves were on edge, I lost about 20 pounds, and my skin broke out. My parents were very upset at my deteriorating physical condition, but no one could convince me to eat animal products." Eventually, Gittleman visited a physician who specialized in nutrition. "He put me on megavitamins and insisted I begin eating chicken. That was the first step on my road back to health" (Gittleman: 62–63).

CONCERN FOR ANIMALS

As has previously been noted, people follow a vegetarian diet for a wide variety of reasons. For some, it is an integral part of their religious beliefs. The Seventh-Day Adventist Church and some Eastern religions, such as Buddhism and Hinduism, promote vegetarian diets (Melina, Davis, and Harrison: 7). Some Jewish people believe that Judaism supports eliminating meat. In a March/April 1999 article in *Tikkun*, Richard H. Schwartz wrote, "God's first dietary law allowed only vegetarian foods. ... Some of the greatest Jewish sages have taught that permission to eat meat was given later only as a grudging concession to people's weakness, and that many prohibitions and restrictions were applied to keep alive a sense of reverence for life" (Schwartz, 1999: 50–51). Further, in *Judaism and Vegetarianism*, Schwartz said that concern for animals is part of the Jewish belief systems. "The Jewish tradition clearly indicates that we are forbidden to be cruel to animals and that we are to treat them with compassion. These concepts are summarized in the Hebrew phrase *tsa'ar ba'alei chayim*, the biblical mandate not to cause pain to any living creature. ... Animals are also God's creatures, possessing sensitivity and the capacity for feeling pain; hence they must be protected and treated with compassion and justice" (Schwartz, 1988: 13–14).

Apart from religion, there are many who are simply against killing animals for food or eating animal-based products. When there are so many alternatives, why should animals die—or be forced to live under terrible circumstances—so that humans may eat? Often, these same people are opposed to various aspects of the meat-producing industry. Some believe that consuming animal products harms the environment.

Raised on a dairy farm in Montana, Howard F. Lyman was the fourth generation of his family to work as a farmer and cattle rancher. For 20 years, he also ran a feedlot. Lyman loved to eat meat. "Sure, I used to enjoy my steaks as much as the next guy," he wrote in *Mad Cowboy* (Lyman with Merzer: 11).

However, Lyman no longer eats any meat. In fact, he went on to become president of the International Vegetarian Union. He explains that the rendering industry uses the parts of slaughtered cows not eaten by humans, along with the entire bodies of diseased cows and other farm animals, euthanized pets, animals captured by animal-control agencies, and animals killed by motor vehicles. The resulting mixture is ground and cooked. The fatty material floating to the top is refined for use in such products as cosmetics, lubricants, soaps, candles, and waxes. The protein material is dried and pulverized into a brown powder. About one-fourth of it consists of fecal material. This powder is used as an additive to pet food and livestock feed.

In August 1997, the FDA issued a regulation banning the feeding of protein from ruminants (cud-chewing animals) to other ruminants. While cattle no longer eat solid parts of other cattle, sheep, or goats, they still are few ground-up parts of other animals and fowls, as well as blood and fecal material of their own species and of chickens (Lyman with Merzer: 11–13).

The environment in which animals live before they are killed may be far from ideal. In *Being a Vegan*, Stefanie Iris Weiss, a writer and longtime vegetarian, writes that animals raised in agribusiness factory farms often live in a harsh, overcrowded environment that has devastating effects on animals. Chickens may try to peck each other to death. To prevent this, they may be debeaked. "Pigs in captivity also have been known to practice self-mutilation in the form of tail biting. Calves intended for slaughter are often kept in pens so small that their muscles are unable to develop properly. This is seen as desirable because veal, the meat that comes from calves, will therefore be more tender." Moreover, Weiss contends that the meat industry wastes natural resources. "It takes 2,500 gallons of water to produce one pound of meat—both to feed the animal and grow the food that the animal consumes. Water is not an endless resource, and much of the ground water left on the earth is contaminated. Factory farming also has contributed to water contamination, for a great deal of animal excrement and pesticide residue has been released into rivers. . . . Cattle raised for meat production consume enough grain to feed 8.7 billion people a year" (Weiss: 14–15).

In *Prisoned Chickens, Poisoned Eggs*, Karen Davis describes standing outside a chicken slaughter plant and watching the trucks with thousands of chickens, who may wait in the trucks for several hours before they are processed. "The killing of birds normally involves three phases: motor paralysis by means of an electric current (inaccurately called "stunning"), throat-cutting, and bleeding. Poultry slaughtered in the United States are neither stunned (rendered unconscious) nor anesthetized (rendered pain-free). Pre-slaughter stunning of poultry is not required by law and is not practiced despite the use of the term "stun" to denote what is really immobilization by means of painful electric shocks" (Davis: 113–114). Davis also details the chickens' pain and suffering: "Like mammals subjected to painful stimuli, chickens show a rapid increase in heart rate and blood pressure, and behavioral changes consistent with those found in mammals indicating pain perception—efforts to escape, distress cries, guarding behavior, and the passive immobility that develops in birds and other animals subjected to traumatic events that are aversive and that continue regardless of attempts by the victim to reduce or eliminate them" (Davis: 113, 122).

Poultry.org, a Web site owned by Farm Sanctuary, an organization dedicated to reducing animal cruelty, outlines other negative aspects of the poultry-farming industry. For example, it notes that almost all the laying hens in the United States live in battery cages, which are "lined up in rows and stacked in tiers inside of huge warehouses." Poultry.org, states that poultry that are bred for eating also have dreadful lives. Most chickens and turkeys are crowded into sheds called "grower houses." Chicken and turkeys bred for meat have been genetically altered to grow faster and larger. This rapid growth rate increases profitability, but also causes health problems, such as legs that cannot support the birds' bodies (Farm Sanctuary Web site, poultry.org).

One might think that free-range chickens have better living conditions, but that is not necessarily the case, according to United Poultry Concerns, a nonprofit organization dedicated to raising public awareness about the poultry industry. "Birds raised in the United States for meat—mainly chickens and turkeys—may be sold as 'range' if they have U.S. Department of Agriculture certified access to the outdoors. No other criteria, such as environmental quality, size of area, number of birds, or space per bird are included in this term. . . . To date, there is no legal or commercial definition of husbandry terms regulating the sale of eggs in the U.S. There are no standards governing the term or the claim 'range' or similar advertisements on egg cartoons, such as 'free running,' 'free roaming,' or 'free walking.' "

Moreover, "free-range hens are debeaked at the hatchery the same as battery-caged hens. Debeaking is a painful mutilation that impairs the hens' ability to eat normally and to preen (practice bodily hygiene). Typically, 2,000 or more hens—each hen having only one to two square feet of floor space—are confined in a shed without access to the outdoors during their lives. If the hens can go outside, the exit usually is very small allowing only the closet hens to get out. The yard may be nothing but a mud yard saturated with droppings and intestinal coccidia and other parasites" (United Poultry Concerns Web site).

Over a period of six years, Sue Coe, a British-born journalist, activist, painter, and printmaker, visited about 30 slaughterhouses. She chroni-

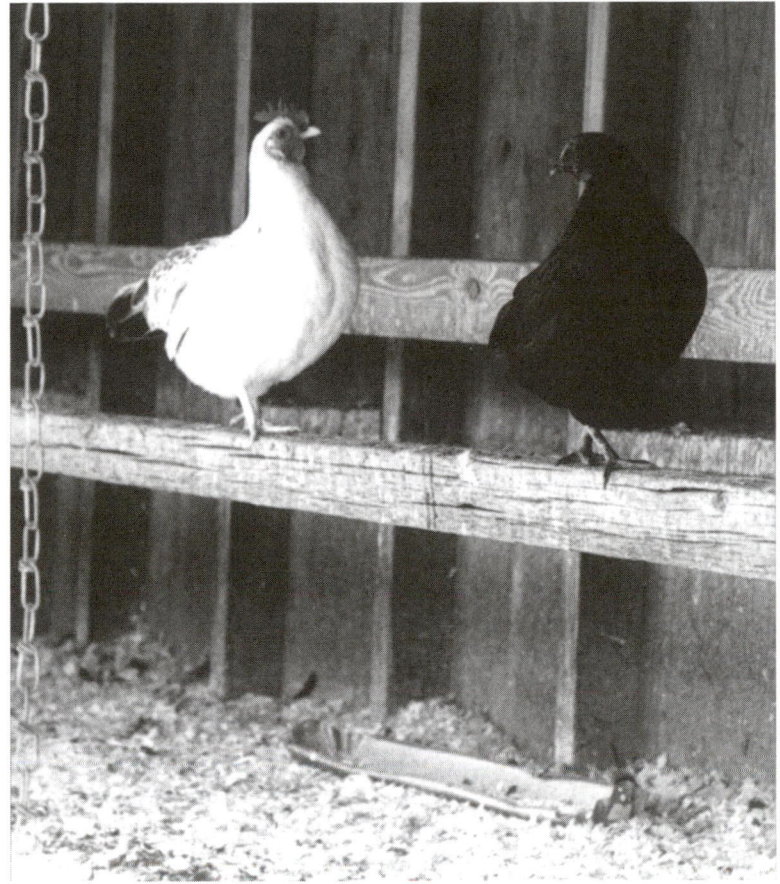

Not all chickens are treated as well as these. Photo by Mark A. Gold-stein.

cled her experiences in a poignant book, filled with her drawings, aptly titled *Dead Meat*. The following is a partial description of a veal slaughterhouse she saw in Montreal:

> Veal calves are slaughtered in lots, each lot containing ten to twenty veals. The calf is three to four months old at slaughter and weighs between 250 and 300 pounds. Veals are kept off feed for eighteen hours before slaughter and handled with care to avoid bruising. Veals have to be dragged to the slaughterhouse, as they are too weak to stand and walk.
> The animals are forced into the restraining pen, two at a time.

The veals can see their comrades having their throats cut. The calves' eyes become practically white. Foam is pouring out of their mouths.

The man with the stun gun waits until there is enough space in the conveyor belt to receive the newly stunned veals. A large metal bolt strikes through the animal's skull. . . . The veal is hung upside down by a chain, and the throat is slit. The animal bleeds to death, which takes up to five minutes, as it moves along the conveyor belt.

The head is taken off. The body is slit open and steam comes out with all the entrails. Hooves come off. The carcass is cut into parts. (Coe: 49)

Here is what Coe observed on slaughter day at an egg factory in North Carolina:

Two men go down the center aisle, grabbing hens by legs, wings, and necks, and stuffing them in crates. The hens are in total dread and terror. They make terrible screeching sounds.

The crates are then thrown on top of each other and are left to wait in the cold for the truck. By the time the hens get to the slaughterhouse, eighty percent of their bones have been broken. The bones are very brittle, as all calcium goes to the eggs. (Coe: 81)

When one considers pigs, it is all too easy to recall the lovable Wilbur in E.B. White's *Charlotte's Web*. For the vast majority of pigs, the reality is far different. In *Vegan*, Erik Marcus, a writer and public speaker, noted that in the 1980s big corporations assumed control over the pig industry and applied the same principles that are in place for poultry farming. For the pigs, the physical living conditions have markedly deteriorated. "Pig sheds are designed to hold the largest number of animals at the lowest cost. Concrete slats are the standard flooring in commercial pig operations. . . . Sleeping on concrete is more than uncomfortable—over time, it creates serious health problems. Joints swell, skin gets scraped off, and the feet get serious abrasions and infections. This adds to the pigs' stress and increases rates of fighting and cannibalism." Many pigs become ill, especially from pneumonia, which may be caused by air that is heavy with dust and smells of ammonia (Marcus: 115–117).

What is life like for a typical pig in a commercial farm? "Shortly after birth, workers snip notches out of each piglet's ear for identification purposes. No anesthetic is used. To reduce injuries caused by fighting, their 'needle' teeth are clipped again without anesthetic. . . . Pigs are raised in as little space as possible. For young 250-pound pigs, operators are advised to allow a little more than one square yard of floor space for each animal. The crowding is not just to save space—crowding also reduces feed costs. . . . A modern pig farmer wants his pigs to stay as motionless as possible—when a pig walks, the farmer sees costly feed wasted to provide the energy for movement instead of being stored as flesh" (Marcus: 119–120). Pigs often panic during the rush to get them loaded on the truck that will transport them to the slaughterhouse. Overloaded trailers cause extra heat, fighting, and stress that kill many pigs (Marcus: 122).

Disputing many of these claims, the American Meat Institute Foundation notes that legal requirements and ethical and economic considerations obligate meat packers to handle livestock in the most humane manner possible. The Humane Slaughter Act of 1978 established strict standards for packing plants that are monitored by federal meat inspectors nationwide. A violation of the act can result in almost immediate shutdown of a plant. The Humane Slaughter Act requires that

- animals be handled and moved through chutes and pens in ways that do not cause stress;
- livestock must be rendered insensible to pain prior to slaughter (the act details the methods that must be used to stun animals);
- animals must have access to water and those kept longer than 24 hours must have access to feed;
- animals kept in pens overnight must be permitted room to lie down; and
- downers or crippled livestock must not be dragged in the stockyards, crowd pen, or stunning chute. (American Meat Institute Foundation Web site)

The American Meat Institute Foundation states that the meat industry has taken a number of initiatives to ensure that animals are handled properly. In 1991, it published *Voluntary Animal Handling Guideline for Meat Packers*, which was translated into Spanish in 1992. In 1997, the industry published *Good Management Practices for Animal Handling and Stunning*. In 1999, the American Meat Institute Foundation held its first-ever Animal Handling and Stunning Conference and released two training tapes: "Good Animal Handling Practices for Beef Processors" and "Good Animal Handling Practices for Pork Processors" (American Meat Institute Foundation Web site).

To the American Meat Institute Foundation, "humane slaughter is an ethical imperative and a common-sense business practice." Plant workers do all that they can to minimize the amount of discomfort animals experience during the slaughter process. "When the slaughter process is performed correctly, the process is so rapid that livestock never feel pain." Further, humane healing makes economic sense. When animals are stressed or treated poorly, the meat is of lesser quality.

CONCLUSION

Health, religion, environmental issues, and animal suffering—there are many reasons to consider a vegetarian diet. It is true that large numbers of people are reducing the amount of meat that they consume and are including more vegetarian options in their diets. Some people regularly plan meatless meals, and restaurants routinely have vegetarian alternatives. It has become a relatively common choice. Should you be a vegetarian? Only you can decide.

TOPICS FOR DISCUSSION

1. Do you eat meat, poultry, and fish? Why or why not?
2. Have you ever considered becoming a vegetarian? Why or why not?
3. Are any of your friends vegetarians? What reasons do they give?
4. Do you believe that vegetarians compromise their health? Why or why not?
5. Has reading this chapter changed any of your beliefs about vegetarianism? How?

REFERENCES AND RESOURCES

Books

Coe, Sue. *Dead Meat*. New York: Four Walls Eight Windows, 1995.

Davis, Karen. *Prisoned Chickens, Poisoned Eggs*. Summertown, Tennessee: Book Publishing Company, 1996.

Eisnitz, Gail A. *Slaughterhouse*. Amherst, New York: Prometheus Books, 1997.

Gittleman, Ann Louise, with James Templeton and Candelora Versace. *Your Body Knows Best*. New York: Pocket Books, 1996.

Havala, Suzanne. *Being Vegetarian*. Minneapolis: Chronimed Publishing, 1996.

Klaper, Michael. *Pregnancy, Children, and the Vegan Diet*. Paia, Maui, Hawaii: Gentle World, 1997.

Klaper, Michael. *Vegan Nutrition: Pure and Simple*. Paia, Maui, Hawaii: Gentle World, 1998.

Kleinman, Ronald E., editor. *Pediatric Nutrition Handbook*. 4th ed. Elk Grove Village, Illinois: American Academy of Pediatrics, 1998.

Lyman, Howard F., with Glen Merzer. *Mad Cowboy*. New York: Scribner, 1998.

Marcus, Erik. *Vegan: The New Ethics of Eating*. Ithaca, New York: McBooks Press, 1998.

Melina, Vesanto, Brenda Davis, and Victoria Harrison. *Becoming Vegetarian*. Summertown, Tennessee: Book Publishing Company. 1995.

Schwartz, Richard H. *Judaism and Vegetarianism*. 2nd ed. Marblehead, Massachusetts: Micah Publications, 1998.

Spock, Benjamin, and Steven J. Parker. *Dr. Spock's Baby and Child Care*. 7th ed. New York: Pocket Books, 1998.

Stepaniak, Joanne. *The Vegan Sourcebook*. Los Angeles: Lowell House, 1998.

Walters, Kerry S., and Lisa Portmess, editors. *Ethical Vegetarianism*. Albany: State University of New York Press, 1999.

Weiss, Stefanie Iris. *Being a Vegan*. New York: Rosen Publishing Group, 2000.

Magazines, Journals, and Newspapers

Ball, Madeline J., and Melinda A. Bartlett. "Dietary Intake and Iron Status of Australian Vegetarian Women." *American Journal of Clinical Nutrition*, September 1999, 70(3): 353.

Brody, Jane E. "Personal Health: Feeding Children off the Spock Menu." *New York Times*, June 30, 1998: Section F, page 7, column 4.

Chipley, Abigail. "Don't Cramp Your Style." *Vegetarian Times*, May 2000, 273: 14.

Coughlin, Carol M. "Nutritional Rx for Aging: What You Need to Know about Vitamins and Minerals." *Vegetarian Times*, February 1991, 234: 30–32.

Drake, Rana, Sheela Reddy, and G. Jill Davies. "Health of Vegetarians during Pregnancy and Pregnancy Outcome." *American Journal of Clinical Nutrition*, September 1999, 70(3): 628S.

Dworkin, Norine. "22 Reasons to Go Vegetarian Right Now." *Vegetarian Times*, April 1999, 260: 90–93.

Hammock, Delia A. "You Know I Don't Eat Meat!" *Good Housekeeping*, April 1996, 222(4): 109–111.

Harbert, Nancy. "The Vegetarian Trap." *Women's Sports and Fitness*, June 1998, 1(9): 104–107.

Hunt, Janet R., Lori A. Matthys, and LuAnn K. Johnson. "Zinc Absorption, Mineral Balance, and Blood Lipids in Women Consuming Controlled Lactoovovegetarian and Omnivorous Diets for 8 Wk." *American Journal of Clinical Nutrition*, March 1998, 67(3): 421–430.

Kjeldsen-Kragh, Jens. "Rheumatoid Arthritis Treated with Vegetarian Diets." *American Journal of Clinical Nutrition*, September 1999, 70(3): 5945–6005.

Labson, Lucy H., Kathryn M. Kolasa, George Poehlman, and Annette I. Peery. "Is a Vegetarian Diet Healthy for Kids?" *Patient Care*, March 15, 2000, 34(5): 111–128.

La Puma, John. "Vegan Diet and Rheumatoid Arthritis." *Internal Medicine Alert*, April 15, 1999, 21(7): 52.

McDougall, John, Vicki Saunders, and Gene A. Spiller. "Rapid Reduction of Serum Cholesterol and Blood Pressure by a 12-d, Very-Low-Fat, Strictly Vegetarian Diet." *American Journal of Clinical Nutrition*, September 1999, 70(3): 625S.

McLaughlin, Lisa. "In Brief: Your Family." *Time*, September 4, 2000, 156(10): 82.

Messina, Virginia K., and Kenneth I. Burke. "Position of American Dietetic Association—Vegetarian Diets." *Journal of the American Dietetic Association*, November 1997, 97(11): 1317–1321.

Neumark-Sztainer, Dianne, Mary Story, Michael D. Resnick, and Robert W. Blum. "Adolescent Vegetarians: A Behavioral Profile of a School-Based Population in Minnesota." *Archives of Pediatrics and Adolescent Medicine*, August 1997, 151(8): 833–838.

O'Connor, Amy. "A Nutritional War on Cancer." *Vegetarian Times*. May 1996, 225: 56–63.

"Omnivorous vs. Vegetarian Diet and Resistance Training–Induced Changes in Body Composition." *Journal of the American Dietetic Association*, May 2000, 100(5): 596.

Schwartz, Richard H. "Vegetarianism: Essential for Jewish Renewal?" *Tikkun*, March–April 1999, 14(2): 50–51.

Turner, Lisa. "Strong Bones without Dairy: 6 Savory Vegan Dishes Packed with Calcium." *Vegetarian Times*, March 1998, 247: 48–53.

Walsh, Teri. "Go Vegan to Curb Cramps." *Prevention*, July 2000, 52(7): 42.

Woo, Jean, Timothy Kwok, Suzanne C. Ho, Aprille Sham, and Edith Lau. "Nutritional Status of Elderly Chinese Vegetarians." *Age and Ageing*, July 1998, 27(4): 455–461.

Organizations to Contact

American Council on Science and Health
1995 Broadway, Second Floor
New York, NY 10023-5860
Phone: 212-363-7044
http://www.acsh.org (September 26, 2000)

American Meat Institute Foundation
Box 3556
Washington, DC 20007
Phone: 703-841-2400
http://amif.org (October 22, 2000)

AMI—American Meat Institute
1700 North Moore Street, Suite 1600
Arlington, VA 22209
Phone: 703-841-2400
http://www.meatami.com (October 22, 2000)

Farm Sanctuary—East
P.O. Box 150
Watkins Glen, NY 14891
Phone: 607-583-2225
Farm Sanctuary—West
P.O. Box 1065
Orland, CA 95963
Phone: 530-865-4617
http://www.farmsanctuary.org, http://www.poultry.org (October 22, 2000)

National Cattlemen's Beef Association
9110 E. Nichols Ave., #300
Centennial, CO 80112
Phone: 303-694-0305
http://www.beef.org, http://www.beefnutrition.org (October 22, 2000)

National Chicken Council
1015 15th St. NW, Suite 930
Washington, DC 20005-2605
Phone: 202-296-2622
http://www.eatchicken.com (October 22, 2000)

National Pork Producers Council
P.O. Box 10383
Des Moines, IA 50306
Phone: 515-223-2600
http://www.porkandhealth.org (October 23, 2000)

Physicians Committee for Responsible Medicine
5100 Wisconsin Ave. NW, Suite 400
Washington, DC 20016
Phone: 202-686-2210
http://www.pcrm.org (October 1, 2000)

United Poultry Concerns, Inc.
P.O. Box 150
Machipongo, VA 23405-0150
Phone: 757-678-7875
http://www.upc-online.org (October 22, 2000)

The Vegetarian Resource Group (VRG)
P.O. Box 1463
Baltimore, MD 21203
Phone: 410-366-VEGE
http://www.vrg.org (September 26, 2000)

4

Animal Growth Hormones

Many of the beef and dairy products that are sold in the United States are produced by using animal growth hormones. Controversy has arisen about whether this practice is safe or is putting consumers at risk.

Do you enjoy a glass of ice-cold milk? How about a grilled medium-rare rib-eye steak? Perhaps you prefer a piece of cheese melted over a hot dog. What do all these foods have in common? They are sources of protein—but also of hormones. For years, most of the food industry has been using hormones to increase the production of meat products and milk. Cattle grow faster and leaner and can be slaughtered sooner. Cows produce more milk. Some contend that the hormones are safe. However, there appears to be an ever-growing movement against the use of hormones. It is not unusual to see supermarkets marketing some of their products as hormone free. Should the public be concerned?

The U.S. Department of Agriculture says that hormones are substances that regulate growth. They are "produced throughout the lifetime of every man, woman and child, and are required for normal physiological functioning and maturation" (U.S. Department of Agriculture Web site)

USE OF HORMONES

According to the National Cattlemen's Beef Association, the beef industry has been using growth-promoting hormones for more than 30 years. It is a simple and very common practice. "The hormones are administered by placing an implant (about the size of a pencil eraser) under the skin behind the animal's ear. Cattle are implanted at a young age while their growth rates are highest. Approximately 63 percent of all cattle and about 90 percent of the fed cattle in the United States are implanted. All manufacturing, marketing and use of implants are regu-

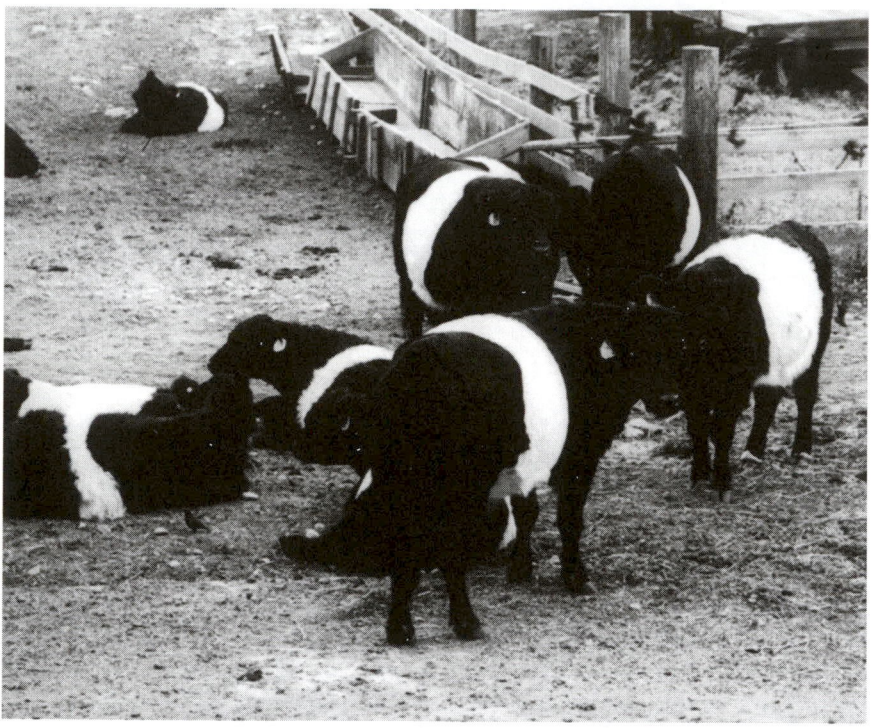

Consumers do not know if cows have been given growth hormones. Photo by Mark A. Goldstein.

lated by the federal government" (National Cattlemen's Beef Association, http://www.beef.org).

The U.S. Department of Agriculture says that "each implant contains a specific, legally authorized dosage of the hormone. The implant itself is inserted into the ear, which is discarded at slaughter and does not enter the human food chain. With an implant, the hormone is released into the bloodstream very slowly, so that the concentration of the hormone remains relatively constant and very low." Farmers have no reason to attempt to use higher dosages. "The prescribed dosage is the level which produces the maximum economic response in the animal. . . . there is no economic incentive for a farmer to use additional implants. A U.S. control system ensures that animals taken to slaughter have normal hormone levels" (U.S. Department of Agriculture Web site).

The National Cattlemen's Beef Association says that the hormones regulate growth and other bodily functions, just as naturally occurring hormones do, and are similar to ones naturally produced in the human body and ones that exist naturally in virtually all foods of plant and animal origin. However, the doses are much smaller than amounts found in humans or in many common foods. "Animals that are implanted with these growth-promoting hormones grow as much as 15 to 20 percent faster than untreated animals. In addition, the cattle produce more lean meat and less fat than cattle raised without the implants, enabling producers to provide consumers with higher quality beef at lower prices" (National Cattlemen's Beef Association Web site, http://www.beef.org).

The National Cattlemen's Beef Association contends that all beef contains natural hormones and that studies have demonstrated that beef produced with growth-promoting hormones does not differ significantly from beef produced without them. The association adds that the human body naturally produces far greater quantities of hormones than it ever consumes by eating beef or any other food. In addition, many everyday foods, such as eggs, have higher amounts of hormone levels than those found in beef (National Cattlemen's Beef Association Web site, http://www.beef.org).

The association claims that there is no reason for people to question the safety of this beef. "There is a worldwide scientific consensus supporting the safety of approved and licensed growth-promoting hormones when used according to good veterinary practice." Moreover, several international scientific bodies have approved hormones, including the World Health Organization, the United Nations' Food and Agricultural Organization, the European Commission Scientific Working Group on Anabolic Agents in Animal Production, and the CODEX Alimentarius Commission (National Cattlemen's Beef Association Web site, http://www.beef.org).

Six hormones are permitted for beef implantation. Estradiol, progesterone, and testosterone "are naturally occurring hormones produced by all humans and food animals." Trenbolone acetate, zeranol, and melengestrol acetate (MGA) are synthetic hormones: trenbolone acetate mimics testosterone, zeranonl mimics estradiol, and MGA mimics progesterone (U.S. Department of Agriculture Web site).

While the U.S. government repeatedly states that the use of these hormones is completely safe, since the late 1980s, the European Union (EU) has banned them. In 1999 the Scientific Committee on Veterinary Measures Relating to Public Health, a European Commission group, concluded that growth hormones present a variety of risks for consumers, ranging from developmental to neurobiological. Estradiol was deemed to be carcinogenic (cancer causing). Children were considered to be at greatest risk (European Commission Web site).

The Bureau Européen des Unions de Consommateurs (BEUC), one of the primary EU consumer groups, supports the continuation of the ban. "EU governments and European consumers consider the potential risk to human health from consuming hormone treated meat to be unacceptable. EU governments are correct to place public health interests above all other interests. EU governments are correct to have taken the precautionary measure of banning the use of hormones in the European food chain and halting the import of hormone treated meat. EU government should maintain this long-standing ban" (Bureau Européen des Unions de Consommateurs Web site.)

A March 2000 article in *Sierra* noted that the European countries and the United States have different attitudes toward food. In the United States, there has been a mass migration to the city. Few people have any link to agriculture or farming. Moreover, fast, highly processed food is ubiquitous. "Europeans, on the other hand, are willing to pay more for their food and to support small farmers and producers" (Rauber: 23). The introduction of beef growth hormones is simply unacceptable to them.

Not all Europeans agree with the ban. In 1999, the United Kingdom–based Society for Endocrinology, which represents about 1,800 endocrinologists, issued a statement declaring that animal growth hormones have little health risk to humans. Commenting on the three naturally occurring hormones, the society said:

- At the point at which the meat from the animals is consumed, the amount of the hormones has dropped to the same level found in untreated cattle, and it is below the levels that occur naturally in beef cattle and bulls.
- The sex hormone levels that are naturally produced by humans are significantly higher than the levels found in treated animals.
- Digestion in the stomach and passage through the liver destroys most of these hormones.

Similarly, there should be no concern about the three synthetic hormones. The society noted that "given current scientific knowledge, and with the doses used for growth promotion, the residues of these hormones in meat are well within the levels regarded as safe" (Society for Endocrinology Web site).

The most vocal U.S. critic is Samuel S. Epstein. In his books, articles, and editorials and as chair of the Cancer Prevention Coalition, Epstein works tirelessly to raise public awareness about the dangers of animal growth hormones. For example, in *The Breast Cancer Prevention Program*, which Epstein cowrote with David Steinman, an investigative journalist, and Suzanne LeVert, an author of several health-related books, the authors note that a random survey in 1986 found that up to half of all cattle sampled had hormone pellets illegally implanted in muscle tissue rather than under the ear, leading to higher absorption of hormones. Even the FDA admitted that the higher residues could have adverse effects. Even when ranchers follow the rules and implant a single pellet under the ear, Epstein and his fellow writers maintain that there is reason for concern. "Levels of estradiol and other hormones in meat and organs are more than triple the levels found in nonimplanted controls. . . . The extent to which hormonal meat contributes to increased breast cancer rates, apart from cancer of the uterus, prostate, and testis, has been virtually ignored. Hormonal beef may also have other endocrine-disruptive effects, such as hastening menarche" (Epstein, Steinman, and LeVert: 194–195).

While the ongoing dispute about beef growth hormones continues, the controversy escalated in the early 1990s when the Monsanto Corporation introduced Posilac, a genetically engineered hormone, which is also known as recombinant bovine growth hormone (rBGH). To avoid using the word *hormone*, Monsanto later said that Posilac was a bovine soma-totropin (bST). Whatever it is called, the product, which is usually re-ferred to as bST by those who support it and rBGH by those who are opposed, was approved for sale in November 1993 and went on the market in early 1994. In this chapter, when not part of a quote, it will be called bST/rBGH, a combination of both names.

ARGUMENTS FOR THE SAFETY OF HORMONES

The FDA insists that bST/rBGH is safe. It notes that separate studies have been conducted by the National Institutes of Health, the World Health Organization, and the Office of the Inspector General of the De-partment of Health and Human Services. Further, reviews of bST/rBGH have appeared in the *Journal of the American Medical Association, Pediatrics*, and the *Journal of the American Dietetic Association*. They have all found bST/rBGH to be safe. In addition, "milk and meat from bST supple-mented cows are safe" (Center for Food Safety and Applied Nutrition Web site).

How does bST/rBGH work? The pituitary glands of dairy cows pro-duce bST/rBGH, but supplemental bST/rBGH may be injected. "Both sources of bST . . . are carried to the liver of the cow via the bloodstream." In the liver, bST/rBGH stimulates the production of insulin-like growth factor (IGF-1), "another protein hormone that plays an important role in helping regulate the conversion of dietary nutrients into milk." Cows who are injected with bST/rBGH produce more milk. Still, the FDA claims that "milk from cows given supplemental bST contains no more bST than milk from cows not given the supplement." It also maintains that there are no real nutrient and sensory differences between milk from bST/rBGH-supplemented cows and nonsupplemented cows (Center for Food Safety and Applied Nutrition Web site). The FDA insists that bST/rBGH must be injected. When ingested by mouth, it is ineffective.

The FDA also states that the amounts of IGF-1 in milk are safe. "The concentration of IGF-1 in milk from supplemented cows is slightly higher than from unsupplemented cows. However, the average increase in concentration in milk is small compared to normal variations in concentration of this compound from cow-to-cow in milk from unsupplemented animals. The average increase of IGF-1 in milk produced by supplemented cows is also small compared to the variation in amount that occur normally from the beginning to end of the cow's lactation period. . . . IGF-1 is normally present in milk. It is a protein hormone and is digested just like any other protein in milk, meat, or other foods that you eat. IGF-1 is not active when consumed by mouth." IGF-1 is also present in human milk. In fact, the average amount of IGF-1 found in human milk is greater than that contained in milk from bST/rBGH-supplemented cows. "IGF-1 is also present in human saliva and the average person consumes IGF-1 from this source each day that is equivalent to the amount consumed from any source of milk" (Center for Food Safety and Applied Nutrition Web site).

The FDA says that bST/rBGH increases milk production by about 10%. "After having a calf, a cow produces milk for about 300 days. The highest daily milk production will occur at about 8 weeks after calving and then the level of milk production per day gradually declines during the rest of the lactation periods. . . . Administration of supplemental bST is started after the peak of milk production occurs and causes the cow to maintain a higher level of milk production per day during the period when milk production is normally declining. Therefore, a cow supplemented with bST will not be producing more milk per day than it produced per day at peak production prior to the start of bST supplements" (Center for Food Safety and Applied Nutrition Web site).

Do the hormones increase the incidence of mastitis (inflammation of the udder) in cows? According to the FDA, "The question of animal health has been reviewed extensively by the FDA and was the subject of a special FDA Expert Advisory Panel hearing on March 31, 1993. The panel reported that based on extensive research results, any increase in mastitis that may result from use of bST is insignificant compared to the increase in mastitis that occurs normally for other reasons, such as seasonal variation, extremes of weather conditions, age of the cow, and stage of lactation."

Nevertheless, treatment of mastitis generally entails giving cows antibiotics. The FDA states that this does not compromise the milk supply. "When a farmer treats a cow with an antibiotic, the milk from that cow is discarded by the farmer for several days, as defined on the label of the antibiotic." If a farmer is concerned that there may be any antibiotics remaining in the milk, he may send a sample for testing. "When milk is picked up at dairy farms, the truck driver must take a sample of milk from the farm bulk tank at every farm before the milk is pumped into the truck. When every truck arrives at a milk processing plant, a milk sample is taken from the milk in the truck and tested for antibiotics." If the milk tests positive for antibiotics, the milk is not unloaded. A second sample is taken and tested for antibiotics. If that is also positive, "then all of the individual farm samples that the driver collected are tested to identify which farm's milk contained the antibiotics. In addition, the dairy plant must notify the local regulatory agency that milk is being discarded, and they need to document the manner in which it was discarded" (Center for Food Safety and Applied Nutrition Web site).

According to the FDA, the consequences are serious for a farmer whose milk contains antibiotics. "There are very large financial penalties imposed on dairy farmers that contaminate a truck load of milk with antibiotics. Many processing plants have offered incentives to their farmers to avoid contamination of tank trucks of milk with antibiotics. If a farmer thinks a mistake has been made and his/her milk is contaminated, he/she can call the plant and have a milk sample picked up and tested. If the tank of milk is positive and the farmer prevented it from contaminating a full truck load, then some plants have a program to pay the farmer for one tank of milk during some period of time."

The FDA believes that bST/rBGH has a positive impact on the environment. Fewer cows produce the same amount of milk. That reduces the amount of animal feed and resulting animal waste. Furthermore, bST/rBGH does not create a milk surplus. "The signal to the dairy farmer to produce more or less milk will continue to be based on the difference between the price paid for milk and the cost of milk production. For the well-managed dairy farm that adopts bST technology (just like any other technology that improves efficiency), profitability should be enhanced" (Center for Food Safety and Applied Nutrition Web site).

In an article that appears on the Web site of the American Council on Science and Health, Terry D. Etherton says that "scientists in academia, government and industry have conducted more than 2,000 scientific studies of bST throughout the world. These studies have clearly shown the efficacy, safety and benefits realized by integrating bST into dairy production. . . . Supplemental administration of bST does not affect the quantity of bST found in milk or milk's composition. Milk and meat derived from bST treated cows are safe for human consumption."

Etherton explains that bST/rBGH is a protein. When digested, it is reduced to single amino acids and tiny peptides. What remains has no hormonal activity. This finding has been confirmed in studies reviewed by the FDA. Thus bST/rBGH cannot be absorbed into the bloodstream.

According to Etherton, bST/rBGH does not negatively impact the health of cows. To ensure the safety of bST/rBGH for dairy cows, the FDA required the establishment of safety margins. To accomplish this goal, cows were treated over a two-week period with 60 times the commercial does for bST/rBGH and up to six times the commercial does for two consecutive lactations. The studies determined that even large doses of bST/rBGH did not affect animal health. With regard to clinical mastitis, Etherton says that a number of factors, such as season, stage of lactation, environment, and milking management, influence a cow's susceptibility to mastitis. He cites a report that evaluated 15 full lactation trials (914 cows) and 70 short-term studies (2,697 cows) and, after accounting for all major factors, found a small positive association between milk yield and mastitis on a per cow basis, but claims that supplementation with bST/rGBH causes no more mastitis than would have occurred with any increase in milk yield. He also thinks that bST/rBGH may help improve the health of cows because somatotropin plays an important role in maintaining the immune system.

Etherton further maintains that bST/rBGH will help to meet the ever-increasing need for food. "The supply of food required to adequately meet human nutritional needs over the next 40 years will be equal to the amount of food previously produced throughout the entire history of humankind. To meet this demand, animal scientists must develop new technologies to increase productive efficiency (that is, the yield of milk or meat per unit of feed), produce leaner animals and provide increased economic return on investment to producers" (American Council on Science and Health Web site).

ARGUMENTS AGAINST THE USE OF HORMONES

Not everyone is this supportive. In *The Breast Cancer Prevention Program*, the book Samuel Epstein cowrote with David Steinman and Suzanne LeVert, Epstein acknowledges that bST/rBGH raises milk production in cows, but he claims that it also has such hazards as increasing fat concentrations in milk, contaminating milk with rBGH, causing udder infections (mastitis) that contaminate milk with pus, bacteria, and the antibiotics used for treatment, and producing milk with high concentrations of insulin-like growth factor (IGF-1) a hormone that regulates cell division and growth. IGF-1 levels in milk are further increased by pasteurization. Because IGF-1 resists digestion, it passes into the bloodstream where it can produce abnormal or premature growth-promoting effects (Epstein, Steinman and LeVert: 197).

Epstein and his coauthors believe that higher levels of IGF-1 place people at greater risk for breast cancer. The hormone fosters the division of cells and encourages normal breast cells to become malignant. "Additionally, IGF-1 helps to maintain the malignancy of breast cancers, increasing their invasiveness and spread, and helps protect cancer cells from self-destructing (a process called apoptosis) in a normal way" (Epstein, Steinman, and LeVert: 197).

On his Cancer Prevention Coalition Web site, Epstein notes that "it is highly likely that IGF-1 promotes transformation of normal breast cellular activity to breast cancers. In addition, IGF-1 maintains the malignancy of human breast cancer cells, including their invasiveness and ability to spread to distant organs. . . . The prenatal and infant breast is particularly susceptible to hormonal influences. Such imprinting by IGF-1 may increase future breast cancer risks, and may also increase the sensitivity of the breast to subsequent unrelated risks such as mammography and the carcinogenic and estrogen-like effects of pesticide residues in food, particularly in premenopausal women" (Cancer Prevention Coalition Web site). Similarly, Epstein thinks that IGF-1 may be associated with colon cancer because it triggers abnormal growth and division of cells that line the surface of the colon (Epstein, Steinman, and LeVert: 198).

Moreover, Epstein says that the hormones harm cows. "Cows injected with rBGH show heavy localization of IGF-1 in beast (udder) epithelial cells. This does not occur in untreated cows." Cows implanted with bST/rBGH show increased rates of mastitis, which contaminates milk with pus. The antibiotics that treat mastitis also leave residues in the milk.

Epstein further claims that the FDA is denying scientific findings. "A 1990 study by Monsanto, the leading maker of rBGH, explicitly revealed statistically significant evidence of growth promoting effects. Feeding relatively low doses of IGF-1 to mature rats for only two weeks results in statistically significant and biologically highly significant systemic effects: increased body weight; increased liver weight; increased bone length; and decreased epiphyseal width. The FDA has failed to investigate the effects of long-term feeding of IGF-1 and treated milk on growth" (Cancer Prevention Coalition Web site).

In *The Politics of Cancer Revisited*, Epstein called for a complete rethinking of U.S. beef-industry policy. "The question we ought to be asking is not why Europe won't buy our hormone-treated meat, but why we allow beef from hormone-treated cattle to be sold to American and Canadian consumers. Untreated meat is currently hard to find and expensive; if it were widely produced and available, the price would come down. At the least, meat produced from hormone-treated animals should be explicitly labeled" (Epstein: 598).

Epstein is not the only person sounding the alarm about animal growth hormones. A 1998 article in the *Ecologist* noted that Monsanto is required to list warnings of the potential ill effects of bST/rBGH on the Posilac label. "The label outlines 21 health problems associated with the use of Posilac, including cystic ovaries, uterine disorders, decrease in gestation length and birth weight of calves, increased twinning rates and retained placenta. Potentially the most serious problem, however, is the increased risk of mastitis" (Kingsnorth: 266–269).

There are other reasons to worry. Antibiotic residues may remain in the milk. When humans consume these, they have the potential to facilitate the development of antibiotic resistance. Thus, humans who require antibiotics may find that they are no longer effective.

A 1996 article published in *Rachel's Environmental and Health News*, a publication of the Environmental Research Foundation, commented that use of bST/rBGH negatively impacts the health of cows. It reduces life expectancy and increases the chance of illness. "Normally for about 12 weeks after a cow calves, she produces milk at the expense of her own tissues. She loses weight, she is infertile, and she is more susceptible to diseases. . . . Eventually her milk output diminishes, her food intake catches up, and she begins to rebuild her body. By injecting rBGH, a farmer can postpone for another 8 to 12 weeks the time when the cow begins rebuilding her body. This means that the cow is stressed for another 8 to 12 weeks and is more susceptible to infection during that period" (Environmental Research Foundation Web site).

In 1998, a report published in the *Lancet* suggested an association between IGF-1 and the incidence of breast cancer in younger women. Researchers compared the levels of IGF-1 in the blood of 397 women who had a history of breast cancer to 620 who did not. "The risk of breast cancer was more than twice as high in premenopausal women with the highest level of IGF-1 compared to those with the lowest level, and more than seven times as high in premenopausal women under 50 years of age." After menopause, no such correlation appeared to exist. The researchers concluded that "there is substantial indirect evidence of a relation between IGF-1 and risk of breast cancer" (Hankinson et al.: 1393–1396).

A study published in 1998 in *Science* examined the connection between levels of IGF-1 and prostate cancer. The investigation, which had 152 cases and 152 controls, found "a strong positive association . . . between IGF-1 levels and prostate cancer risk" (Chan et al.: 563–566). Men with high levels of IGF-1 had "four times the risk of prostate cancer as men with lower levels" (Grady: Section A, page 14, column 1). It should be noted that while men with higher levels of IGF-1 appear to be at significantly greater risk, they are not necessarily fated to get the disease.

Another study, published in 1999 in the *Journal of the National Cancer Institute*, collected plasma samples from 14,916 men without diagnosed cancer. During the 14-year follow-up, 193 men were found to have colorectal cancer. Men with higher levels of IGF-1 were more likely to have colorectal cancer than were men with lower levels. The researchers concluded that elevated levels of IGF-1 may place people at increased risk for colorectal cancer (Ma et al.: 620–625).

Though the link is still unproven, there is concern that growth hormones may play a role in the premature sexual development of young girls. A 1997 article in *Pediatrics* theorized that "American girls may be entering puberty at younger ages than current standards indicate." Researchers asked 225 pediatricians to evaluate the sexual maturation of 17,077 girls between the ages of 3 and 12 years. More than 90% of the girls were white; fewer than 10% were African American. The results were quite striking. "African-American girls began development before white girls. The average age of breast development was 8.87 years for African-American girls and 9.96 years for white girls. Menstruation began at 12.16 years in African-Americans and 12.88 years in white girls. White girls seem to be developing six months to one year earlier than current standards suggest." Additionally, there were some unsettling findings. "At age 3, 3% of African-American girls and 1% of the white girls showed breast and/or pubic hair development, with proportions increasing to 27.2% and 6.7%, respectively, at 7 years of age. At age 8, 48.3% of African-American girls and 14.7% of white girls had begun development" (Herman-Giddens et al.: 505–512). Though no one is certain why this is happening, one of the possible explanations is the use of animal growth hormones. "The list of potential triggers includes growth hormones in meat and milk, estrogen-like substances in dental sealants used on children, and the plastic wrap used on sandwiches for kids' lunches" (Gillette: 42–43).

In view of these findings, Paul B. Kaplowitz and Sharon E. Oberfield, two pediatric endocrinologists, reviewed the subject and issued conclusions in a 1999 *Pediatrics* article. They were, in part, as follows:

- The current recommendation that breast development before age 8 is precocious is based on outdated studies. Until 1997, no data on pubertal staging in U.S. girls were available that could have documented a trend to earlier maturation.

- The 1997 study indicates that stage 2 of breast and pubic hair development is being achieved—1 year earlier in white girls and 2 years earlier in African-American girls than previous studies have shown.

- New guidelines propose that girls with either breast development or pubic hair should be evaluated if this occurs before age 7 in white girls and before age 6 in African-American girls. No changes in the current guidelines for evaluating boys (signs of puberty at younger than 9 years) can be made at this time. (Kaplowitz and Oberfield: 936–941)

After this article was published, eight pediatric endocrinologists submitted a letter to the editor in which they noted that it was premature to change any of the current guidelines. They said that such alterations would be based on the single study published in 1997, a study that had "a fundamental flaw: the prevalence of the early signs of puberty was not ascertained in a sample of children drawn at random from the general population." Commenting on this statement, some of the authors of the 1997 study noted that "the large numbers of girls studied would make it unlikely that they were different from the population as a whole" (Rosenfield et al.: 622–623).

CONCLUSION

Are animal growth hormones really safe? If so, why have other countries banned their use? Is there reason for concern? Are they serving as a catalyst for premature puberty or deadly diseases such as breast cancer? Are they potentially dangerous? There are no clear and definitive answers to these questions. As a result, there are many worried consumers who are paying extra for foods that have been prepared without the use of hormones. Clearly, there is a great need for more research in this field. Consumers want to know if the foods they are eating have the potential to compromise their health as well as the well-being of their family members.

TOPICS FOR DISCUSSION

1. Before reading this chapter, were you aware that farmers used implants to increase the rate of cattle growth? If not, has this information changed how you feel about eating beef?
2. Has the European Union overreacted by banning animal growth hormones? Why or why not?
3. Should farmers use bST/rBGH to increase milk production? Are you comfortable drinking milk that was produced with this hormone?
4. Are you concerned that dairy products may contain antibiotics? Do you believe that this may pose a long-term public health problem, such as the development of a resistance to antibiotics?
5. Do you believe that Epstein has a reason to be concerned? Should people listen to what he has to say?

ACKNOWLEDGMENT

Material from the American Council on Science and Health (ACSH) Web site reprinted with permission of "The Efficacy, Safety and Benefits of Bovine Somatotropin and Porcine Somatotropin," a publication of the ACSH. For more information on ACSH or to obtain a copy of the publication, visit www.acsh.org.

REFERENCES AND RESOURCES

Books

Berkson, D. Lindsey. *Hormone Deception*. Chicago: Contemporary Books, 2000.

Epstein, Samuel S. *The Politics of Cancer Revisited*. Fremont Center, New York: East Ridge Press, 1998.

Epstein, Samuel S., and David Steinman, with Suzanne LeVert. *The Breast Cancer Prevention Program*. New York: Macmillan, 1997.

Magazines, Journals, and Newspapers

Barinaga, Marcia. "Study Suggests New Way to Gauge Prostate Cancer Risk." *Science*, January 23, 1998, 279(5350): 475.

Bellow, Daniel. "Vermont, the Pure-Food State." *Nation*, March 8, 1999, 268(9): 18–21.

Chan, J.M., M.J. Stampfer, E. Giovannucci, P.H. Gann, J. Ma, P. Wilkinson, C.H. Hennekens, and M. Pollak. "Plasma Insulin-Like Growth Factor-1 and Prostate Cancer Risk: A Prospective Study." *Science*. January 23, 1998, 279(5350): 563–566.

Epstein, Samuel S., and Liza Gross. "The High Stakes of Cancer Prevention." *Tikkun*, November 2000, 15(6): 33.

Gillette, Becky. "Premature Puberty: Is Early Sexual Development the Price of Pollution?" *F.*, November/December 1997, 8(6): 42–43.

Grady, Denise. "Hormone Seen as Risk Factor for Cancer of the Prostate." *New York Times*, January 23, 1998: Section A, page 14, column 1.

Hankinson, Susan E., Walter C. Willett, Graham A. Colditz, David J. Hunter, Dominique S. Michaud, Bonnie Deroo, Bernard Rosner, Frank E. Speizer, and Michael Pollak. "Circulating Concentrations of Insulin-Like Growth Factor-1 and Risk of Breast Cancer." *Lancet*, May 9, 1998, 351(9113): 1393–1396.

Herman-Giddens, Marcia E., Eric J. Slora, Richard C. Wasserman, Carlos J. Bourdony, Manju V. Bhapkar, Gary G. Koch, and Cynthia M. Hasemeier. "Secondary Sexual Characteristics and Menses in Young Girls Seen in Office Practice: A Study from the Pediatrics Research in Office Settings Network." *Pediatrics*, April 1997, 99(4): 505–512.

Kaplowitz, Paul B., and Sharon E. Oberfield. "Reexamination of the Age Limit for Defining When Puberty Is Precocious in Girls in the United States." *Pediatrics*, October 1999, 104(4): 936–941.

Kingsnorth, Paul. "Bovine Growth Hormones." *Ecologist*, September/October 1998, 28(5): 266–269.

Ma, Jing, Michael N. Pollak, Edward Giovannucci, June M. Chan, Yuzhen Tao, Charles H. Hennekens, and Meir J. Stampfer. "Prospective Study of Colorectal Cancer Risk in Men and Plasma Levels of Insulin-Like Growth Factor (IGF)-1 and IGF-Binding Protein-3." *Journal of the National Cancer Institute*, April 7, 1999, 91(7): 620–625.

Rauber, Paul. "Raging Hormones." *Sierra*, March 2000, 85(2): 23.

Rosenfield, Robert L., Laura K. Bachrach, Steven D. Chernausek, Joseph M. Gertner, Michael Gottschalk, Dana S. Hardin, Ora H. Pescovitz, Paul Saegner, Marcia E. Herman-Giddens, Eric Slora, and Richard Wasserman. "Current Age of Onset of Puberty." *Pediatrics*, September 2000, 106(3): 622–623.

Watson, Rory. "EU Says Growth Hormones Pose Health Risks." *British Medical Journal*, May 29, 1999, 318(7196): 1442.

Organizations to Contact

American Council on Science and Health
1995 Broadway, Second Floor
New York, NY 10023-5860
Phone: 212-362-7044
http://www.acsh.org (February 25, 2001)

BEUC The European Consumers' Organization
Avenue de Tervueren 36, Bte 4
B-1040 Brussels
Phone: 0032 2 743 1590
http://www.beuc.org (March 14, 2001)

Cancer Prevention Coalition
School of Public Health
University of Illinois at Chicago
2121 W. Taylor St.
Chicago, IL 60612
Phone: 312-996-2297
http://www.preventcancer.com (March 14, 2001)

Center for Food Safety and Applied Nutrition
Food and Drug Administration
5100 Paint Branch Parkway
College Park, MD 20740-3835
Phone: 1-888-SAFEFOOD
http://vm.cfsan.fda.gov/list.html (March 1, 2001)

Environmental Research Foundation
P.O. Box 5036
Annapolis, MD 21403-7036
Phone: 410-263-1584
http://www.rachel.org (March 16, 2001)

European Commission
B-1049 Brussels
Belgium
Phone: 00 32 2 299 11 11
http://europa.eu.int/comm (March 14, 2001)

National Cattlemen's Beef Association
9110 E. Nichols Ave., #300
Centennial, CO 80112
Phone: 303-694-0305
http://www.beef.org (February 25, 2001); also http://www.
  beefnutrition.org

Organic Consumers Association
6101 Cliff Estate Road
Little Marais, MN 55614
Phone: 218-226-4164
http://www.purefood.org (March 27, 2001)

Society for Endocrinology
17/18 The Courtyard, Woodlands, Bradley Stoke
Bristol BS32 4NQ, UK
Phone: +44 (0) 1454 642200
http://www.endocrinology.org (March 2, 2001)

United States Department of Agriculture
14th and Independence Ave. SW
Washington, DC 20250-1300
202-720-2791
http://www.usda.gov (February 25, 2001)

5

Imported Food

Ever-increasing amounts of food are imported into the United States. It is not always certain whether all of this food is safe to eat. Serious lapses in the inspection of food within the United States have resulted in people becoming sick from tainted foods. During the mid-1990s, when one batch of pasteurized ice cream was transported in tanker trailers that had previously carried unpasteurized liquid eggs, 224,000 people became ill with *Salmonella enteritidis*. Around the same time, a California producer of unpasteurized juices was not sufficiently careful, and a sixteen-month-old toddler died in Colorado of E. coli. Thirteen other children had to be hospitalized. Perhaps one of the best-known cases occurred in 1993 when four children died from hamburgers contaminated with E. coli 0157:H7 purchased at a restaurant in the Northwest. Many hundreds more became ill (Brody: Section F, page 5, column 1).

The situation is even more risky because much of the food that is consumed in the United States has been produced in other countries where there may be different food-safety standards. In 1980, about 24% of the fresh fruit consumed in the United States came from other countries; in 1995, that figure was 33%. During the same period of time, the percentage of seafood purchased from other countries rose from 45% to 55%. Even so, no more than a tiny fraction of this food is checked for safety. A study published in 1998 by the General Accounting Office (GAO), the investigative arm of Congress, said that in 1997 only 1.7% of imported produce was inspected. A few years earlier, in 1992, that figure was 8% (Allen: 23).

Since so little of the imported food is examined, many people think that there is a significant risk of the transmission of foodborne illness. Because about one-third of all cases of acute gastrointestinal illness are believed to be caused by foodborne organisms (Brody: Section F, page

5, column 1), unchecked, tainted food from other countries may introduce uncommon pathogens into the United States. According to the GAO, these could include strains of salmonella and the cyclospora parasite.

Such incidents have already occurred. "In 1996 and 1997, outbreaks of foodborne illness linked with the Cyclospora parasite in raspberries from Guatemala affected nearly 2,500 people in the United States and Canada, causing prolonged gastrointestinal distress and other painful symptoms" (United States General Accounting Office Web site). Imported foods also have the potential to contain pathogens like hepatitis A, which are difficult to detect either through direct examination or laboratory analysis. In a January 2001 article in the *New York Times*, Jane E. Brody wrote that over the past decade there have also been food-poisoning outbreaks caused by "carrots from Peru, mangoes from South America, strawberries, scallions and cantaloupes from Mexico, coconut milk from Thailand, canned mushrooms from China, a snack food from Israel, and alfalfa sprouts from several countries" (Brody: Section F, page 5, column 1).

REGULATION OF IMPORTED FOOD

The GAO noted that the Food Safety and Inspection Service (FSIS) monitors meat, poultry, and some egg products, while the Food and Drug Administration controls all the other foods. Before a shipment of imported food is released into U.S. commerce, it is sent from customs to the FSIS or FDA for review. When there are outbreaks of foodborne illness, the Centers for Disease Control and Prevention (CDC) becomes involved and joins with state and local health departments to determine what happened.

According to the GAO report, the Clinton administration and federal lawmakers were responsible for failing to take action to correct the overall situation. The GAO contended that "the U.S. food safety system is characterized by a fragmented organizational structure with numerous agencies implementing a hodgepodge of inconsistent regulations and laws." Not surprisingly, such an approach could not provide adequate protection for the food supply within the United States. "That same fragmented structure and inconsistent regulatory approach is being used to ensure the safety of imported foods as well." It was failing to guarantee the safety of either the internal supply of food or food imported from other countries.

On May 14, 1998, speaking before the Permanent Subcommittee on Investigations of the Committee on Governmental Affairs of the U.S. Senate, Robert E. Robertson, the associate director of the Food and Agriculture Issues, Resources, Community, and Economic Development Division of the GAO, summarized some of the most serious problems with imported food. He said that the FDA does not have the legal authority to require countries that export food to the United States to maintain equivalent food-safety systems. The FSIS has this authority and uses it. Since the FDA does not have this power, in its attempt to locate and ban unsafe food, it is usually forced to rely on port-of-entry inspections. However, these covered less than 2% of the shipments in 1997. This approach is generally thought to be inadequate.

Robertson said that if they focused on those shipments that had the highest safety risk, the FDA and the FSIS could use their available resources in a better and more efficient manner. He added that the FDA's procedures were subject to abuse from "unscrupulous importers." He explained that importers usually retain control over their shipments until they are released by the agency. If importers transfer their shipments into U.S. commerce before they have been inspected by the FDA or before they have been deemed safe by laboratory testing, then the FDA has no means to force the importers to return the shipments for inspection, destruction, or reexport. Further, when the FDA has questioned the safety of a shipment, it has permitted the importer to select the laboratory that conducts the testing.

Commenting on the testimony, Republican Senator Susan M. Collins of Maine, the head of the committee, said that "the safety of food imports is literally a life-and-death issue for many Americans. . . . The GAO's report represents a very serious indictment of our current regulatory structure." She noted that in many instances inspectors give far greater weight to "whether paperwork was filled out correctly than with whether or not the shipment was actually safe" (Shulman: 40).

In view of the limitations of the lax laws and inadequate implementation, it should not be surprising to read stories that significant amounts of unsafe food are making their way into U.S. commerce. An article that was published in *FDA Consumer* in 1997 reported that three executives had been found guilty of various crimes for selling about $4.5 million of decomposed imported shrimp. After the shrimp had been treated with a solution of chlorine and copper sulfate, they had been said to be "fresh frozen." The shrimp had also been obtained from an unapproved packer. Normally, such an action would place the shipment on "automatic detection, prohibiting the shipments entry into the country until the shipper or importer proves the product meets FDA standards." However, in this instance, the importing company "used false invoices with the names of approved packers to avoid detention." Apparently, the company "had imported more than 50 shipments of shrimp with false labels over a two or three year period" (Segal: 32–34).

Meanwhile, a 1998 article in *U.S. News and World Report* described how a federal food inspector in San Francisco who was a 35-year veteran of the U.S. Food and Drug Administration—a man whose job it was to help ensure that imported food was not contaminated with bacteria, insects, chemicals, or pesticides—had been the recipient of thousands of dollars in bribes. According to authorities, the 65-year-old man had received a minimum of $200,000 in payoffs from at least five importers. The man's codefendant, who had been an inspector for 17 years, "accepted bribes to look the other way." The story noted that during the previous year, "an import broker and another FDA inspector were found guilty of bribery and smuggling restricted foods into Los Angeles" (Spake: 28–30).

On the other hand, in still another case, the attempts to corrupt an inspector failed. A 1996 article in *FDA Consumer* noted that a New York seafood importer had been fined $5,000 and sentenced to 18 months' probation for offering a gratuity to a compliance officer in the New York district office of the FDA. Offering a gratuity to a government official is illegal. Apparently, the importer was hoping to have a shipment of contaminated imitation scallops cleared for sale. A laboratory analysis of the scallops found that they were contaminated with *Listeria monocytogenes*, a bacterium that has the potential to cause serious illness. Cooking food kills listeria. However, these imitation scallops were a cooked processed product. Cooked processed products are often served without any further cooking in salad bars (Janiger: 32).

Deliberate misrepresentation appears not to be uncommon. One company was accused of trying to pass off swordfish as whitefish. Officials in the company were concerned that the swordfish would be tested for methyl mercury, a toxic metal that is found in higher concentrations in swordfish. Methyl mercury is not retained by whitefish. No one would bother to test whitefish for the presence of methyl mercury.

Cases of falsification are numerous. Good food may be used to camouflage food that is in less desirable condition. Thus importers, assuming that inspectors will only scrutinize the food on top layers, will place inferior food under the better food. Sometimes, when notified that their food will be inspected, importers send over cases of fish that have already passed inspection. Because fish is used from food in a fish "bank," this is called "banking" (Spake: 28–30). The sample that the FDA examines obviously passes, and the shipment of fish that was actually never inspected is sold. In one instance, six West Coast importers were found to have shared the same "bank" sample.

Apart from these serious illegalities, the FDA has other concerns, such as insufficient resources with which to complete its responsibilities. The previously mentioned *U.S. News and World Report* story noted that there were only 309 inspectors to cover 330 ports. The amount of work for each inspector had almost tripled in five years. To compensate for the lack of inspectors, the FDA employs computers to screen shipments. "This automated system allowed 56 percent of incoming shipments to enter because the product, the country of origin, or the exporter's history posed little risk." The computer or paper records of an additional 42.3% of shipments were actually checked, but only about 3 to 10 minutes were spent on each one. As was earlier noted, the remaining 1.7% of the shipments were examined. This figure stands in contrast to the number of shipments reviewed by the FSIS. In 1997, it checked 118,000. All were examined for damage and labeling. About 20% were sent to the lab for testing (Spake: 28–30).

Another questionable FDA practice is permitting food that is tainted to be "reconditioned." Let's say that shrimp is found to be contaminated with salmonella. One would think that the shrimp should be discarded. But salmonella is killed by cooking, so the FDA allows the shrimp to be sent to a plant where it is cooked. Then the shrimp may be sold as cooked shrimp. Fortunately, the FDA does require that the cooked shrimp be retested.

Hoping to address these problems, on December 11, 1999, President Bill Clinton ordered the implementation of a multistage plan to improve the safety of imported food. The FDA and customs were charged with enforcing strict rules for importers who have repeatedly distributed imported food before release by the FDA or who have given false or misleading information to the U.S. government. These importers will be required to store their shipments in secure, independently owned facilities until the shipments have been reviewed and released by the FDA. If the FDA determines that the food should not be released, then the importer can remove the food, which may be exported or destroyed. All storage costs would be paid by the importer (U.S. Department of Health and Human Services Web site). Meanwhile, unless it is exported within 90 days, the secretary of the Treasury must arrange the destruction of any food that is refused admission into the Unites States. In these cases, the government pays the costs of storage and destruction.

With the assistance of customs, the FDA must prohibit any attempt to reimport food that has previously been denied admission into the United States. To assist this process, whenever possible, the outside of the containers should display a permanent mark to facilitate the identification of previously refused food products. All related paperwork should show the mark.

The FDA was also told to consider standards for private laboratories that collect and analyze the imported food, and customs was asked to increase the amount of bond that importers must post on their food. Finally, there should be greater outreach to both the public and the trade. It is believed that these changes will likely serve as a deterrent to those who may wish to sidestep U.S. laws and bring unsafe or contaminated food into the country.

In 2000, Rhona S. Applebaum, executive vice president of Scientific and Regulatory Affairs of the National Food Processors Association, submitted comments on the new proposals. She noted that her organization was generally pleased with the FDA and customs plan "that targets the few problem importers without unfairly putting burdens on the large numbers of importers who consistently meet the U.S. requirements." Still, she underscored the belief that the "vast majority of foods imported into the United States are safe and enter the country legally." Applebaum did not deny that there are loopholes. "It is true that the system is vulnerable to unscrupulous importers and that adulterated, misbranded and, on occasion, unsafe products may bypass existing controls."

Regardless, Applebaum said that by dealing with food safety at the point of entry into the United States, the proposals do not sufficiently address prevention. She advised the FDA "to emphasize the development of equivalence agreements with foreign governments to assure that foods exported to the U.S. meet U.S. safety standards." Further, she would like to see "more on-site reviews of foreign systems to assure that the foreign government has the authority and has set (and is enforcing) appropriate standards and that the country has the infrastructure to justify a determination of equivalence" (National Food Processors Web site).

MAD COW DISEASE

Bovine spongiform encephalopathy (BSE) or mad cow disease is not a new illness. Rather, it is considered a "new variant of Creutzfeldt-Jakob disease," a sickness in humans that leaves brain tissue filled with holes. It has horrendous clinical manifestations. "First come mood swings and numbness, then hallucinations, uncontrolled body movements and finally a progressive dementia that destroys the mind as thoroughly as Alzheimer's disease—except that this illness can strike at any age" (Graff and Park: 58+). At the end stages of the disease, the memories of the victims have been destroyed and they are unable to complete even the most basic activities such as feeding themselves, speaking, or seeing (Schardt and Schmidt: 1). A March 2001 article in *FDA Consumer* described the last few weeks of one of the victims, a 14-year-old from Manchester, England: "The ordeal . . . began more than two years earlier. First she cried for two weeks, then came the hallucinations and continuous screaming. As the disease progressed, the pain in her legs worsened until she couldn't walk. Bedridden, her brain wasting away, she was reduced to communicating through moans and grunts" (Bren: 12).

In the 1980s, mad cow disease began to appear in British cattle. After his cow became ill, Peter Stent, a South Downs, England, dairyman, didn't know what to do. He had never seen anything quite like it. The cow had trouble with balance and lost weight. "When the vet came to investigate, the animal was acting completely crazy—drooling, arching

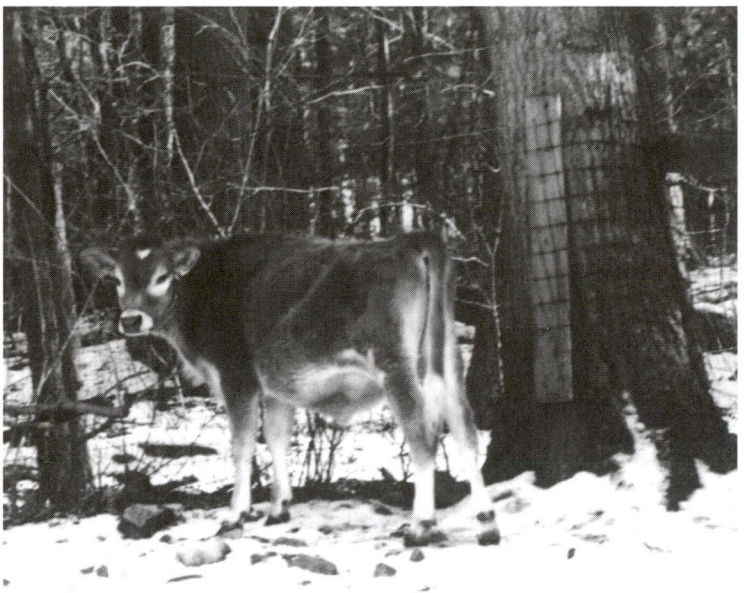

Could this cow have mad cow disease? Photo by Mark A. Goldstein.

its back, waving its head, threatening its peers" (Cowley: 52–61) The sickness quickly spread to other cows. More reports of this strange malady soon appeared.

The British were slow to respond. It was not until 1988 that they ordered the destruction of sick cows and stopped using these cows and other sick animals to make cattle feed. Farm animals do eat other animals, "usually in the form of meat-and-bonemeal protein supplements, which are made by rendering (boiling and grinding up) the carcasses of sheep, cattle, pigs, poultry, road kill, whatever. Just about anything not removed at the slaughterhouse—bones, brains, internal organs—goes into the renderer's pot" (Schardt and Schmidt: 1). A July–August 2001 article in *E* noted that this practice produced "a cannibalistic feeding loop." "Common sense might dictate that this practice is a bad idea, but the scientists and farmers who used this material genuinely believed it would be safe" (Rampton: 34–39).

Since many infected cows appeared outwardly healthy, it was not always easy to tell which cows were ill. Furthermore, instead of seizing all feed that might be tainted, the government gave farmers five weeks to deplete their inventories and only prohibited feeding the tainted feed to cows. Farmers could feed it to their pigs and chickens. With the animals all mingling on the same farms, the food probably also ended up in the mouths of the cows. Besides, the regulations did not inhibit ex-portation of the cattle feed. From 1988 to 1996, "Britain's banned cattle feed flooded other countries" (Cowley: 52–61).

Meanwhile, the British people kept eating beef, and there were reports of BSE appearing in other noncattle animals. Late in 1990, a number of cow parts deemed highly infectious—brain, spinal cord, spleen, thymus, tonsils, and intestines—were banned from animal and human food products. Still, the government insisted that humans were safe, but by the mid-1990s, evidence to the contrary could no longer be denied. Pathologists examining the brains of several dead young adults knew that the cause of death was BSE. At some point, mad cow disease had crossed the species barrier. Procrastination was no longer an option. Farm animals could not be recycled; meat-based cattle feed could not be exported.

Since 1995, more than 80 Britons have died from mad cow disease, and it has traveled to other European countries. About 200,000 British and European cattle have died from the sickness. Before the imposition of the bans, cattle feed made from the BSE-infected cows was shipped throughout the world, to approximately 80 countries (Cowley: 52–61).

BSE is caused by prions (pronounced PREE-ons), which are incredibly resistant abnormal, infectious proteins that destroy tissue from the nervous system. They are able to withstand harsh solvents and extreme temperatures; they are not destroyed by cooking or even by radiation. One article noted that "you can freeze them, boil them, soak them in formaldehyde or carbolic acid or chloroform, and most will emerge no less deadly than they were" (Cowley: 52–61). The incubation period seems to vary from a few years to as long as decades. Most victims die within two years after the first symptoms appear (Baker: 28).

In all probability, mad cow disease in humans is caused by eating beef that has brain or spinal tissues from mad cows. "Scientists believe it was spread in Europe by farmers feeding brains and spinal cords from infected cows and sheep to cattle as a protein supplement" (Kaufman, February 9, 2001: Page A03). It has also appeared in young adults who received the past versions of growth hormone injections during their childhood, not the currently used synthetic growth hormone.

During the winter of 2000–2001, the popular press was filled with reports of outbreaks of mad cow disease throughout Europe. Europeans greatly reduced their consumption of beef. In Germany alone, it was estimated that beef consumption dropped by 80 percent (Came: 20). "The disease has decimated the European beef industry—millions of cattle have been destroyed" (Kaufman, June 5, 2001: Page A19).

The heightened concern continued. Could the infected meat make its way to the United States? "The fact that British, and later European, health officials misunderstood the disease for years, and didn't stop its early spread, has made the job of keeping it out of the United States even more pressing" (Kaufman, June 5, 2001: Page A19). Imports of British animals had been against U.S. law since 1989, and imports of European animals had been prohibited since 1997. "The 500 or so animals that were imported from those countries before 1997 . . . have almost all been quarantined or purchased and killed" (Enserink: 1639). Likewise, the FDA has taken a number of additional actions to reduce the risk of importing the disease. For example, in December 2000, the Animal and Plant Health Inspection Service of the U.S. Department of Agriculture barred the importation of rendered animal proteins from more than 30 countries that have found BSE in their cattle. At the same time, the FDA permitted the detention of shipments from these countries if they contain "animal feed (including pet food), animal feed ingredients, and certain other products of animal origin intended for animal use" (Bren: 12). However, as has been noted earlier in this chapter, illegal imported foods are making their way into U.S. commerce. Hoping to quell some of the fears, the National Cattlemen's Beef Association and other groups "pledged strict enforcement of import restrictions" (Kaufman, February 9, 2001: Page A03). The U.S. government even banned people who had spent more than six months in Britain between 1980 and 1996 from donating blood.

The U.S. Department of Agriculture looks for mad cow disease by testing dead cattle that show evidence of a neurological problem. At the same time, the Centers for Disease Control and Prevention tracks death certificates, looking for people who may have died from this new variant of Creutzfeldt-Jakob disease. In those instances where there is a suspicion of Creutzfeldt-Jakob disease, "the person's brain tissue is sent to a special laboratory for examination" (Baker: 28). Thus there is a multilayered approach to looking for the disease in the United States.

It is far too early to say if the United States will be spared the ravages of BSE. There are simply too many opportunities for slipups in the system. For example, during the winter of 2000—2001, a feedlot in Texas accidentally fed meat and bonemeal that was reserved for pigs and poultry to more than 1,200 cattle (Schardt and Schmidt: 1). Fortunately, the owner responded to the situation. "The company purchased all the animals and promptly removed them from the food chain" ("Mad Cow Safeguards": 26). There are problems in some of the manufacturing plants. "A March 2001 FDA inspection report showed that about one in seven feed mills and rendering plants didn't have adequate procedures to prevent commingling; many haven't been inspected yet" (Enserink: 1639–1641).

There is also the risk of infection from mechanically separated meat or meat paste that is produced from the carcass of an animal. Such a product may contain tissue from the brain and spinal cord of an animal, common areas of prion infection. While a piece of filet mignon might be perfectly safe, a hot dog, which has mechanically separated meat, may not. Luckily, mechanically separated meat is believed to be fairly uncommon in the United States, and the food that does contain such products should mention it on the label. Still, much of today's food is eaten away from home, where there are generally no labels, so it is possible that consumers could eat food that contains spinal-cord tissue.

A number of U.S. meat processors have replaced mechanically separated meat with advanced meat recovery (AMR). The primary difference between the two processes is that AMR does not crush the bones. The resulting product is not a paste and is not identified on the label. Before placing an animal through the machine, processors are supposed to remove the brains and spinal cords. However, on occasion, some spinal-cord tissue remains.

A June 2001 article in *Nutrition Action Healthletter* offered some advice to meat eaters. Eating all forms of meat in countries in which BSE has not been found is viewed as safe. In countries where cases of BSE have been identified, it is better to eat muscle meats such as boneless steaks and roasts. It may be desirable to avoid processed meats such as burgers, even in countries with BSE, fish, pork, lamb, mutton, poultry, and dairy products are thought to be safe (Schardt and Schmidt: 1). An October/ November 2001 article in *Natural Health* advises meat eaters to limit themselves to organic meats. "Mad cow disease has never been found in cows raised their entire lives on organic farms, including those in Britain. ... The USDA's National Organic Standards require that certified organic animals be fed a plant-based diet" (Lohn: 131).

There are less obvious sources of meat. For example, gelatin is derived from the hides and bones of pigs and cows. It is used in a number of foods such as Jell-O and some yogurts and ice creams and is found in the capsules that cover a variety of over-the-counter supplements and medications. Indeed, many supplements contain animal parts, including brain tissue. The FDA has asked manufacturers to refrain from using products that have been obtained from countries in which cases of BSE have been identified. However, since 1994, when Congress deregulated dietary supplements, the FDA has been unable to enforce such requests. If at all possible, it is probably best to avoid supplements that have been determined to have animal brains, glands, or eyes, but since the amount of labeling may vary, that may not always be practical. It is known that dietary supplements called glandulars "can contain freeze-dried brain and spinal cord from cows" (Burros: Section F, page 7, column 2).

An article in a May 2001 issue of the *New York Times* outlined additional flaws in the U.S. system that make it at risk for mad cow disease. "The United States lags behind Europe in testing for the disease, and regulations to prevent prion contamination of animal feed are unevenly enforced." Additionally, there are insufficient inspections to keep infected meat from crossing U.S. borders. "An Agriculture Department official who spoke on the condition of anonymity said the agency was 'very short-staffed and the number of people in the field keeps going down.' " Only a tiny fraction of the 45 million pounds of meat that are mechanically stripped each year is tested. In the year 2000, only 27 samples were taken. Of these, one was found to be positive for tiny amounts of nerve tissue (Burros: Section F, page 7, column 2). The article concludes with comments from William D. Hueston, professor and chair of Veterinary Medicine and associate dean of the Maryland Campus of the Virginia-Maryland Regional College of Veterinary Medicine, who was formerly an official with the Department of Agriculture. He calls for the expansion of the surveillance programs. If one is forced to deal with a disease like BSE, one should not be constrained by inadequate resources.

An August 2001 story in the *Houston Chronicle* highlighted differences in inspection practices between the European Union and the USDA. It noted that during the first six months of 2001, more than 3.2 million cows were tested by the European Union. This stands in sharp contrast to the 13,000 cow brains analyzed by the USDA during the last decade of the twentieth century. That number is a miniscule portion of the 68 million slaughtered cattle (Christian: Section A, page 37).

Despite the potential problems, Americans are eating record amounts of meat. In fact, beef eating has been increasing since 1999. Even during the first quarter of 2001, when the media were filled with reports of mad cow disease, beef consumption was up 2%. An August 2001 article in the *Denver Post* said, "Americans are expected to gobble up $55.3 billion worth of beef this year, up $2.4 billion from last year's record" (McGhee: Business section, page C-01). Around the same time, an article that appeared in the *Boston Herald* quoted a spokesperson from the National Cattlemen's Beef Association as saying, "I think Americans are, for the most part, confident that our beef is safe." According to a recent study, the spokesperson added, "consumer awareness of mad cow is at an all-time high, confidence is also at an all-time high" (Dornbusch: Page 043).

In the last chapter of *Mad Cow U.S.A.*, authors Sheldon Rampton, an investigative journalist, and John Stauber, founder and executive director of the nonprofit Center for Media and Democracy, discuss whether mad cow disease could break out in the United States. Clearly, they noted, "farmers and governments have an obvious incentive to conceal the true incidence of BSE in their countries." That makes it more likely that mad cow will "slip into the United States." Further, "even the best executed surveillance would only detect the disease *after* it has arrived in the United States, by which time the damage would already have been done." It is almost impossible to scrutinize all the avenues that mad cow disease could spread. "The number of hypothetical risks from these novel disease agents seems endless. They could pop up in medicines, in organ transplants, in gelatin (which is used in everything from dessert mixes to medicine gel-caps), or in garden fertilizer made from rendered bone meal.... There are too many bullets to dodge, and the shots may be blanks anyway." That is why Rampton and Stauber advise more effective preventive action. "If we let industry set the rules ... there will literally be no limit to what we'll swallow, and the nightmare of mad cow disease—or something just as bad, or worse—not only *can* happen here, but almost certainly *will*" (Rampton and Stauber: 209, 210, 218, 220).

FOOT-AND-MOUTH DISEASE

During the winter of 2000–2001, while Europe was attempting to deal with the ravages of mad cow disease, it was hit with another contagious animal illness known as foot-and-mouth disease. After twenty years since the last breakout in England, it reappeared. Highly contagious, it "strikes cloven-hoofed animals like sheep, cows, goats and pigs" (Lyall: Section 1, page 3, column 1). Though it is rarely fatal to adult animals, it does debilitate them and render them unfit for the market. Young animals may succumb to the infection, which generally lasts for a few weeks, though it may continue for months. It is believed that only in the rarest of instances does foot-and-mouth disease infect humans. In the United Kingdom, the last documented case in humans occurred in 1967. "The farm worker affected was thought to have been infected by drinking contaminated milk. His symptoms included a mild fever, sore throat, blisters on the palms of his hands, and weals on his tongue.... The man recovered within a few weeks and had no lasting health effects" (Mayor: 1085).

Hoping to contain the epidemic, the British ordered the slaughter of millions of animals. The slaughter was not limited to sick animals. Rather, healthy animals on farms up to a few miles from the diseased animals were also killed. The loss devastated the British economy. As a result of all the negative publicity, tourism plummeted. Business that depended upon tourists, such as bed-and-breakfasts, barely stayed open or closed altogether. Though the government compensated the farmers for their loss, there was no assistance offered to the owners of these related industries.

Soon it was evident that foot-and-mouth disease was appearing in other European countries such as France and Holland. "Foot-and-mouth disease can spread by the mud on a person's boots, the meat or milk from contaminated cattle or simply the wind that turns windmills on both sides of the Dutch-German border" (Andrews: Section A, page 4, column 3).

Although imports of animals and animal products from European Union countries were banned by the U.S. government in mid-March

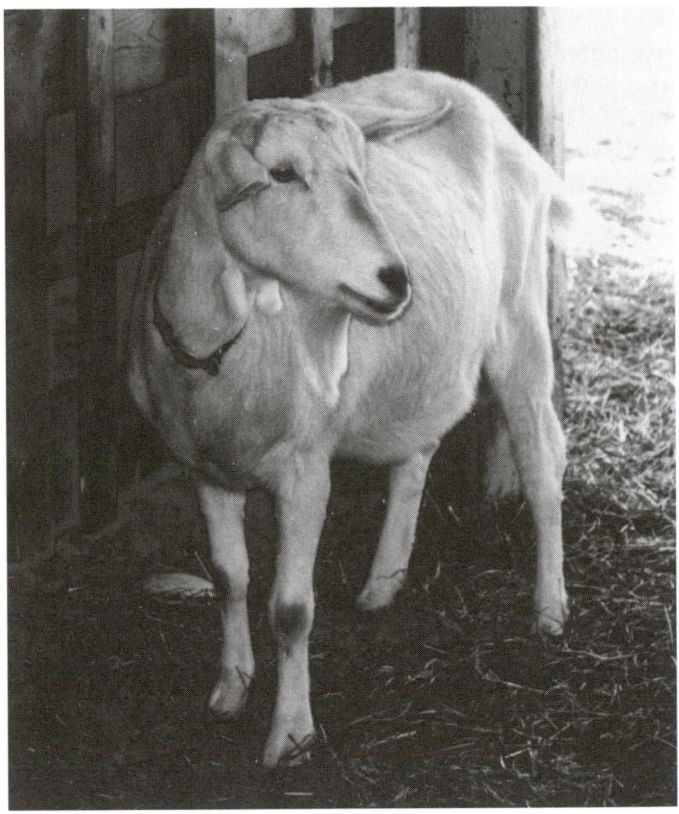

Is this goat at risk for foot-and-mouth disease? Photo by Mark
A. Goldstein.

2001, the concern remained that foot-and-mouth disease could still make
its way into the country. Humans can carry the virus on their clothing,
shoes, body (particularly throat and nasal passages), and personal items.
The U.S. Department of Agriculture advised travelers to take preventive
action. Travelers were asked to avoid farms, sale barns, stockyards, animal laboratories, packing houses, zoos, fairs, or other animal facilities
for five days prior to travel. Moreover, before returning to the United
States, travelers were asked to launder or dry-clean all clothing and out-
erwear and remove all dirt and soil from shoes. In addition, for five days
after arrival in the United States, travelers should avoid contact with
livestock or wildlife. Extra precautionary measures should be taken for
people traveling from farms in infected locales to visit or work on farms
in the United States.

Despite the precautions, potentially unsafe food made its way into the
United States. In mid-August 2001, an article in the *New York Times* re-

ported that "at the height of the foot-and-mouth epidemic in Europe at least three quarters of a million pounds of prohibited meat found its way into inspection warehouses in the United States" (Becker: Section A, page 12, column 1). This was not a single situation confined to one location. The inspection houses were located in different states, including New Jersey, Maryland, and Texas.

CONTAMINATED MELONS

In the spring of 2001, while news reports were expressing serious anxiety about mad cow disease and foot-and-mouth disease, there were stories of an outbreak of an uncommon form of salmonella from cantaloupes imported from Mexico. The fruit was believed to have been shipped to 14 states and eaten between April 6 and May 4. Since many people self-diagnose their symptoms as stomach flu rather than food poisoning, the exact number of people who became ill is unknown, but at least two people died from eating the melons. "Because of the rough texture of its skin, cantaloupe can be contaminated in the field by human or animal waste" (Pimentel: News, page A17). To minimize the risk, health officials advised consumers to wash the melons with a brush and clean water. After cutting cantaloupes, consumers should also wash their knives.

CONCLUSION

The vast majority of foods that consumers purchase and eat are safe. However, at least a portion has the potential to carry and spread disease. Some of these products originate outside the U.S. borders and are imported into the country. Hopefully, continued improvements in the systems that monitor foods will translate into more rigorous inspections and the closer scrutiny of potential hazards. In addition to more inspectors, there is a need for more rigorous tracking and inspections of importers who have a history of attempting to import tainted food.

TOPICS FOR DISCUSSION

1. Why do you think so little imported food is checked? Do you think it is primarily a function of economics?
2. Could there be other reasons why more food is not examined? If so, what could they be?
3. Do you think that the plan offered by the Clinton administration to improve the safety of imported food will help? Why or why not?

4. Do you think that the United States is at risk for mad cow disease? Explain your answer.

5. Since the mad cow disease scare, have you altered your meat-eating habits? Why or why not?

REFERENCES AND RESOURCES

Book

Rampton, Sheldon, and John Stauber. *Mad Cow U.S.A.* Monroe, Maine: Common Courage Press, 1997.

Magazines, Journals, and Newspapers

Allen, Robin Lee. "No Couch Potato, GAO Proposes Plan to Provide Safer Fish, Foreign Produce." *Nation's Restaurant News*, July 13, 1998, 32(28): 23.

Andrews, Edmund L. "Dutch Farmers Facing Mass Foot-and-Mouth Slaughter." *New York Times*, April 6, 2001: Section A, page 4, column 3.

Baker, Chris. "A Beef with Beef." *Insight on the News*, March 12, 2001, 17(10): 28.

Becker, Elizabeth. "Prohibited Meat Entered U.S., a Report Finds." *New York Times*, August 14, 2001: Section A, page 12, column 1.

Bren, Linda. "Trying to Keep 'Mad Cow Disease' out of U.S. Herds." *FDA Consumer*, March 2001, 35(2): 12.

Brody, Jane E. "A World of Food Choices, and a World of Infectious Organisms." *New York Times*, January 30, 2001: Section F, page 5, column 1.

Burros, Marian. "Experts See Flaws in U.S. Mad Cow Safeguards." *New York Times*, May 8, 2001: Section F, page 7, column 2.

Came, Barry. "Up in Smoke: A Total Ban on Farm Animal Movement Was Imposed in Hopes of Curbing a Disease So Contagious That It Can Spread on a Gust of Wind." *Maclean's*, March 12, 2001, 114(11): 20–22.

Christian, Carol. "Mad Cow Disease: Could It Be Here?" *Houston Chronicle*, August 5, 2001: Section A, page 37.

Cowell, Alan. "Trying to Stem Foot-and-Mouth, Britain Buries Carcasses." *New York Times*, March 27, 2001: Section A, page 3, column 1.

Cowley, Geoffrey. "Cannibals to Cows: The Path of a Deadly Disease." *Newsweek*, March 12, 2001, 137(11): 52–60.

Dornbusch, Jane. "The Beef Goes On: Despite Mad Cow Headlines, Americans Still Have a Stake in Steak." *Boston Herald*, July 18, 2001: Page 043.

Dulen, Jacqueline. "Produce under Spotlight." *Restaurants and Institutions*, November 1, 1997, 107(26): 86.

Elvin, John. "More to Mad Cow than Burgers, Steaks." *Insight on the News*, July 2–July 9, 2001, 17(25): 35.

Enserink, Martin. "Is the U.S. Doing Enough to Prevent Mad Cow Disease?" *Science*, June 1, 2001, 292(5522): 1639–1641.

Fulmer, Melinda. "Tainted Cantaloupes Kill 1, Sicken 30." *Los Angeles Times*, May 16, 2001: Business, part 3, page 1.

Graff, James L., and Alice Park. "Can It Happen Here? Panic over Mad Cow Has Already Infected Europe. Now It's Our Turn." *Time*, January 29, 2001, 157(4): 58+.

Hayasaki, Erika, and Nedra Rhone. "Melons Blamed in Second Death." *Los Angeles Times*, May 26, 2001: California, part 2, page 1.

Janiger, Herman. "Importer Convicted of Attempted Bribery." *FDA Consumer*, September 1996, 30(7): 32.

Kaufman, Marc. "Moving to Keep the Beef out of Disease Shadow: FDA, Industry Work to Bolster Mad Cow Safeguards." *Washington Post*, February 9, 2001: Page A03.

Kaufman, Marc. "On the USDA's Front Line against Mad-Cow Disease: Detwiler Key to Keeping Illness out of Country." *Washington Post*, June 5, 2001: Page A19.

Lindner, Lawrence. "We Know What You'll Eat This Summer, and Most of It— Okay, Some of It—Is Absolutely Safe." *Washington Post*, July 3, 2001: Page T12.

Lohn, Martiga. "Why Mad Cow Could Happen in America." *Natural Health*, October/November 2001, 31(8): 76–79, 128–131.

Lyall, Sarah. "A Tenacious Disease Finds New Victims in British Herds." *New York Times*, August 5, 2001: Section 1, page 3, column 1.

"Mad Cow Safeguards to Help U.S. Beef Exports." *Successful Farming*, March 2001, 99(4): 26.

Marquis, Christopher, and Donald G. McNeil, Jr. "Meat from Europe Is Banned by U.S. as Illness Spreads." *New York Times*, March 14, 2001: Section A, page 1, column 3.

Mayor, Susan. "UK Investigates Possible Human Cases of Foot and Mouth Disease." *British Medical Journal*, May 5, 2001, 322(729): 1085.

McGhee, Tom. "Americans' Taste for Beef Spurs Bell-Ringing Sales." *Denver Post*, August 7, 2001: Business section, page C-01.

Nulty, Thom. "When Traveling Abroad, Protect Yourself from Dangerous FMD." *Memphis Business Journal*, May 25, 2001, 23(4): 26.

Pimentel, Benjamin. "Cantaloupe Salmonella Warning." *San Francisco Chronicle*, May 17, 2001: News, page A17.

"A Primer on 'Mad Cow' and Related Diseases." *Consumers' Research Magazine*, March 2001, 84(3): 22.

Prusiner, Stanley B. "Neurodegenerative Diseases and Prions." *New England Journal of Medicine*, May 17, 2001, 344(20): 1516–1526.

Rampton, Sheldon. "It Can Happen Here." *E*, July–August 2001, 12(4): 34–39.

Rather, John. "Epicenter of Foot-and-Mouth Research." *New York Times*, April 1, 2001: Section 14LI, page 9, column 1.

Schardt, David, and Stephen Schmidt. "How Now Mad Cow?" *Nutrition Action Healthletter*, June 2001, 28(5): 1.

Segal, Marian. "Importer, Executives Convicted of Selling Substandard Shrimp." *FDA Consumer*, April 1997, 31(3): 32–34.

Shulman, Andrew. "Are Imports Safe to Eat?" *Insight on the News*, September 28–October 5, 1998, 14(36): 40.

Spake, Amanda. "Sick of Mean Cuisine: As Food Imports Increase, So Do

Schemes to Avoid Inspection." *U.S. News and World Report*, September 14, 1998, 125(10): 28–30.

Winter, Greg. "Contaminated Food Makes Millions Ill Despite Advances." *New York Times*, March 18, 2001: Section 1, page 1, column 6.

Organizations to Contact

EarthSave International
1509 Seabright Avenue, Suite B1
Santa Cruz, CA 95062
Phone: 831-423-0293
http://www.earthsave.org/ (August 5, 2001)

National Food Processors Association
1350 I Street, Suite 300
Washington, DC 20005
Phone: 202-639-5900
http://www.nfpa-food.org/ (May 22, 2001)

United States Department of Agriculture
14th and Independence Avenue SW
Washington, DC 20250-1300
Phone: 202-720-2791
http://www.usda.gov/ (August 25, 2001)

United States Department of Health and Human Services
200 Independence Avenue SW
Washington, DC 20201
Phone: 877-696-6775
http://www.hhs.gov/ (June 13, 2001)

United States General Accounting Office
441 G Street NW
Washington, DC 20548
Phone: 202-512-4800
http://www.gao.gov/ (May 25, 2001)

6

Life-Enhancing/Life-Threatening Foods

Not all food is healthful. Some is downright dangerous. It is not always clear which is which. A clear and undeniable correlation exists between food and illness. Eating certain foods on a regular basis will tend to make you healthier. Not surprisingly, other foods have the opposite effect. Eating too many of these may well have long-term negative consequences. Foods may be deceptive. Something may appear to be healthful when, in fact, it is not. Another food may seem to be a poor choice when it is actually a better alternative.

Even the healthiest food may carry a foodborne disease if it is handled improperly or inadequately prepared (see the previous chapter). Such foods have the potential to cause serious illness or death. There are also people who have food allergies and intolerances. For them, the ingestion of seemingly harmless items may have profoundly negative effects. There are "miracle" foods that are believed to help heal a variety of medical problems. The relationship between food and well-being is far more complicated than it may initially appear to be.

DIETARY RECOMMENDATIONS OF THE DEPARTMENT OF AGRICULTURE

From the Web site of the U.S. Department of Agriculture, one may download a publication entitled "Dietary Guidelines for Americans, 2000." It presents a number of principles that are useful in the food-selection process. According to the guidelines, people should consume daily between 6 and 11 servings from the bread, cereal, rice, and pasta group; every day they should eat between 3 and 5 servings from the vegetable group and 2 to 4 from the fruit group. The milk, yogurt, and cheese group and the meat, poultry, fish, dry beans, eggs, and nuts group should each comprise 2 to 3 servings. Fats, oils, and sweets should be consumed sparingly. Here are some examples of serving sizes:

- Bread, cereal, rice, and pasta group: 1 slice of bread or 1 cup of ready-to-eat cereal or ½ cooked cereal, rice, or pasta
- Vegetable group: 1 cup raw leafy vegetables or ½ cup of other vegetables or ¾ cup of vegetable juice
- Fruit group: one medium apple, banana, orange, or pear or ½ cup of chopped, cooked, or canned fruit or ¾ cup of fruit juice
- Milk, yogurt, and cheese group: ½ cup milk or yogurt or 1½ ounces of natural cheese or 2 ounces of processed cheese
- Meat, poultry, fish, dry beans, eggs, and nuts group: 2 to 3 ounces of cooked lean meat, poultry, or fish or a meat alternative as follows (each item counts as 1 ounce of lean meat): ½ cup of cooked dry beans, ½ cup of tofu, a 2½ ounce soyburger, 1 egg, 2 tablespoons of peanut butter, or ⅓ cup of nuts (U.S. Department of Agriculture Web site)

Within each group, how does one select the better alternatives? The guidelines say to organize meals around plant foods. "Eating a variety of grains (especially whole grain foods), fruits, and vegetables is the basis of healthy eating. Enjoy meals that have rice, pasta, tortillas, or whole grain bread as the center of the plate, accompanied by plenty of fruits and vegetables and a moderate amount of low-fat foods from the milk group and the meat and beans group. Go easy on foods high in fats or sugars" (U.S. Department of Agriculture Web site).

While the guidelines advise consuming only "moderate" amounts of fat, they acknowledge that not all fats are alike. Saturated fats tend to raise blood cholesterol. Such fats are found in high-fat dairy products, fatty fresh and processed meats, the skin and fat of poultry, lard, palm oil, and coconut oil. Limit your intake of these foods. Foods high in cholesterol, such as liver and other organ meats, egg yolks, and dairy fats, also tend raise blood cholesterol. Trans fatty acids, which tend to raise blood cholesterol, are found in many hard margarines and shortenings, which are common ingredients in some commercially fried foods and some bakery goods.

Unsaturated fats (oils), which do not raise blood cholesterol, occur in vegetable oils, most nuts, olives, avocados, and fatty fish like salmon. Olive, canola, sunflower, and peanut oils are high in monounsaturated fats. Soybean, corn, and cottonseed oils and many kinds of nuts are sources of polyunsaturated fats. Salmon, tuna, and mackerel contain omega-3 fatty acids. These are being studied to determine if they protect against heart disease. Eat moderate amounts of foods high in unsaturated fats, taking care to avoid excess calories (U.S. Department of Agriculture Web site).

The following U.S. Department of Agriculture list (from its Web site) compares the saturated fat content of some foods:

Food	Portion	Saturated Fat Content in Grams
Cheese		
Regular cheddar cheese	1 oz.	6.0
Low-fat cheddar cheese	1 oz.	1.2
Ground Beef		
Regular ground beef	3 oz. cooked	7.2
Extralean ground beef	3 oz. cooked	5.3
Milk		
Whole milk	1 cup	5.1
Low-fat (1%) milk	1 cup	1.6
Breads		
Bread	1 medium slice	6.6
Bagel	1 medium	0.1
Frozen Desserts		
Regular ice cream	½ cup	4.5
Frozen yogurt	½ cup	2.5
Table Spreads		
Butter	1 tsp.	2.4
Soft margarine	1 tsp.	0.7

It is important to remember that fat content may be hard to detect. In *Heart Fitness for Life*, Mary P. McGowan and Jo McGowan Chopra note, "Many people are aware of butter, cream, margarine, salad dressing, red meats, and mayonnaise as rich sources of fat. But fat is also found in muffins, chocolate, potato and tortilla chips, cookies, peanut butter, all vegetable oils, crackers, and ice cream. Restaurant food is famous for hidden fats: a burger and a small order of fries can contain 35 to 40 grams of fat—more than a day's allowance for most adults" (McGowan and Chopra: 42).

SUGAR

Like fat, dietary sugars should be limited. In the United States, the major sources of added sugar are soft drinks, cakes, cookies, pies, drinks such as punch and lemonades, dairy desserts, and candy. Added sugar comes in a variety of forms and under names such as brown sugar, corn sweetener, corn syrup, dextrose, and fructose. "Consuming excess calories from these foods may contribute to weight gain or lower consumption of more nutritious foods" (U.S. Department of Agriculture Web site). In *Heart Fitness for Life*, McGowan and Chopra write that the physiological consequences of consuming a high-sugar diet can be quite serious. When there is excess sugar in the bloodstream, the pancreas releases large amounts of insulin. Insulin then increases the release of the lipoprotein lipase, an enzyme that facilitates the transfer of fat from the bloodstream into fat cells. When fat is in the cells, it is more difficult to remove. Further, insulin plays a direct role in the production of cholesterol. "The higher the level of circulating insulin, the more cholesterol a person's liver produces." There is also some indication that insulin levels help determine where an individual stores excess body fat. "High levels of insulin promote abdominal weight gain, often called 'central obesity,' the very type of fat that increases the risk of developing cardiac disease" (McGowan and Chopra: 49).

SALT

There should be similar constraints on the intake of salt. Often the problem is not the added salt from a salt shaker but the salt contained in processed foods. The following list includes some of the major sources of dietary sodium:

Canned soups

Canned vegetables, unless labeled "no salt added" or "low sodium"

Processed meats—luncheon meats, hot dogs, ham, sausage

Broth or bouillon, unless labeled "low sodium"

Meat tenderizers

Seasoned salts

Soy sauce

Pickles, relishes, and olives

Sauerkraut

Frozen dinners

Fast-food cooking wines (McGowan and Chopra: 187)

Read nutrition labels carefully.

AMERICAN HEART ASSOCIATION GUIDELINES

The American Heart Association offers similar suggestions, although they are presented in a different format. While total fat should be no more than 30% of calories, saturated fat intake should be 7–10% of calories, polyunsaturated fat should be up to 10% of calories, and mono-unsaturated fat should comprise no more than 15% of calories. Cholesterol should be less than 300 milligrams a day, and sodium or salt should not exceed 2,400 milligrams each day. About 55 to 60% of the calories should come from carbohydrates, especially complex carbohydrates. "The guideline applies to total calories eaten over several days, such as a week. If it's applied to single foods, the '30 percent of calories from fat' guideline will cause many foods that fit into a well-balanced eating plan to be excluded. Examples of these foods include oil and margarine (100% of calories from fat), regular and low-calorie salad dressings (75–100% of calories from fat), dark chicken meat without skin (43 % of calories from fat), salmon (35% of calories from fat), lower-fat meals like turkey ham (34% of calories from fat), as well as many nuts and seeds (75–90% of calories from fat." The association adds that "these guidelines were developed for the U.S. population; however, persons with a history of heart disease and/or high cholesterol need to reduce their saturated fat intake to less than seven percent of total calories and keep their total cholesterol intake to less than 200 mg per day. Reducing excess body weight and regular exercise are also extremely important for people at high risk for coronary heart disease and stroke" (American Heart Association Web site).

Mediterranean populations are known to have lower rates of heart disease and some cancers than people in the United States. Many believe that this is because of the foods that the people tend to eat. The Mediterranean diet includes "mostly fruits, vegetables, cereals, canola and olive oil with low intake of cholesterol, saturated and polyunsaturated" (American Cancer Society Web site). It "contains less cholesterol, less polyunsaturated and saturated fats and more fiber and more vitamin C" than the American Heart Association diet (American Cancer Society Web site).

An important article on the Mediterranean diet appeared in 1998 in the *Archives of Internal Medicine*. Researchers in Lyon, France, studied 605 men and women, with an average age of 53, who had coronary heart disease. Participants in the control group ate a diet recommended by the American Heart Association; the second group adhered to the Mediterranean diet. During a four-year period, the two groups experienced a total of 38 deaths, 24 in the control group versus 14 in the experimental group. There were also 24 cancer diagnoses. "After adjustment for age, sex, smoking, leukocyte count, cholesterol level, and aspirin use, the reduction of risk in experimental subjects compared with control subjects was 56% . . . for total deaths, 61% . . . for cancers, and 56% . . . for the combination of deaths and cancers." The researchers concluded that "patients following a cardioprotective Mediterranean diet have a prolonged survival and may also be protected against cancer" (De Lorgeril et al.: 1181–1187).

A study published in 2000 in *JAMA: The Journal of the American Medical Association* reported that people who ate higher amounts of fruits, vegetables, and whole-grain foods and lower amounts of sugars, fats, and oils have lower mortality rates. More than 40,000 women were followed for an average of 5.6 years. Those who were most willing to eat fruits, vegetables, and whole-grain foods "had mortality rates that were 30% lower than the rate in the women who were least compliant." Commenting on their observations, the researchers noted that their "results provide evidence in support of the prevailing food-based dietary guidelines and suggest that diets complying with current dietary recommendations are indeed associated with improved health outcome. The potential public health implications of these findings are considerable; despite increased public awareness of the importance of diet in decreasing the risk of chronic disease, large gaps remain in food-based recommendations and actual dietary practices of the U.S. population" (Kant et al.: 2109–2115).

Early in 2000, the *Journal of the National Cancer Institute* published a report on the connection between diet and prostate cancer. The researchers noted that in the past, when this relationship has been studied, there have been conflicting results. In this investigation, the researchers compared 628 men under the age of 65 who were newly diagnosed with prostate cancer to 602 men "from the same underlying population and frequently matched to case participants by age." The men's diets were chronicled over a three- to five-year period. While no association was found between the intake of fruit and prostate cancer, the researchers did observe a correlation with the consumption of vegetables, especially cruciferous vegetables. "Men consuming 28 or more servings of vegetables per week showed a 35% decreased risk for prostate cancer when compared with those eating fewer than 14 servings per week. There was also a 41% decreased risk among men eating three or more servings of cruciferous vegetables per week compared with those eating less than one serving per week, even after controlling for total vegetable intake" (Cohen, Kristal, and Stanford: 61–68).

FOOD CONTAMINATION

Sometimes perfectly healthful food, such as produce, becomes contaminated. S.T.O.P or Safe Tables Our Priority, a nonprofit organization of victims of foodborne illnesses and others concerned with contamination to the food supply, describes several ways this can happen.

Wild animals and birds can contaminate produce on a farm on orchard with their feces. Water from wells or streams and rainwater runoff can contaminate crops. Manure from cattle or poultry can contain pathogens.

Humans who handle produce during harvesting can spread human pathogens such as hepatitis A or get contaminated dirt on the produce. Processing facilities can be vunerable to contamination from dust or animals. Dirt floors and unclean water are further risks.

Alfalfa sprouts are usually thought to be healthful. Unfortunately, they are particularly risky because the conditions that foster their growth also promote bacterial growth. "For approximately three days, sprout seeds are warmed, kept moist and given a lot of light in order to encourage growth. If contaminated seed comes into a sprout growing facility, it can enable an organism to 'set up shop' in a location within the facility, thereby enabling multiple batches to be contaminated" (S.T.O.P.—Safe Tables Our Priority Web site). A January 1999 article in *FDA Consumer* noted, "Since 1995, health officials have attributed 13 food-borne disease outbreaks worldwide to sprouts. Ten of these outbreaks occurred in the United States, resulting in illnesses in at least 956 Americans and at least one death" (Kurtzweil: 18).

While we tend to hear more about food poisoning from poultry, meat, and fish, other products such as grains, flours, spices, and herbs could be sources. For example, an outbreak of salmonellosis in Germany between April and September 1993 was traced to the paprika powder that coated a company's potato chips (Satin: 90).

Food can become spoiled in many ways. There are "more than 200 known diseases transmitted through food." These are caused by a variety of factors such as "viruses, bacteria, parasites, toxins, metals, and prions." Symptoms range "from mild gastroenteritis to life-threatening neurologic, hepatic, and renal syndromes" (Mead et al.: 607–625). Writing in *FDA Consumer*, Audrey Hingley noted, "The sad fact is that food-borne illness can be very serious. . . . Food-borne infections can cause spontaneous abortion, reactive arthritis, Guillain-Barre syndrome (the most common cause of acute paralysis in both children and adults), and HUS (hemolytic uremic syndrome), which can lead to kidney failure and death" (Hingley: 7–9).

In *Food Alert!* Morton Satin, a molecular biologist who is an expert on food safety, wrote that just about any food—whether eaten at home or away from home—has the potential to cause illness. "Food-borne diseases are certainly not limited to restaurants, cafeterias or fast-food outlets. Improper handling or cooking of foods in the home can be equally fatal and very often is. Both the frequency and severity of food-borne disease outbreaks are on the rise—trends that will most probably continue because of the proportionate increase in the population of older and immunocompromised consumers" (Satin: xi).

Satin said that there are a number of errors made by people in their own kitchens that result in food poisoning. These may be characterized as "critical" or "major." The most common critical violation is cross-contamination, chiefly caused by overlooked hand washing. "Other reasons are (a) storing raw materials directly over foods ready to be consumed; (b) putting utensils used for tasting back into the food being prepared; (c) using a dirty sink; (d) putting washed produce back into the original soiled container; (e) using unclean utensils to prepare foods; (f) not decontaminating cutting boards between uses; (g) using unclean scissors to open food bags; and (h) negligence in washing fresh produce." Additional critical violations are improper cooling of leftovers, improper labeling and storage of kitchen chemicals, incomplete cooking of food, improper refrigeration temperature, improper holding of cooked foods, neglecting appropriate use of gloves, use of severely damaged cans, and preparing food while ill. In order of their frequency of occurrence, the following are some of the major violations: misuse of cloths, towels, or sponges, neglect of thermometer, products used past the labeled "use-by" date, smoking, eating, or chewing gum while handling food, products stored uncovered, improper thawing practice, evidence of infestation, and the unavailability of hand towels (Satin: 39).

A January 1998 article in *Better Homes and Gardens* offered additional hints on avoiding foodborne illness in the home. Meat and eggs should be cooked to 160 degrees, and poultry should be cooked to 180 degrees. Take care with kitchen sponges on surfaces that hold food particles and bacteria. "Your efforts to scrub your kitchen clean and shiny may be spreading harmful bacteria throughout the kitchen. Similarly, moist dishcloths can transfer contaminants from spills to clean tabletops or dishes. After daily use, throw your sponge in the dishwasher and toss your dirty dishrag in the laundry. Discard sponges every few weeks and replace worn-out dishrags" (Gallo: 66–70).

In *Safe Eating*, David W.K. Acheson, a doctor, and Robin K. Levinson, a journalist who specializes in health, science, and fitness, list a number of ways that grocery store consumers can increase their chances of bringing home safe food. Some of these are as follows:

- Select frozen food that is stored below the frost line.
- Packages of meat or chicken should be well-sealed. Select those at the bottom of the case, where it is colder.
- To minimize the possibility of cross-contamination, keep seafood, meat, and poultry items separate.
- Stay away from meat or poultry packages that are dripping. If your hands become wet with from meat or poultry juice, wash them.

- Don't buy raw fish that has an odor. Fresh fish should not smell "fishy."
- Cooked fish, such as cooked shrimp, should not be stored in the same case with raw fish.
- Before purchasing deli meats, check to see if the deli equipment is clean.
- Select frozen foods, produce and dairy products at the end of the shopping trip.

Following the 40–140 rule is a good way to keep food safe. Keeping hot foods above 140 degrees and cold foods below 40 degrees prevents most bacteria from multiplying. Hot leftovers should be refrigerated quickly, preferably in a container with a large surface area to promote fast cooling. Foods left out in the open between 40 and 140 degrees are fertile breeding grounds for bacteria and viruses. Keep foods between these temperatures for no longer than two hours, and be especially careful with such protein foods as ham, chicken, and egg salad (Salter: 92).

Despite the problems, there is still a measure of control within the home setting. When you are away from home, that is much less the case. The National Restaurant Association notes that "almost 50 billion meals are eaten in restaurants and school and work cafeterias each year." Further, "in 1998, almost half of all adults (46 percent) were restaurant patrons on a typical day, and 21 percent of U.S. households used some form of takeout or delivery" (National Restaurant Association Web site).

In *It Was Probably Something You Ate*, Nicols Fox, a journalist, wrote, "When you eat away from home, the safety of your food is in someone else's hands. . . . And those hands, in all probability, belong to someone making minimum wage, who doesn't have sick leave either. You cannot be sure they are clean hands, or that the person they are connected to has had any training in food safety, or even that the restaurant owner has a clear understanding of how foodborne microbes get into food. In short, eating out, from a food-safety perspective, involves risk" (Fox, 1999: 127).

There are ways to reduce the risk. It is important to use care and common sense when selecting a restaurant. First and foremost, look for cleanliness. "The more expensive and the better the reputation a restaurant has, the more likely the chef will have had good training in food safety at a culinary institute. On the other hand, it is no guarantee. The most expensive restaurant may unknowingly purchase food already contaminated" (Fox, 1999: 129).

Special caution should be used when consuming food from buffets. With so much chopping and peeling, many sets of hands may be involved. There is also the potential for cross-contamination if vegetables are cut on a surface that was used to prepare raw meat. Foods may not be maintained at proper temperature and can be contaminated by customers. "If a salad bar or buffet is your only choice, go for foods that have had a heavy dose of vinegar (a microbe inhibitor), such as bean salads, or choose hot foods that are obviously hot. Absolutely avoid any that might be tempting for hands, such as bowls of loose raisins" (Fox, 1999: 129–130).

FOOD ALLERGIES AND INTOLERANCES

There are still other ways in which food may make us ill. Some people have allergies and/or intolerances to foods or non-nutrient products added to foods. An allergic response is an adverse reaction of the body's immune system to even a tiny amount of a particular food (usually some form of protein) or an environmental agent such as an animal enzyme or plant pollen. Allergic reactions are out of proportion to the amount of alien material taken into the body and can even be fatal. On the other hand, an intolerance response takes place when the body is unable to "detoxify" certain elements of something that is ingested. There is no involvement of the immune system. The item may be a non-nutrient to be gotten rid of as quickly as possible, or it may be a nutrient that the person lacks the enzymes necessary to digest because of his or her genetic makeup (Emsley and Fell: 1–2).

Allergic reactions may be immediate and intense or develop over a relatively brief period of time. Intolerances are generally slower in coming. "The culprits in food intolerance are foods that are eaten very regularly, especially items such as wheat and milk that are consumed at almost every meal. . . . Food intolerance . . . may well disappear if the food is not eaten for a few months. But it will tend to recur if the food is ever eaten regularly again" (Brostoff and Gamlin: 14–15).

In *Was It Something You Ate?* John Emsley, a science writer, and Peter Fell, a doctor, note that "about 90% of food allergies are caused by proteins in certain foods, particularly milk, eggs, fish, crab, shrimp, lobster, peanuts, tree nuts, soybeans, and wheat. . . . The vast majority of people (99%) are not allergic to their food, although many are intolerant of something in their diet" (Emsley and Fell: 40).

In *Food Allergies and Food Intolerance*, Jonathan Brostoff and Linda Gamlin describe the experiences of Jane, a person with an allergy to peanuts. When Jane was a child, her mouth and tongue swelled enormously on one or two occasions, and she had to be rushed to the hospital. Her mother concluded that peanuts were the cause, and prick tests confirmed that Jane was allergic to peanuts. Jane carefully avoided peanuts, but one day, when she was about eight, she handed a bowl of nuts to the guests at a party her parents were giving. Later, she rubbed her eyelids, and they began to swell and itch. Years later, Jane had a career that involved much traveling and eating out. On one occasion, she ordered some cheesecake. The waiter assured her that the brown powder on the dessert was pure chocolate. Unfortunately, the supply of chocolate had run out, and the chef had used finely grated nuts, including peanuts. As soon as Jane ate her first bite of cheesecake, her mouth began to itch. Her tongue swelled and blocked her windpipe. She soon collapsed on the floor. A doctor happened to be at the next table, and he managed to unblock her windpipe. Someone else telephoned the hospital, and another doctor brought the life-saving medicines Jane needed (Brostoff and Gamlin: 1–2).

Brostoff and Gamlin note some of the common symptoms of food intolerance: headache, migraine, fatigue, depression/anxiety, hyperactivity (in children), recurrent mouth ulcers, aching muscles, vomiting, nausea, stomach ulcers, duodenal ulcers, diarrhea, irritable bowel syndrome, constipation, flatulence, bloating, Crohn's disease, joint pain, rheumatoid arthritis, and edema (water retention) (Brostoff and Gamlin: 15). Generally, an elimination diet, "a regime in which specific elements are removed while keeping the remainder of the diet unchanged" (Emsley and Fell: 122), is used to detect the problematic foods.

At least a portion of the people who suffer from food intolerance probably have celiac disease, a autoimmune disorder in which the body cannot tolerate gluten, a protein found in wheat, oats, barley, and rye. Until recently, celiac disease was thought to be quite rare. Researchers now think that about 1 in every 250 Americans has it (National Institute of Diabetes and Digestive and Kidney Diseases Web site). "More recent studies appearing in the *Lancet* have reported a prevalence of one in 122 of the Irish, one in 85 of the Finnish, one in 70 of the Italians in Northern Sardinia, and one in 18 Algerian Saharawi refugee children." It is believed that of every 20 people with celiac disease, 19 are unaware that they have it (Braly: 43). "When people with celiac disease eat foods containing gluten, their immune system responds by damaging the small intestine. Specifically, tiny fingerlike protrusions, called villi, on the lining of the small intestine are lost. Nutrients from food are absorbed into the bloodstream through these villi. Without villi, a person becomes malnourished—regardless of the quantity of food eaten" (National Institute of Diabetes and Digestive and Kidney Disease Web site). In *Food Allergies*, William E. Walsh notes that celiac disease is different from food allergies. While they may have a devastating effect on the body, food allergies do not harm body tissues. People with celiac disease are physically harmed when they eat gluten. "In gluten-sensitive people, it [gluten] strips away the inner layer of the intestine like sandpaper. The 'sandpapered' intestine handles food poorly; it struggles to absorb the proteins, carbohydrates, and vitamins from food, and this poor absorption can lead to malnutrition. It poorly absorbs water and other dietary components necessary for health. Much of what a sufferer eats and drinks passes through the intestine and ends up uselessly in the stool" (Walsh: 218).

Since celiac disease is genetically linked, it tends to run in families. "Seventy percent of identical twins both get it (175 times more prevalent than in the general population), while the number of siblings and off-spring who get the disease exceeds 12 percent (thirty times more prevalent than in the general population" (Braly: 43). It may appear in childhood or anytime in adulthood. Even elderly people are diagnosed. "Sometimes the disease is triggered—or becomes active for the first time—after surgery, pregnancy, childbirth, viral infection, or severe emotional stress" (National Institute of Diabetes and Digestive and Kidney Diseases Web site).

Symptoms vary from person to person. They "may or may not occur in the digestive system. For example, one person might have diarrhea and abdominal pain, while another person has irritability or depression. In fact, irritability is one of the most common symptoms in children." Other symptoms are as follows:

- Recurring abdominal bloating and pain
- Chronic diarrhea
- Weight loss
- Pale, foul-smelling stool
- Unexplained anemia (low count of red blood cells)
- Gas
- Bone pain
- Behavior changes
- Muscle cramps
- Fatigue
- Delayed growth
- Failure to thrive in infants
- Pain in the joints
- Seizures
- Tingling numbness in the legs (from nerve damage)
- Pale sores inside the mouth, called aphthus ulcers
- Painful skin rash, called dermatitis herpetiformis
- Tooth discoloration or loss of enamel

- Missed menstrual periods (often because of excessive weight loss) (National Institute of Diabetes and Digestive and Kidney Disease Web site)

It is not uncommon for people with celiac disease to have another autoimmune disorder such as diabetes or thyroid disease. "Many thyroid specialty clinics in Europe are beginning to routinely test all autoimmune thyroid-diseased patients for gluten sensitivity and celiac disease" (Braly: 44).

Testing for celiac disease usually begins by determining the levels of antibodies to gluten contained in the blood. If the tests are positive, physicians may decide to use a long, thin tube, known as an endoscope, to take tissue samples from the small intestine. Still, in the United States, where there is little recognition of the prevalence of celiac disease, there is no universal screening. That stands in sharp contrast to Italy, where all children are screened by age six. As a result, asymptomatic cases are detected early. "In addition, Italians of any age are tested for the disease as soon as they show symptoms. As a result of this vigilance, the time between when symptoms begin and the disease is diagnosed is usually only 2 to 3 weeks. In the United States, the time between the first symptoms and diagnosis averages about 10 years" (National Institute of Diabetes and Digestive and Kidney Disease Web site).

Celiac disease is treated by following a gluten-free diet. This is not as easy as it may initially appear to be. Gluten is not only found in such obvious foods as bread and pasta, but is hidden in a host of prepared foods such as salad dressings and soups. It is also found in some medications and supplements. "People with celiac disease have to be extremely careful about what they buy for lunch at school or work, eat at cocktail parties, or grab from the refrigerator for a midnight snack. Eating out can be a challenge as the person with celiac disease learns to scrutinize the menu for foods with gluten and question the waiter or chef about possible hidden sources of gluten. However, with practice, screening for gluten becomes second nature and people learn to recognize which foods are safe and which are off limits" (National Institute of Diabetes and Digestive and Kidney Diseases Web site).

In *Kids with Celiac Disease*, Danna Korn, the mother of a celiac child and founder of Raising Our Celiac Kids (ROCK), an international support group, listed some additional items of unease:

- Rice and soy beverages, because their production process utilizes barley enzymes.
- Bad advice from health-food-store employees (e.g., that spelt is safe for celiacs).

- Cross-contamination between bins in food stores selling raw flours and grains (usually via the scoops).
- Wheat-bread crumbs in butter and jams, in the toaster, on the counter, and the like.
- Stamps, envelopes, or other gummed labels.
- Toothpaste and mouthwash.
- Medicines, many of which contain gluten.
- Cereals, most of which contain malt flavoring or some other non-gluten-free ingredient.
- Some brands of rice paper.
- Sauce mixes and sauces such as soy sauce, fish sauce, catsup, mustard, and mayonnaise.
- Ice cream.
- Packet and canned soups.
- Dried meals and gravy mixes.
- Laxatives.
- Grilled restaurant food, because the grill may be contaminated with gluten.
- Fried restaurant foods, because the grease may be contaminated with gluten.
- Ground spices, in which wheat flour is commonly used to prevent clumping. (Korn: 66)

James Braly, an expert on food allergy, says that for a person with celiac disease, "eating in restaurants lies somewhere between a challenge and an impossibility." "Even meals that seem gluten-free may contain wheat flour used to thicken a sauce or gravy. Your best bet: Avoid eating in restaurants. But if you must, eat simply. Eat single, whole foods without sauces, coatings, or gravies, such as steamed vegetables, fresh fruits, and simply prepared baked or grilled fish, meats, or chicken" (Braly: 46).

HEALING FOODS

There are foods that are naturally healing. While the list is too long to mention all of them, it may be useful to discuss a few. In *Healing Foods*, Michio Kushi, a pioneer in macrobiotic practice and an advocate of natural foods, presents 55 foods that prevent and relieve common medical problems. One of these is broccoli, which is high in fiber, beta-carotene, calcium and vitamin C. It reduces the risk of cancer and heart disease. Another is brown rice, which Kushi believes "contains a nearly perfect balance of energy and nutrients." Cauliflower is supportive of healthy lungs and large intestinal functions and useful again cancer and heart disease. It is high in vitamin C and beta-carotene. One food that you may not have heard about is kale, which is "an excellent source of calcium and iron" and "creates strong bones and teeth and helps prevent osteoporosis" (Kushi: 5, 14, 15, 20).

In *Healing Foods*, Miriam Polunin, a professional writer and food enthusiast, describes "50 foods with outstanding benefits, supported by scientific and traditional evidence" (Polunin: 28). Included in the group are cranberries. They are useful for preventing and treating urinary-tract infections. "The most common bacteria causing urinary tract infections, *Escherichia coli*, thrives by attaching itself to the walls of the intestines and bladder. An unidentified substance in cranberry discourages the adhesion. In tests, drinking commercial cranberry juice regularly reduced the amount of *E. coli* in urine." Cranberries do even more. "Cranberries are antiviral and anti-fungal (but not against *Candida albicans*, which causes yeast infections). . . . For those with kidney stones, small amounts of cranberries may help lower levels of calcium in urine, so less is present for stone formation" (Polunin: 39).

Pineapples, which contain bromelain enzymes, are an additional multipurpose food that facilitates healing, reduces inflammation, and assists in digestion. "The anti-inflammatory action of pineapples is not understood; one theory is that bromelain enzymes block the prostaglandins that play a part in swelling. These enzymes have been used with dramatic success to treat rheumatoid arthritis and to speed tissue repair as a result of injuries, diabetic ulcers, and general surgery. . . . Pineapple enzymes act specifically to break down protein, helping to ease digestion. . . . [They] reduce blood clotting and may also help remove plaque from arterial walls" (Polunin: 41).

Bananas have a number of healing properties. In *Smart Guide to Healing Foods*, Katharine Colton, a professional writer and editor, noted that bananas "help lower blood pressure, boost energy levels, help improve mood, relieve constipation and diarrhea, relieve acid indigestion and may help prevent ulcers, [and] may lower risk of heart disease and stroke." According to Colton, "Bananas are known as nature's perfect fast food, and with good reason. Delicious, nutritious, and a great source of long-lasting energy, they're a favorite with everyone from infants to iron-pumping athletes" (Colton: 60).

There is also garlic. In *Healing with Whole Foods*, Paul Pitchford, a healer and educator, wrote that garlic "promotes circulation and sweating; removes abdominal obstructions and stagnant food; inhibits the common cold virus as well as viruses, amoebae, and other microorganisms associated with degenerative diseases such as cancer. Eliminates worms, unfavorable bacteria, and yeasts including *Candida albicans*; promotes the growth of healthy intestinal flora; used for dysentery, pneumonia, tuberculosis, asthma, hay fever, diarrhea, snake bite, warts, abscesses, and hepatitis" (Pitchford: 506). A May 2000 article in *Better Nutrition* noted, "When it comes to maintaining long-term health, the expression really should be 'a clove a day keeps the doctor away,' since almost everyone can benefit from a bit of garlic daily" (Starbuck: 46).

Finally, we should note the healing powers of ginger. While ginger is probably best known for helping relieve nausea and motion sickness, it has a number of added properties. It is believed to assist with indigestion and reduce flatulence and to aid circulation and fight colds and coughs. Research has found that it prevents blood clots. "In tests, ginger is even more effective than garlic or onion in discouraging the formation of blood clots, causing stroke or heart attack" (Polunin: 44).

A March 1999 article in *Consumer Reports on Health* advises caution. Foods that are considered healthful seem to come and go. "One reason for those dizzying swings is that virtually all individual foods have at most only a modest effect on health, since any one item makes up only a small part of the total diet.... And for most foods, studies have only suggested a benefit, they haven't proved it" ("Disease-Fighting Foods?": 8–9).

CONCLUSION

It is not always clear which foods are healthful and which are not. A food that may be beneficial for one person has the potential to harm or even kill another. What could be wrong with a slice of whole wheat toast? Nutritionists have been telling us to eat whole wheat products for years. Yet, a person with celiac disease may become quite ill from even trace amounts of wheat. And, what could be wrong with a single peanut? For someone with a peanut allergy, it could be deadly. Every day, people become sick from food that is not handled properly. It is important to educate oneself on the ways to ensure the safe handling of food. On the other hand, there are foods that appear to be natural healers. Although more medical research needs to be conducted on these, as often as possible, they should be included in your diet.

TOPICS FOR DISCUSSION

1. Do you believe that there is a strong correlation between diet and illness? Why or why not?
2. Should you be concerned if your diet is high in fat, sugar, or salt? Why? What are some things you can do?

3. If you develop food poisoning from food served at a restaurant, should you hold that restaurant accountable? Should there be stricter regulations? If not, what do you think should be done?

4. Since some people are extremely sensitive to certain foods, do you think that the government should require ingredient labeling that says, "No Peanuts" or "No Glutens"? Why or why not?

5. Do you believe in the power of healing foods? Why or why not?

REFERENCES AND RESOURCES

Books

Acheson, David W.K., and Robin K. Levinson. *Safe Eating*. New York: Dell, 1998.

Braly, James, with Jim Thompson. *Food Allergy Relief*, Lincolnwood, Illinois: Keats Publishing, 2000.

Brostoff, Jonathan, and Linda Gamlin. *Food Allergies and Food Intolerance*. Rochester, Vermont: Healing Arts Press, 2000.

Colton, Katharine. *Smart Guide to Healing Foods*. New York: John Wiley and Sons, 1999.

Emsley, John, and Peter Fell. *Was It Something You Ate?* New York: Oxford University Press, 1999.

Fox, Nicols. *It Was Probably Something You Ate*. New York: Penguin Books, 1999.

Fox, Nicols. *Spoiled*. New York: BasicBooks, 1997.

Korn, Danna. *Kids with Celiac Disease*. Bethesda, Maryland: Woodbine House, 2001.

Kushi, Michio. *Healing Foods*. Becket, Massachusetts: One Peaceful World Press, 1998.

McGowan, Mary P., and Jo McGowan Chopra. *Heart Fitness for Life*. New York: Oxford University Press, 1997.

Pitchford, Paul. *Healing with Whole Foods*. Berkeley, California: North Atlantic Books, 1993.

Polunin, Miriam. *Healing Foods*. New York: DK Publishing, 1997.

Rampton, Sheldon, and John Stauber. *Mad Cow U.S.A*. Monroe, Maine: Common Courage Press, 1997.

Rhodes, Richard. *Deadly Feasts*. New York: Simon and Schuster, 1997.

Salter, Charles A. *Food Risks and Controversies*. Brookfield, Connecticut: Millbrook Press, 1993.

Satin, Morton. *Food Alert!* New York: Checkmark Books, 1999.

Thom, Dick. *Coping with Food Intolerances*. Portland, Oregon: JELD Publications, 1995.

Walsh, William E. *Food Allergies*. New York: John Wiley and Sons, 2000.

Wedman–St. Louis, Betty. *Living with Food Allergies*. Lincolnwood, Illinois: Contemporary Books, 1999.

Wood, Marion N. *Coping with the Gluten-Free Diet*. Springfield, Illinois: Charles C. Thomas, 1982.

Magazines and Journals

Andrews, N.J., C.P. Farrington, S.N. Cousens, P.G. Smith, H. Ward, R.S.G. Knight, J.W. Ironside, and R.G. Will. "Incidence of Variant Creutzfeldt-Jakob Disease in the UK." *Lancet*, August 5, 2000, 356(9228): 481.

Chipley, Abigail. "Mad Cow Disease Update." *Vegetarian Times*, November 2000, 279: 19.

Cohen, Jennifer H., Alan R. Kristal, and Janet L. Stanford. "Fruit and Vegetable Intakes and Prostate Cancer Risk." *Journal of the National Cancer Institute*, January 5, 2000, 92(1): 61–68.

De Lorgeril, Michel, Patricia Salen, Jean-Louis Martin, Isabelle Monjaud, Philippe Boucher, and Nicolle Mamelle. "Mediterranean Dietary Pattern in a Randomized Trial: Prolonged Survival and Possible Reduced Cancer Rate." *Archives of Internal Medicine*, June 8, 1998, 158(11): 1181–1187.

"Disease-Fighting Foods? (Many Are Overhyped, but All Offer Important Lessons about Good Nutrition)." *Consumer Reports on Health*, March 1999, 11(3): 8–9.

Gallo, Nick. "Are You Safe at the Plate?" *Better Homes and Gardens*, January 1998, 76(1): 66–70.

Gormley, James J. "Ginger May Improve Digestive Complaints and Motion Sickness." *Better Nutrition*, January 1, 1996, 58(1): 34–35.

Hingley, Audrey. "Rallying the Troops to Fight Food-Borne Illness." *FDA Consumer*, November–December 1997, 31(7): 7–9.

Kant, Ashima K., Arthur Schatzkin, Barry I. Graubard, and Catherine Schairer. "A Prospective Study of Diet Quality and Mortality in Women." *JAMA: The Journal of the American Medical Association*, April 26, 2000, 283(16): 2109–2115.

Kurtzweil, Paula. "Questions Keep Sprouting about Sprouts." *FDA Consumer*, January 1999, 33(1): 18.

Mead, Paul S., Laurence Slutsker, Vance Dietz, Linda F. McCaig, Joseph S. Bresee, Craig Shapiro, Patricia M. Griffin, and Robert V. Tauxe. "Food-Related Illness and Death in the United States." *Emerging Infectious Diseases*, September–October 1999, 5(5): 607–625.

Starbuck, Jamison. "Garlic Powerful (Pungent) Medicine." *Better Nutrition*, May 2000, 62(5): 46.

Organizations to Contact

American Cancer Society
1599 Clifton Road NE
Atlanta, GA 30329-4251
Phone: 800-ACS-2345, 404-320-3333
http://www.cancer.org/ (October 30, 2000)

American Heart Association
National Center
7272 Greenville Avenue

Dallas, TX 75231
Phone: 800-AHA-USA1
http://www.americanheart.org/ (October 30, 2000)

Center for Food Safety and Applied Nutrition
Food and Drug Administration
5100 Paint Branch Parkway
College Park, MD 20740-3835
Phone: 1-888-SAFEFOOD
http://vm.cfsan.fda.gov/list.html (October 30, 2000)

National Institute of Allergy and Infectious Diseases
Office of Communications and Public Liaison
Building 31, Room 7A50
31 Center Drive, MSC 2520
Bethesda, MD 20892-2520
Phone: 301-496-5717
http://www.niaid.nih.gov/ (October 28, 2000)

National Institute of Diabetes and Digestive and Kidney Diseases
Office of Communications and Public Liaison
NIH
Building 31, Room 9A04
31 Center Drive, MSC 2560
Bethesda, MD 20892-2560
Phone: 301-496-3583
http://www.niddk.nih.gov/ (October 30, 2000)

National Restaurant Association
1200 Seventeenth Street NW
Washington, DC 20036
Phone: 800-424-5156, 202-331-5900
http://www.restaurant.org/ (November 2, 2000)

S.T.O.P.—Safe Tables Our Priority
P.O. Box 4352
Burlington, VT 05406
Phone: 1-800-350-STOP, 802-863-0555
http://www.stop-usa.org/ (October 30, 2000)

United States Department of Agriculture
14th and Independence Ave. SW
Washington, DC 20250
Phone: 202-720-2791
http://www.usda.gov/ (October 30, 2000)

7

Food Labeling

Food labels may be a tremendous assistance for people who carefully monitor what they eat, but some labels may present inaccurate or incomplete information. In the mid-1980s, the role of diet in the development of chronic illness was better understood than before, but there were laws that prevented manufacturers from placing nutritional information on food labels. Everything changed in October 1984 when the Kellogg Company and the National Cancer Institute (NCI) joined together to launch a promotional campaign for All-Bran, a high-fiber breakfast cereal. The cereal package carried an explicit health claim for bran cereals in the diet and offered tips from the NCI to reduce the risk of cancer. Although such labeling was against the law, the U.S. Food and Drug Administration took no regulatory action. Other cereal manufacturers soon began to make similar health claims on their products.

These actions triggered a host of controversies between the scientific community, food manufacturers, and regulators. Were these labels appropriate? Were they valid? Did they assist consumers? Amid all the dissension, consumers did not know whom or what to believe.

Nevertheless, the actions of these cereal manufacturers proved to be a catalyst for change. The federal government acted quickly. In just a few years, the food-labeling landscape changed dramatically. Food labels now contain a great deal of information. Consumers appear to be responding. While results vary, about half of consumers use food labels when making product choices (Geiger: 1312–1322). Consumers most often use product labels as the source for nutritional information.

A 1998 article in the *Journal of the American Dietetic Association* stated, "One of the most valuable real estate locations in the food marketing environment is the food label—a very hot property." An average supermarket may have 30,000 items. Every day, manufacturers add another

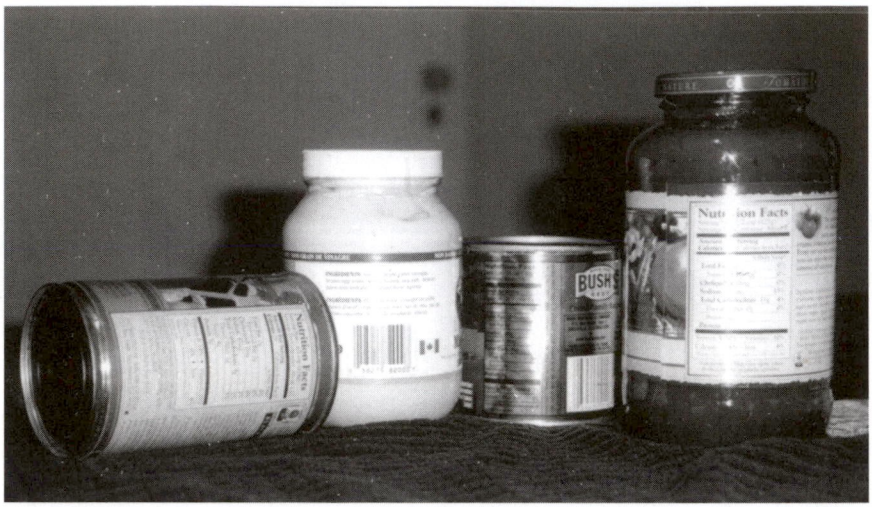

It is important to read carefully the ingredients on food labels. Photo by Mark A. Goldstein.

34 products. "The challenge for nutrition educators and food marketers is to determine and evaluate which information helps consumers decide—in the blink of an eye—which products will move off the shelves" (Coulston: 1470). Still, while studies have shown that more consumers are interested in nutrient information and reading labels, large numbers of people appear indifferent (Burke, Milberg, and Moe: 242–255).

According to the International Food Information Council, "food labeling is a broad term that encompasses several items required on food packages by federal law and regulations." These include "product identity, statement of net contents, name and address of manufacturer, ingredient and nutrition labeling, and nutrition and food claims" (International Food Information Council Web site). Food labeling is controlled by several federal government agencies. Most packaged foods, produce, seafood, milk, and eggs are regulated by the Food and Drug Administration (FDA) in the U.S. Department of Health and Human Services. Meat and poultry products are regulated by the Food Safety and Inspection Service (FSIS) in the U.S. Department of Agriculture (USDA). At the same time, the U.S. Federal Trade Commission (FTC) is in charge of food advertising. Throughout the years, a number of acts have formed the basis of food and nutrition labeling. These include the Meat Inspection Act of 1906, the Federal Food, Drug and Cosmetic Act of 1938, the Poultry Products Inspection Act of 1957, and the Wholesome Meat Act of 1967. Over the years, they have been amended many times.

Ingredient labeling is not the same as nutrition labeling. A food's ingredient label lists the composition of a food. "Federal food, meat and poultry laws require a statement of ingredients on most food labels. Both FDA and USDA regulations require that ingredients be listed in order of their predominance in a food and by their common, specific names." On the other hand, nutrition labeling provides information on the nutritional content of foods. The need to offer more information on nutrient values gained momentum in the late 1960s. In 1973, the FDA began the process to establish the current food-labeling system. A standard format was devised. Though food labeling was voluntary for most products until 1990, "nutrition labeling was mandatory on any food for which a nutrient was added (i.e., enriched with Vitamin C) or for which a nutrition claim was made (i.e., low fat)" (International Food Information Council Web site).

During the 1980s, as evidence of the role diet played in health and well-being increased, greater numbers of people began asking for changes in the nutrition-labeling law. Finally, the Nutrition Labeling and Education Act of 1990 (NLEA) was passed. This law required the federal government to participate in activities to educate consumers about use of the improved label information in making dietary choices. The NLEA has done much more. All products regulated by the FDA are required to have food labels. Since May 8, 1994, all packaged food must have labeling, and fresh fruits, vegetables, and seafood must have point-of-purchase information. Since July 6, 1994, the USDA requires nutrition labeling on packaged meat and poultry. The labeling of fresh meat and poultry remains voluntary. Meanwhile, in order to focus on the nutrients of greatest public health concern, there were modifications in the mandated listing of nutrients and food components on the new "Nutrition Facts" panel. The following nutrients and food components per serving are now listed on the label: total fat, calories from fat, energy as calories, sodium, cholesterol, dietary fiber, total carbohydrate, protein, sugars, vitamins A and C, and minerals iron and calcium. The information is based on a diet of 2,000 calories and the exact specified serving size.

While each individual has unique nutritional needs, the information on the "Nutrition Facts" panel "is based on a 2,000 calorie diet and the specific serving size." And, "the daily value percentage on the Nutrition Facts panel reflects how much of a specific nutrient that a food contains relative to a recommended amount for an entire day" (International Food Information Council Web site). Additionally, the new rules standardize serving sizes and offer definitions for nutrition claims such as free, low, light or "lite," reduced, less, and high. For instance, the term "high" can be used for foods containing 20% or more of the daily value of a particular nutrient per serving, and "good source" means one serving of a food contains 10 to 19% of the daily value of a particular nutrient. (See the Center for Food Safety and Applied Nutrition Web site for detailed definitions of many other terms.) The rules permit statements describing the amount and percentage of nutrients in a food and present criteria for claiming a relationship between a food and a health benefit. "Examples are calcium and osteoporosis, dietary fat and heart disease, dietary fiber and heart disease, soluble fiber from psyllium seed husk or whole oats and coronary heart disease, sodium and high blood pressure, and folic acid and neural tube defects" (International Food Information Council Web site). Other health claims correlate dietary sugar with increased risk of dental cavities and soy protein with preventing heart disease.

These health claims are made in a variety of ways. One method is through a third-party reference such as the National Cancer Institute. There may also be statements, symbols (such as a heart), and vignettes or descriptions. However the health claims are presented, they must meet certain requirements. They may not claim a degree of risk reduction, and they may only say that the food "may" or "might" play a role in reducing the incidence of an illness. Further, the label must note that there are other contributory factors to the particular disease (Center for Food Safety and Applied Nutrition Web site).

There are specific values for the common nutrition claims. A product may be considered calorie free if it has less than 5 calories per serving. A low-calorie item must be less than 40 calories. Similarly, a fat-free food can have no more than 0.5 g of fat. To be considered low fat, a food should have no more than 3 g of fat (Rubin: 58).

The Center for Food Safety and Applied Nutrition of the Food and Drug Administration notes that labels may contain health claims and structure/function claims, and there is a difference between the two. "Manufacturers may make statements about a food substance's effect on the structure or function of the body—for example, 'calcium builds strong bones.' Unlike health claims, structure/function claims do not deal with disease risk reduction." The FDA has no authority over structure/function claims. Instead, when structure/function claims are used by a manufacturer, it is the responsibility of the company to assure that the statements are truthful and not deceptive (Center for Food Safety and Applied Nutrition Web site).

An article in the July 1999 issue of the *Tufts University Health and Nutrition Letter* states that structure/function claims give companies a greater amount of marketing latitude. "For instance, Golden Temple Vanilla Crisp cereal, which contains the herb ginkgo, promises to 'support mental alertness.' That's true enough. But a Twinkie, as well as any other food that contains calories and therefore provides energy to the brain, supports 'mental alertness,' too, and could legally make the same claim" ("Who's Minding Health Claims on Food?": 1).

As a result of the government rulings, about 90% of processed food has nutritional labeling. Exemptions include plain coffee, tea, some spices and flavorings, ready-to-eat food that is prepared on-site, restaurant food, bulk food that is not resold, and food produced by small businesses. While the FDA defines a small business as one in which there is no more than $50,000 in annual food sales or total sales of less than $500,000, the FSIS considers a small business to be one that employs 500 or fewer people and produces no more than a certain poundage of products. Foods that do not make nutrition claims and are in small packages, such as the size of a package of Life Savers or less than half an ounce of meat or poultry, are also excluded. Even so, FDA-regulated foods are required to list a telephone number or address where consumers may obtain nutrition information (Center for Food Safety and Applied Nutrition Web site). For many fresh fruits, vegetables, and fresh fish, nutrition labeling is voluntary. Nevertheless, "if a nutrient or health claim is made (e.g., low calorie), then nutrition information must be available" (Rubin: 58).

USE OF FOOD LABELS

While food labeling is useful for just about anyone, it may be of particular value to certain people, such as those who are trying to lose weight. The labels of lower-calorie and lower-fat foods must compare the difference between their caloric or fat content and the amount in a regular-calorie or regular-fat product. For example, the label of a container of low-fat cottage cheese might state that one serving has 80 calories and 1.5 grams of fat, but it would also compare this to the 120 calories and 5 grams of fat per serving in regular cottage cheese (Center for Food Safety and Applied Nutrition Web site). However, some foods such as cookies and cakes may have lower amounts of fat, but high levels of sugar.

Additionally, food labels are valuable for people trying to prevent heart disease. It is well known that higher intakes of saturated fat and cholesterol are correlated with elevated amounts of cholesterol in the blood. High blood cholesterol levels are, in turn, associated with a greater risk for coronary heart disease (CHD). The most common form of heart disease, CHD is a direct result of the narrowing of the arteries to the heart. The Dietary Guidelines for Americans advises fat intake to be 30% or less of the total daily caloric intake. Saturated fat should be even more restricted—no more than 10% of the daily calories. The daily values used in food labeling follow these guidelines.

Those searching for heart-healthier alternatives can also check fiber content on labels. There is a considerable amount of evidence that dietary fiber or fiber from foods such as fruits, vegetables, and grains lowers the risk of heart disease. "The Daily Value for fiber is 25 g. This is based roughly on FDA and USDA reference amounts of 11.5 g of fiber per 1,000 calories." Similarly, people may wish to review the amount of sodium in foods. In some people, sodium has been found to raise blood pressure. High blood pressure is another risk factor for heart disease. Under the new regulations, sodium has a daily value of 2,4000 mg (Center for Food Safety and Applied Nutrition Web site).

A report published in 1998 in *Family Economics and Nutrition Review* noted that large numbers of Americans consume too much salt. (There are about 2,000 mg of sodium in every teaspoon of salt.) The majority of Americans eat more than the recommended limit, and around two-thirds add salt to their food at the table. About 75% of the sodium that people consume with their diets has been added during food processing (Saltos and Bowman: 49). Detecting sodium is not always easy. It is unseen in a number of foods and processed products and is found in preservatives, flavorings, and stabilizers and in kosher meats such as beef, lamb, and chicken. Furthermore, "sodium also is present naturally in some foods, such as milk, cheese, meat, fish, and some vegetables" (Center for Food Safety and Applied Nutrition Web site).

Since implementation of the regulations, more people seem to be reading food labels. A study published in 1998 in the *American Journal of Public Health* reviewed the pre- and postregulation use of food labels. Data from a 1993 survey of 1,001 men and women were compared to a 1996 survey of 1,450 men and women. Researchers found that consumers significantly increased their use of food labels, by 8.5% among women and 11.3% among men. Greater numbers of people found that they were looking for information on fat content. Fewer neglected to read labels because they were confusing or required too much time. The researchers concluded that the "use of food labels and satisfaction with their content have increased, but 70% of adults still want labels to be easier to understand" (Kristal et al.: 1212–1215).

Another study reported in a 1997 issue of *Journal of Public Policy and Marketing* found that governmental attempts to educate consumers about a diet high in fiber were by and large unsuccessful, but after cereal companies were permitted to advertise this information, awareness rose to 32%. "This implies that consumers acquire much of their nutritional knowledge from packaging and advertising. In fact, brands that supply more product information generally enjoy more favorable consumer attitudes" (Burke, Milberg, and Moe: 242–255).

A survey of residents of Washington State found that label reading was higher among women, people under the age of 35, and those with more than a high-school education. After demographic factors were controlled, researchers concluded that the people most likely to read labels believed in the value of eating a low-fat diet and in the relationship between diet and cancer. Some were following the maintenance stage of a low-fat diet (Neuhouser, Kristal, and Patterson: 45–50).

A report published in 1999 in the *Journal of the American Dietetic Association* determined that food labels may help middle-aged women with type 2 diabetes mellitus manage their illness. Although it is well known that "nutrition therapy is an essential component of successful diabetes management," previous research has determined that women with diabetes tend not to read food labels. In this study, more than 40 women between the ages of 40 and 60 who lived in a rural community in Pennsylvania were divided into two groups. The experimental group received nine weekly educational sessions on nutrition and food labels. Participants in the control group were sent the same information in the mail. There was no significant difference between the two groups in the pretest knowledge scores. Though both groups had a relatively poor knowledge about food labels, there was noteworthy improvement among those who participated in the experimental group. The researchers concluded that there are large numbers of women with type 2 diabetes who would benefit from more training in food labels. "Education about the label should be a primary component of practice guidelines for medical nutrition therapy for people with diabetes" (Miller, Jensen, and Achterberg: 323–328).

Popular thinking contends that college food is often higher in fat. It is not uncommon for college students to joke about the 15 pounds gained during the freshman year. However, college students may be lacking nutrients for other reasons as well. Students may eat on the run or skip meals entirely. They may have limited access to healthier choices. Female students are known to consume inadequate intakes of calcium, iron, and vitamin A (Marietta, Welshimer, and Anderson: 445–449).

Initial results of a study appear to show that, when given the option, at least some college students read food labels. Two hundred and eight students enrolled in a basic life science course at Southeast Missouri State University, Cape Girardeau, participated in an investigation. There were 141 women and 67 men, ranging in age from 17 to 53 years. The study found that 44% of the students used the label for first-time purchases, but they were only concerned with certain aspects of the label such as total fat, calories, calories from fat, and serving sizes. Far less attention was paid to calcium, iron, and vitamin A. There were limitations. "Students were able to obtain basic facts from the labels but were less successful at performing more complex tasks such as finding which one of four labels contained the most fat and fiber" (Marietta, Welshimer, and Anderson: 445–449). Moreover, many of the students questioned the validity of the nutrition claims such as "fat free," "good source," and "reduced calories" that were noted on the label. This is only one study at one school. The findings should not be generalized to include all college students.

CONTROVERSIES SURROUNDING FOOD LABELING

While food labeling has many supporters, it has generated some controversy. In "Food Labeling—The Problems of Mandated Information for Biotechnology," Frances B. Smith, executive director of Consumer Alert, a nonprofit, nonpartisan consumer group, wrote that the government requirements for labeling fail to distinguish between the "broadcast" versus the "narrow" uses of information. In the broadcast approach of food labeling, everyone is given the same information, whether or not it is relevant to their lives. Smith wonders if this is the best method. For example, there are people who are lactose intolerant. When they consume dairy products, especially those that are higher in lactose, they may experience some undesirable symptoms such as upset stomach, bloating, and diarrhea. "Yet foods containing lactose do not carry a specific information label going to the general public that notes that fact or points out the risk/discomfort of lactose for those who are intolerant of that ingredient. Rather, the minority of people who are sensitive to lactose seek out lactose-free, acidophilus milk and other products" (Consumer Alert Web site).

Moreover, Smith continued, when manufacturers are required to list a host of different label information, there may be little room for other crucial items. When a great deal of information is noted, it is harder for consumers to locate what they need to know. Someone who is obese may be more interested in the calorie- and fat-related values; someone on a sodium-restricted diet probably would want to check the sodium content. Other essential items, such as how a food should be prepared or whether it should be refrigerated, may be less visible or harder to locate, but lack of knowledge about these items can increase the risks of foodborne disease. "Too much information often means too little—in the sense that little information is read or important information is overlooked or cannot readily be found" (Consumer Alert Web site).

Consumers may also misunderstand or misinterpret food labels. A 1997 article in the *Journal of Public Policy and Marketing* wondered whether "consumers will use information provided by one brand about a common but previously neglected attribute to infer that the other brands in the product category do not possess the attribute" (Burke, Milberg, and Moe: 242–255). For example, if the label on a bottle of corn oil indicates that the product is free of cholesterol, consumers may believe, incorrectly, that other brands of corn oil contain cholesterol. Corn oil is a plant-based food, and cholesterol is only found in animal-based foods. Nevertheless, without such labeling, some consumers may not realize that corn oil is free of cholesterol and therefore a healthier alternative than an oil filled with cholesterol. The authors propose using "broader 'nutrient free' claims (that suggest the typicality of the health benefit in the product category)" (Burke, Milberg, and Moi: 242–255). To the authors, these better convey the necessary information without misleading the consumer.

A 1997 article in *Nutrition Today* noted the following problems with food labels:

- Photographs are often more appealing than actual appearance.
- "No preservatives" claims on the front make people uneasy when the ingredients list on the back contains numerous chemical-sounding names, even though they are not preservatives, but other additives with different legal definitions.
- "Lemonade" (in big type) followed by "flavor" (in small) might leave some people feeling tricked when they find no lemons in the ingredients list.
- "Natural" and "fresh" sound wrong for anything that is produced in a manufacturing plant.
- "New" and "improved" might make a consumer ask: If something is new, how can it be improved? If something is improved, how can it be new?
- Some food labeling is too puzzling for most people to understand. For example, a product may indicate that it contains less sugar or fat, but there is little or no reduction in calories. Most people do not realize that manufacturers use various carbohydrates to "provide the sweetness of sugar or the mouth-feel of fat." (McNutt: 252–256)

On occasion, a food label may be incorrect. A 1999 story in *Family Practice* reported that there have been at least three children who had life-threatening anaphylactic reactions to dark chocolate with "pareve" labeling, a kosher designation that means, in part, the absence of milk. The children experienced a number of serious reactions such as coughing, congestion, asthma, hives, itching, angioedema, bronchospasm, diarrhea, vomiting, wheezing, and nonresponsiveness. All were transported to medical facilities to receive emergency treatment with epinephrine. The child who was nonresponsive required intubation. "The reason milk can be present in dark chocolate certified to be made without milk is that it is made on the same processing equipment as milk chocolate" (Worcester: 54). Cross-contamination obviously occurred.

As noted in the previous chapter, cross-contamination is a worry for people with celiac disease, an autoimmune disorder. Celiacs are unable to eat the gluten found in wheat, oats, barley, and rye. While the ingredients in a corn cereal, as noted on the label, may be perfectly safe, if the cereal is processed on the same machinery as the gluten-containing cereals, there may well be cross-contamination. Celiacs often check directly with manufacturers to determine if the food is safe for them to eat. In *Kids with Celiac Disease*, Danna Korn writes that celiacs need to become good food-label readers. If any of the following foods appear on an ingredient label, the food may contain gluten:

- Brown rice syrup (frequently made from barley)
- Caramel color
- Dextrin (usually corn, but sometimes derived from wheat)
- Flour or cereal products
- Hydrolyzed vegetable protein (HVP), vegetable protein, hydrolyzed plant protein (HPP), or textured vegetable protein (TVP)
- Malt or malt flavoring (usually made from barley; okay if made from corn)
- Malt vinegar
- Modified food starch or modified starch from an unspecified or forbidden source
- Mono- and diglycerides (in dry products only)
- Flavorings in meat products
- Soy sauce or soy sauce solids (many soy sauces contain wheat)
- Vegetable gum (Korn: 212–213)

Some people oppose the American Heart Association logo that appears on a number of foods. When the logo is on a food item, it means that the food is low in fat (3 grams or less), low in saturated fat (1 gram or less), low in cholesterol (20 milligrams or less), and moderate in sodium (480 milligrams or less). Moreover, the food provides at least 10% of the daily value for one or more of the following nutrients: protein, vitamin A, vitamin C, calcium, iron, or fiber (American Heart Association Web site). Use of the logo is expensive. There is an initial charge, followed by annual fees. Many smaller companies that produce heart-healthy foods do not have the resources to participate in the program. While their foods might be just as healthful, or even more so, they are unable to display the logo.

Some have expressed concern that labeling fails to distinguish the different forms of sugar. According to an article published in *Environmental Nutrition* in 2000, Americans eat the equivalent of 20 teaspoons of sugar each day, twice the amount recommended by the government and health groups. Sugar is found naturally in many foods, but it is also added to products. To enhance their flavor, fat-free foods may have high amounts of sugar. While acknowledging that scientists see little variation between the types of sugar, the author of the article contends that there are important differences. "Naturally occurring sugars are accompanied by vitamins, minerals and phytochemicals. For instance, the fructose in an orange keeps company with vitamin C, folate and fiber. . . . In contrast, added sugar, such as table sugar (sucrose) or high fructose corn syrup, is a loner, adding nothing but empty calories" (Neville: 2).

Food labels have the potential to be confusing. The FDA requires that all labeling be "truthful and not misleading," but the FDA cannot monitor all products, and it cannot stop marketers from slightly bending the rules. In a March 14, 2001, article in the *New York Times*, Marian Burros wrote that she enjoys reading egg cartons. The label of one carton noted that the hens are "cage-free." Burros wondered what that really meant. Are the chickens free-range? Or are they not in cages, "but in large enclosed areas where they stand beak to beak"? One of Burros's favorite labels is used by a chicken producer who indicates that his birds have "no artificial hormones." Commenting on the label, Burros wrote, "A double asterisk beside the statement leads to this notice: 'U.S.D.A. regulations prohibit the use of artificial growth stimulates and hormones in this product.' The company is making a virtue out of not doing what it is not permitted to do" (Burros: Section F, page 2, column 1).

A 1997 article in *Consumers' Research Magazine* said that when the FDA examined 300 food products, it found that the amounts of fat, sodium, vitamins, and other nutrients were accurate approximately 91% of the time. While the total fat content was correct 96% of the time, only 69% of the time did the labels give the exact amount of iron. For people who are at risk for an iron overload—a condition known as hemochromatosis—this is crucial. Other information was also problematic. "Only 80% of the values listed were accurate for cholesterol, dietary fiber, vitamin C, and calcium. Cholesterol in some frozen seafood products was significantly understated" (Hunter: 8–9). Clearly, there is much room for improvement in food labeling.

CONCLUSION

It is becoming increasingly evident that many people are concerned about what is contained in the food that they eat. How much fat does it contain? Cholesterol? Sodium? This is important information, especially if you have a medical problem. One of the most obvious ways to learn what is in the food is to read food labels. Thanks to changes in federal laws, it is now quite easy to read labels. Still, large numbers of people rarely do or never bother. Further, not everyone supports the current labeling requirements. Some believe that they are often confusing, misleading or inaccurate.

TOPICS FOR DISCUSSION

1. Do you read food labels? Why or why not?
2. If you do read labels, what are you looking for? Why?
3. If you were developing food and nutrition labels for a box of cereal, what would you include? What would you delete? Why?
4. Has a food label ever caused you to buy a product? Describe the experience and what triggered the sale.
5. Do you think that food labels are overcrowded with information? Why or why not?

REFERENCES AND RESOURCES

Books

Koerner, Celide Barnes, and Anne Muñoz-Furlong. *Food Allergies*. Minneapolis: Chronimed Publishing, 1998.

Korn, Danna. *Kids with Celiac Disease*. Bethesda, Maryland: Woodbine House, 2001.

Magazines, Journals, and Newspapers

Burke, Sandra J., Sandra J. Milberg, and Wendy W. Moe. "Displaying Common But Previously Neglected Health Claims on Product Labels: Understanding Competitive Advantages, Deception, and Education." *Journal of Public Policy and Marketing*, Fall 1997, 16(2): 242–255.

Burros, Marian. "Eating Well: The Truth behind the Feel-Good Labels." *New York Times*, March 14, 2001: Section F, page 2, column 1.

Coulston, Ann M. "President's Page: Nutrition Messages on Food Packages—Location, Location, Location." *Journal of the American Dietetic Association*, December 1998, 98(12): 1470.

Geiger, Constance J. "Health Claims: History, Current Regulatory Status, and Consumer Research." *Journal of the American Dietetic Association*, November 1998, 98(11): 1312.

Hunter, Beatrice Trum. "Nutritional Labeling Revisited." *Consumers' Research Magazine*, May 1997, 80(5): 8–9.

Kristal, Alan R., Lisa Levy, Ruth E. Patterson, Sue S. Li, and Emily White. "Trends in Food Label Use Associated with New Nutrition Labeling Regulations." *American Journal of Public Health*, August 1998, 88(8): 1212–1215.

Marietta, Anne B., Kathleen J. Welshimer, and Sara Long Anderson. "Knowledge,

Attitudes, and Behaviors of College Students Regarding the 1990 Nutrition Labeling Education Act Food Labels." *Journal of the American Dietetic Association*, April 1999, 99(4): 445–449.

McNutt, Kristen. "Why Some Consumers Don't Believe Some Nutrition Claims." *Nutrition Today*, November/December 1997, 32(6): 252–256.

Miller, Carla K., Gordon L. Jensen, and Cheryl L. Achterberg. "Evaluation of Food Label Nutrition Intervention for Women with Type 2 Diabetes Mellitus." *Journal of the American Dietetic Association*, March 1999, 99(3): 323–328.

Neuhouser, Marian L., Alan R. Kristal, and Ruth E. Patterson. "Use of Food Nutrition Label Is Associated with Lower Fat Intake." *Journal of the American Dietetic Association*, January 1999, 99(1): 45–50.

Neville, Kerry. "Sugar: How Do I Disguise Thee? Let Me Count the Ways." *Environmental Nutrition*, March 2000, 23(3):2.

Rubin, Karen Wilk. "Terms and Definitions: Food Labeling." *Food Service Director*, January 15, 2001, 14(1): 58.

Saltos, Etta, and Shanthy Bowman. "Dietary Guidance on Sodium: Should We Take It with a Grain of Salt?" *Family Economics and Nutrition Review*, Fall 1998, 11(4):49.

Stapleton, Stephanie. "Group Wants More Informative Nutrition Labels." *American Medical News*, August 23, 1999, 42(32): 27.

"Who's Minding Health Claims on Food?" *Tufts University Health and Nutrition Letter*, July 1999, 17(5): 1.

Worcester, Sharon. "Pareve Labeling Doesn't Always Mean Milk Free." *Family Practice News*, May 1, 1999, 29(9): 54.

Organizations to Contact

American Heart Association
National Center
7272 Greenville Avenue
Dallas, TX 75231
Phone: 800-AHA-USA1
http://americanheart.org/ (April 18, 2001)

Center for Food Safety and Applied Nutrition
Food and Drug Administration
5100 Paint Branch Parkway
College Park, MD 20740-3835
Phone: 1-888-SAFEFOOD
http://vm.cfsan.fda.gov/list.html (April 5, 2001)

Consumer Alert
1001 Connecticut Avenue NW, Suite 1128
Washington, DC 20036
Phone: 202-467-5809
http://www.consumeralert.org/ (April 5, 2001)

International Food Information Council
1100 Connecticut Avenue NW, Suite 430
Washington, DC 20036
Phone: 202-296-6540
http://www.ific.org/ (April 5, 2001)

8

Hidden Ingredients in Food

Sometimes it is a challenge to determine what ingredients are in certain foods. Foods often contain hidden ingredients that may threaten the health and well-being of some people. By design or by accident, many types of foods may contain ingredients not listed on the label. The Food and Drug Administration (FDA) allows trace amounts of natural products to be omitted from the label. It also takes no exception to the failure of manufacturers to mention the small amounts of insects, mold, and rodent filth that make their way into foods during processing. For example, the FDA permits cochineal, an insect that spends its life sucking on plants, to be used as red coloring, and frozen broccoli may have "up to 60 aphids, thrips or mites" (American-Asian Kashrus Service Web site).

NATURAL FLAVORINGS

Let's begin with natural flavorings. The American-Asian Kashrus Services (an extensive Web site on kosher food, run by a rabbi) notes on its Web site: "When it comes to flavourings, it has long been the industry's policy to mask the true nature of the additive under the generic term 'Natural flavourings.' This sounds very gentle and downright healthy. However, using the example of the flavourings, we learn that the source of this additive is from the sperm whale. Yet another such example is 'Civet absolute,' which is derived from the civet cat. These additives are offered to the unsuspecting consumer as 'natural flavours,' which of course, they actually are!" (American-Asian Kashrus Services Web site).

The Code of Federal Regulations defines natural flavors and flavorings as follows: "The term natural flavor or natural flavoring means the essential oil, oleoresin, essence or extractive, protein hydrolysate, distillate, or any product of roasting, heating or enzymolysis, which contains the flavoring constituents derived from a spice, fruit or fruit juice, vegetable or vegetable juice, edible yeast, herb, bark, bud, root, leaf or similar plant material, meat, seafood, poultry, eggs, dairy products, or fermentation products thereof, whose significant function in food is flavoring rather than nutritional" (Center for Food Safety and Applied Nutrition Web site). The Vegetarian Resource Group notes, "Natural flavors can be pretty much anything approved for use in food." As a result, unless a company specifically lists the source of its natural ingredients on the label, the consumer is left without a clue. A few, primarily smaller, companies list sources, but the vast majority do not. Most consumers probably do not realize the types of hidden ingredients that may be in their food.

In *Fast Food Nation*, a 2001 best-seller that describes the impact of the fast-food industry on life in the United States, Eric Schlosser noted that a number of fast-food products obtain their flavors from unexpected sources. For example, the Grilled Chicken Sandwich sold at Wendy's contains beef extracts, and the BK Broiler Chicken Breast Patty sold at Burger King has "natural smoke flavor." Schlosser says that Red Arrow Products Company "manufactures natural smoke flavor by charring sawdust and capturing the aroma chemicals released into the air. Then the firm turns this smoke into liquid with a solvent" (Schlosser: 128).

Foods may also contain insects, molds, and rodent filth. How many of these hidden ingredients might be in a typical meal? The Web site of the American-Asian Kashrus Services notes the following examples: "coffee beans: up to 10% can be insect infected; tomato juice: up to 10 fly eggs per 100 grams; cereal: up to 9 milligrams of rodent excreta and 50 insect fragments per 50 grams."

The FDA contends that "it is economically impractical to grow, harvest, or process raw products that are totally free of non-hazardous, naturally occurring, unavoidable defects" (Center for Food Safety and Applied Nutrition Web site). The FDA does set limits, and it is against the law for manufacturers to exceed these. The limits are listed in a report more than 30 pages long entitled *The Food Defect Action Levels* that may be found on the Web site of the Center for Food Safety and Applied Nutrition of the U.S. Food and Drug Administration (http://vm.cfsan. fda.gov/~dma/dalbook.html). The FDA maintains that manufacturers do not simply attempt to remain slightly below the permissible level. "The defect levels do not represent an average of the defects that occur in any of the products—the averages are actually much lower. The levels represent limits at which FDA will regard the food product 'adulterated' and subject to enforcement action" (Center for Food Safety and Applied Nutrition Web site).

By becoming a diligent reader of food labels, one may try to avoid foods with natural flavorings, especially those in which the natural flavorings are not identified. While this is difficult and time-consuming, it may work with products purchased at a store, but vigilant label reading is of little assistance with restaurant or take-out foods. It is of no help with processed foods that may contain FDA-permissible amounts of insects, mold, and rodent filth.

Would organic foods be less likely to be tainted? As is noted in the chapter on organic foods, the term *organic* relates to the way in which the food is grown and produced, not the method in which it is processed. Like other foods, natural flavorings would be listed as an ingredient of processed organic foods. As long as they remain within FDA limits, they may have the same contaminants.

AVOIDING HIDDEN INGREDIENTS

As a result of concerns about hidden ingredients, a number of Jewish and non-Jewish people are eating more kosher products. According to Rabbi Eliezer Eidlitz, who maintains the Web site KosherQuest, many people believe that "kosher certification is their best guarantee that the product and its ingredients are being watched carefully. . . . In the U.S. alone, there appear to be at least five million people who buy products based on their being kosher" (KosherQuest Web site). There are no hidden ingredients in kosher foods. All ingredients are clearly labeled. The American-Asian Kashrus Services Web site notes that "close to 100,000 products and ingredients in the U.S. today are certified Kosher." That means that "millions of Americans from all religions and walks of life are looking to kosher certified foods as the only real guarantee as to the true nature of what they are eating."

More people are also reducing their intake of processed foods. A newly washed fresh tomato is exactly that—a tomato. However, the FDA allows canned tomatoes to have no more than 10 or more drosophila fly eggs per 500 grams or 5 or more drosophila fly eggs and 1 or more maggots per 500 grams or 2 or more maggots per 500 grams (Center for Food Safety and Applied Nutrition Web site). Fresh fruit may also contain some insects. An August 2000 article in the *Christian Science Monitor* noted that 500 grams of berries may have 4 larvae or 10 whole insects (Huntington: Page 18).

Although some people will only be shocked to learn what might be in their food, other people who have food allergies and intolerances may have significant negative reactions to the food they eat because of these unnamed ingredients. Even small amounts of certain foods hidden in other foods may make them ill. A reaction from a food allergy may actually kill someone. Allergic reactions are not uncommon occurrences. Seven million Americans are believed to have food allergies (Winter:

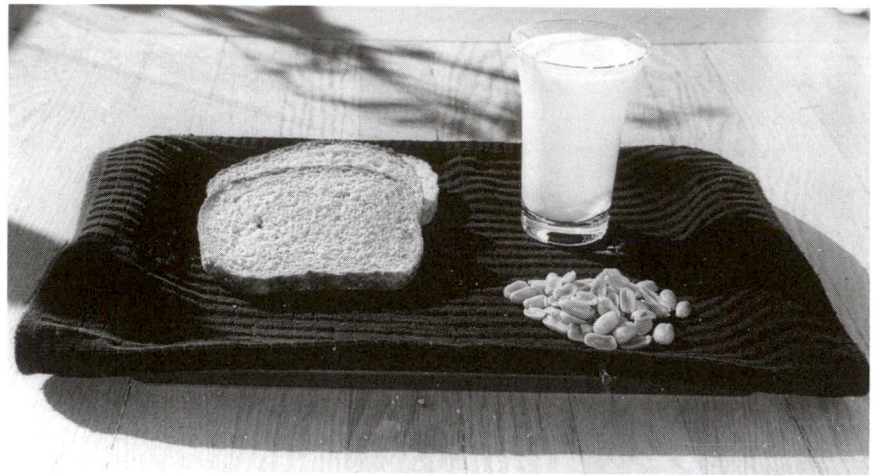

Some common foods may have life-threatening or disease-producing ingredients. Photo by Mark A. Goldstein.

Section C, page 1, column 2). "Every year some 30,000 people are rushed to emergency rooms with allergic reactions to foods" ("Dangerous Omissions on Food Labels": Section A, page 28, column 1). For an additional discussion of this topic, see the previous chapter.

Those who are allergic have no choice but to avoid the allergen. They should begin by reading ingredient labels. If there is no ingredient label, allergic people may attempt to contact the manufacturer. Unless an allergic person is able to determine that all the ingredients are safe, the food should not be consumed.

That is sometimes easier to say than to do. Hoping to study the situation, in October 1998, the Food and Drug Administration formed a partnership with the Minnesota Department of Agriculture and the Wisconsin Department of Agriculture. They decided to begin a two-year investigation of the eight foods that cause 90% of the severe life-threatening reactions: peanuts, eggs, milk and milk products, wheat, tree nuts, soy, fish, and shellfish. "Although this Partnership looked at control of all food allergens, the Partnership focused on peanut and egg allergens. Ice cream, bakery and candy manufacturers were selected for coverage. Selection was made randomly of small, medium, and large establishments" (Center for Food Safety and Applied Nutrition Web site). In total, 85 companies were examined.

For those with food allergies, the findings were disturbing. "As many as 25 percent of manufacturers failed to list common ingredients that can cause potentially fatal allergic reactions.... A quarter of the companies made products with raw ingredients like nuts, but omitted them from the labels describing the food." Also shocking was the fact that "only slightly more than half of the manufacturers checked their products to ensure that all of the ingredients were accurately reflected on the labels." Some of the problems arose because of the manufacturing process. A number of bakers cross-contaminated foods because they used the same utensils for different mixes or reused baking sheets without washing them. Parchment papers were sometimes used as many as 10 times before replacement. One conveyor belt that coated candies in chocolate was cleaned only once a year (Winter: Section C, page 1, column 2).

Cross-contamination may occur in many places. Lisa Cipriano Collins, a marriage and family therapist who has a son with severe peanut and tree-nut allergies, observed in *Caring for Your Child with Severe Food Allergies*: "You need to imagine the production of foods and consider the possibility that cross-contamination can occur in raw material containers, processing machinery, packaging machinery, and display cases. Many times a label will be free of an allergen, but your common sense will tell you that the probability of cross-contamination is high. . . . For example, my common sense told me that granola bars without nuts listed on the label were not the best choice for my son when there were five other varieties of nut-containing granola bars available from the same manufacturer" (Collins: 31).

Marianne S. Barber, the mother of a food-allergic child, an award-winning copywriter, and a founding member of the Connecticut chapter of the Food Allergy Initiative, Maryanne Bartoszek Scott, and Elinor Greenberg note in *The Parent's Guide to Food Allergies* that cross-contamination with ice cream containing nuts is a risk in ice-cream parlors. At a deli counter, a child who is highly allergic to dairy is at risk if ham or turkey has been sliced with a blade just used for cheese. (An establishment that adheres strictly to kosher rules will have separate slicers for meats and cheeses.) Similarly, at a salad bar, tongs may have just held shredded cheese or other salad ingredients containing milk products. "When eating in restaurants, it's best either to bring a safe meal with you or order the simplest meal possible: plain grilled meat or chicken, baked potato, and salad or vegetable. Be sure to ask about the grilled meat. Anytime you are dealing with more than one ingredient, keep your antennae up. If your child loves hamburgers, you'll have to find out if the patties are 100 percent beef—there could be soy, wheat, even egg or other fillers hiding in there. If the allergy is to milk, egg, soy, wheat, peanut, or nuts, bring your own dessert" (Barber, Scott, and Greenberg: 118–119).

In *The Peanut Allergy Answer Book*, Michael C. Young notes that because of its ability to add flavor and texture, peanut butter is added to a host of different cooked foods. "Peanut butter is often used as a shortening or oil in recipes for many gravies. It can give a smoother texture to sauces and gravies. It is used as a thickener for many recipes. Peanut butter has adhesive properties that allow it to be used to 'glue down' the ends of egg rolls to keep them from coming apart." Additionally, peanuts, peanut oil, and peanut butter are included in a variety of international foods such as Chinese, Japanese, Indian, Ethiopian, Vietnamese, and Thai. Peanuts are hidden in many prepared products. "Sauces and toppings can have finely crushed peanuts mixed in without any visible sign of them. Peanut sauce is often included as a hidden ingredient in chicken marinade. . . . Peanut flour is used in certain brands of frozen dinners. 'Slivered almonds' found on some baked goods may actually be made from raw peanuts because they are much cheaper" (Young: 55–56).

A 1997 article in *Dairy Foods* explains how the Kellogg Company described Rice Krispie Treats prepared with margarine as a safe snack for children with milk allergies. When the company began to sell Rice Krispie Treat Cereal, it was deemed milk free. However, after eating the dry cereal, a consumer with milk allergies had a reaction. Upon investigating the matter, Kellogg learned that the flavors used in the cereal that were described as "natural and artificial flavors" had tiny amounts of an allergenic butter flavor. The ingredient label was quickly changed to read "natural & artificial butter flavor' " (Gorski: 31–33).

"Reworking" is also an issue. Reworking is a process by which ice cream may be made. A manufacturer may begin by making a variety with nuts. While a subsequent variety may not contain nuts, there may be leftover nuts from the previous batch. "This method is used to enhance the flavor of the ice cream not containing nuts" (Collins: 28).

There are other ways that hidden food allergens may contaminate seemingly safe food. For example, restaurants with deep fryers may fry a variety of foods in the same oil. If you are allergic to shellfish and another patron's shrimp is fried in the same oil as your eggplant, you might well become ill. Restaurants may be dangerous for other reasons as well. An article that appeared in 1997 in *Restaurant and Institutions* recalled how, hoping to prevent food-allergy problems, Anne Muñoz-Furlong, founder of the Food Allergy and Anaphylaxis Network, selected a first-class resort hotel for her family's vacation. She even explained her daughter's medical concerns to the restaurant manager. "On the first evening, Muñoz-Furlong carefully ordered a plain, unsauced meal for her daughter. The toddler was ill that night. Next day: same meal, same reaction. Muñoz-Furlong summoned the chef, who sheepishly admitted that he'd felt sorry for the little girl dining on such austere fare and had added a pat of butter to her rice" (Rousseau: 78).

Chefs and their assistants do not necessarily understand that the foods causing allergic reactions must have no contact with the food that will be eaten by the allergic patron. It is not appropriate to simply take away the nuts from a salad that has been returned. Someone who is sensitive to nuts may still have a reaction, even after the nuts have been removed. A new, nutless salad must be prepared. An individual who is sensitive to wheat cannot eat wheatless pancakes that have been made on the same griddle as wheat-based pancakes. "Some people are so sensitive that simply inhaling invisible airborne particles from someone else's meal or snack could precipitate an attack, which is why some airlines have decided to stop serving peanuts" (Brody: Section F, page 8, column 1).

Lisa Cipriano Collins describes one case of an allergic reaction that was the basis for a lawsuit against a large restaurant chain. A woman who was allergic to nuts asked the waitress at the restaurant to list the ingredients of the pesto sauce. Since nuts were not on the list, she ordered it. When the dish was brought, she asked the waitress directly if the sauce had nuts in it. The waitress allegedly stated that no nuts were in the sauce, but it contained both pine nuts and walnuts. The woman went into anaphylactic shock and later died (Collins: 27).

The Food Allergy Initiative advises people with food allergies to carry a card that lists their specific food allergies. Before ordering food at a restaurant, the card should be shown to the chef, manager, or waiter. The card should state, "Please let me know if any of the food items, sauces or garnishes have these ingredients or if there is a risk that they can 'contaminate' my food during preparation" (Food Allergy Initiative Web site).

In *Food Allergies*, a book written for the American Dietetic Association by Celide Barnes Koerner and Anne Muñoz-Furlong, the authors discuss cross-contamination in detail. They note that the following products are risky for those with certain allergies, especially dairy products, tree nuts, and peanuts: candy bars, baking pieces, chocolate bars, and other candies; mixed products or products that contain multiple ingredients, such as granola bars; and nut butters. All of these products are commonly run on shared production lines (Koerner and Muñoz-Furlong: 46).

Cross-contamination may easily occur in the grocery store. Bulk-food bins rarely list the ingredients of the foods and are at high risk for cross-contamination from other foods if they are not thoroughly cleaned between uses. Deli cheeses and meats that contain dairy products such as casein (a milk protein often used as a binder in ham) can cause cross-contamination if they are sliced on the same equipment as the other deli meats. Juices from allergy-causing foods can leak onto other foods in the grocery cart. Any such food should be tightly wrapped in a plastic bag before it is placed in the cart (Koerner and Muñoz-Furlong: 47–48).

There is similar concern about the contamination of pareve foods. Although the exact origin of the word is unknown, pareve essentially means that the food lies between the extremes of meat and dairy. Pareve foods, which contain a label with a U in a circle or the word *pareve*, have no meat or dairy derivatives. They have not been cooked or mixed with any meat or dairy foods and may be eaten with both meat and milk foods. Eggs, fish, fruit, vegetables, grains, and juices in their natural, unprocessed state are common pareve foods. Other pareve foods include pasta, soft drinks, coffee and tea, and many types of candy and snacks. During processing, however, the pareve designation may be rendered meaningless. Pareve foods may lose their pareve status if they are processed on dairy equipment or when additives are used. The label may give no indication of this processing. Some pareve foods may not be safe for people with dairy allergies. The Food Allergy and Anaphylaxis Network Web site contains a warning about pareve foods: "Pareve-labeled products indicate that the products are considered milk-free *according to religious specifications*. . . . These may contain enough milk protein to cause an allergic reaction to those with milk allergy." The network warns against relying on a kosher symbol to ensure a milk-free product. Persons with allergies should also be concerned about another kosher designation, "D.E.," which is an abbreviation for dairy equipment. Food that is labeled D.E. may well be dairy free, but it is processed on equipment that is used to make dairy products. The kosher labeling "D" means that the food is a dairy food.

Though they may have different reasons for discomfort, vegetarians, who do not eat animal foods but do eat dairy products, and vegans, who eliminate animal and dairy products, worry about hidden ingredients in their foods. Vegetarians and vegans may have various motivations for choosing their diets—animal rights and/or personal health—but they do not want to eat a seemingly vegan food, such as guacamole, that contains food from an animal, such as gelatin, or hash browns that have been fried in the same oil as meat or seafood products. To assist its readership, a few years ago, the *Vegetarian Journal*, a publication of the Vegetarian Resource Group, printed two articles listing acceptable and unacceptable items in more than 100 fast-food and family-style restaurants. One example is the description of Hardee's: "The sourdough bread and specialty bun at Hardee's are vegan. Hardee's no longer offers a garden salad as a menu item but does offer a vegan side salad consisting of lettuce, tomatoes, cucumbers, carrots, and purple cabbage. However, no vegan dressings are available" (Bartas, 1997: 16–19). Those who are uneasy about hidden animal products in their food may wish to investigate the Web site of the Vegetarian Resource Group.

The North American Vegetarian Society has further tackled this problem. On its Web site, it warns of inaccurate labeling. Manufacturers may contend that their products contain no animal ingredients when, in fact, they have foods such as honey, whey, casein, bone, rennet, and gelatin, all of which are from animals. For example, rennet, which is made from the lining of the stomach of calves, is used to solidify hard cheese, and gelatin, which is made from ground skin and bones, is used for Jell-O and supplements. The site notes that "hidden animal ingredients may not be visible to the naked eye. They may be hard to detect on a product label and even harder to taste" (North American Vegetarian Society Web site).

In *Being Vegan*, Joanne Stepaniak, who has written extensively on vegan living, writes that there are a number of ingredients found in commercially prepared food that are usually animal based. Some of the most common are lactate, lactose, albumin, pepsin, royal jelly, suet, tallow, lard, and whey. Sometimes manufacturers are simply unaware "if their ingredients are from animal or nonanimal sources, because buyers frequently alternate among suppliers, depending on who has the lowest market price" (Stepaniak, 2000: 163–164).

In another of Stepaniak's books, *The Vegan Sourcebook*, she addresses the challenge of hidden animal ingredients in restaurant foods. Some examples she gives are beans and tortillas that contain lard, French fries cooked in animal fat, fresh and dried pastas made with eggs, and bread and rolls made with eggs, butter, cow's milk, or whey. Salad dressings and sauces may contain dairy products or gelatin. Chicken broth or beef bouillon are often used in preparing soups and gravies. "Even vinaigrette dressings are frequently spiked with Parmesan cheese" (Stepaniak, 1998: 199–200).

In Eric Schlosser's *Fast Food Nation*, he describes the French fries sold at McDonald's restaurants. The McDonald's Corporation has refused to disclose the source of the natural flavor used in the fries. However, "in response to inquiries from *Vegetarian Journal* . . . McDonald's did acknowledge that its fries derive some of their characteristic flavor from 'animal products' " (Schlosser: 128).

A 2001 article in the *New York Times* describes how some New York City chefs were adding hidden ingredients such as tripe, pork jowls, and pigs' feet and calling them "secret spices." "Rather than risk offending the squeamish, they follow a silent rule: if you can't see it on the plate, you don't have to mention it on the menu." Clearly, this is not possible with some menu items. "Menu editing works with ingredients that disappear in the dish or are served on the side, but not with foods that are the main part of a dish, like snails" (Clark: Section F, page 3, column 1).

Despite the many advances, there is a growing awareness that some ingredients are still not listed on food labels. A number of national organizations and countless Internet sites can provide information. Most fast-food restaurants post lists of all the ingredients in their products. Whenever possible, these include the "hidden ones." These lists may also be obtained on the Internet. Certainly, in the better restaurants, when a customer notifies a member of the waitstaff of a food allergy or intolerance, the server will quickly provide information or check with the chef. Chefs and the members of their staff are becoming increasingly aware of the problem and adjusting their meals to suit the needs of their customers.

CONCLUSION

While it is no longer necessary for people with food allergies and intolerances to avoid eating away from home, they must, nevertheless, always be cautious. They should veer in the direction of eating plain foods with fewer ingredients. They should ask for food that has been kept separate and prepared in a carefully washed pan. They should support and patronize restaurants and stores that cater to their needs. Above all, they should continue to speak out, raise public awareness, and write letters to their congressional representatives asking for stricter food standards. If legislators believe that there is a strong constituency for these issues, they will respond with new laws and increased resources.

TOPICS FOR DISCUSSION

1. Before reading this chapter, did you realize what natural flavorings were? Has the chapter influenced how you feel about them? Why or why not?

2. Do you have any friends who have food allergies? Has your school made adequate provisions for them? Are there ways the school could improve what it does?

3. Pretend you are allergic to peanuts. Think of five ways that you could reduce your chances of cross-contamination in a restaurant.

4. What are some of the ways that restaurant personnel may be better educated about the seriousness of food allergies? Devise a few strategies.

5. What should be the FDA's role regarding standards for food? Are the current standards sufficient? Why or why not?

REFERENCES AND RESOURCES

Books

Adelman, Todd, and Jodi Behrend. *Special Foods for Special Kids*. San Francisco: Robert D. Reed Publishers, 1999.
Astor, Stephen. *Hidden Food Allergies*. Garden City Park, New York: Avery Publishing Group, 1997.
Barber, Marianne S., Maryanne Bartoszek Scott, and Elinor Greenberg. *The Parent's Guide to Food Allergies*. New York: Henry Holt and Company, 2001.

Collins, Lisa Cipriano. *Caring for Your Child with Severe Food Allergies*. New York: John Wiley and Sons, 2000.

Joneja, Janice Vickerstaff. *Dietary Management of Food Allergies and Intolerances: A Comprehensive Guide*. Vancouver, British Columbia, Canada: J.A. Hall Publications, 1998.

Koerner, Celide Barnes, and Anne Muñoz-Furlong. *Food Allergies*. Minneapolis: Chronimed Publishing, 1998.

Korn, Danna. *Kids with Celiac Disease*. Bethesda, Maryland: Woodbine House, 2001.

Schlosser, Eric. *Fast Food Nation*. Boston: Houghton Mifflin Company, 2001.

Stepaniak, Joanne. *Being Vegan*. Los Angeles: Lowell House, 2000.

Stepaniak, Joanne. *The Vegan Sourcebook*. Los Angeles: Lowell House, 1998.

Young, Michael C. *The Peanut Allergy Answer Book*. Gloucester, Massachusetts: Fair Winds Press, 2001.

Magazines, Journals, and Newspapers

Bartas, Jeanne-Marie. "Vegan Menu Items at Fast Food and Family-Style Restaurants, Part I." *Vegetarian Journal*, November/December 1997, 16(6): 16–19.

Bartas, Jeanne-Marie. "Vegan Menu Items at Fast Food and Family-Style Restaurants, Part II." *Vegetarian Journal*, January/February 1998, 17(1): 24–29.

Brody, Jane E. "Personal Health: Ways to Stop Extreme Allergic Reactions." *New York Times*, August 22, 2000: Section F, page 8, column 1.

Clark, Melissa. "Menus That Don't Tell the Whole Story." *New York Times*, January 24, 2001: Section F, page 3, column 1.

"Dangerous Omissions on Food Labels." *New York Times*, April 12, 2001: Section A, page 28, column 1.

"Dietitians Face the Challenge of Food Allergies." *Journal of the American Dietetic Association*, January 2000, 100(1): 13.

Dominus, Susan. "The Allergy Prison." *New York Times Magazine*, June 10, 2001: Pages 62–67, 78–80, 113, 121.

Gorski, Donna. "Reducing Allergen Risks." *Dairy Foods*, February 1997, 98(2): 31–33.

Hingley, Audrey T. "Food Allergies: When Eating Is Risky." *FDA Consumer*, December 1993, 27(10): 26–31.

Huntington, Sharon. "You're Already Eating Insects." *Christian Science Monitor*, August 8, 2000: Page 18.

Kleiner, Susan M. "Sense and Food Sensitivity." *Physician and Sportsmedicine*, May 1998, 26(5): 105.

O'Toole, Christine. "Fatal Fare: Allergies to Foods, Especially Nuts, Can Be Life-Changing and Life-Threatening." *Pittsburgh Post-Gazette*, April 21, 1998: Page D-1.

Peiper, Howard, and Nina Anderson. "What You Need to Know about Your Food Allergies." *Better Nutrition*, March 2000, 62(3): 36.

Rousseau, Rita. "Food Safety for the Few: Ordinary Foods Can Be Poison for People with Allergies." *Restaurants and Institutions*, February 1, 1997, 107(3): 78.

Winter, Greg. "F.D.A. Survey Finds Faulty Listings of Possible Food Allergens." *New York Times*, April 3, 2001: Section C, page 1, column 2.

Organizations to Contact

American-Asian Kashrus Services
37 Deans Way
Edgware, Middlesex, UK
HA8 9NH
No phone listing; e-mail: rmeyer@kashrus.org
http://www.kashrus.org/ (April 25, 2001)

Center for Food Safety and Applied Nutrition
Food and Drug Administration
5100 Point Branch Parkway
College Park, MD 20740-3835
Phone: 1-888-SAFEFOOD
http://vm.cfsan.fda.gov/list.html/ (April 30 2001)

The Food Allergy and Anaphylaxis Network
10400 Eaton Place, Suite 107
Fairfax, VA 22030-2208
Phone: 800-929-4040
http://foodallergy.org/ (April 26, 2001)

Food Allergy Initiative
625 Madison Avenue
New York, NY 10022
Phone: 212-527-5835
http://foodallergyinitiative.org/ (June 7, 2001)

KosherQuest
Kosher Information Bureau
12753 Chandler Boulevard
North Hollywood, CA 91607
Phone: 818-762-3197
http://kosherquest.org/ (July 20, 2001)

National Institute of Allergy and Infections Diseases
Office of Communications and Public Liaison
Building 31, Room 7A50
31 Center Drive, MSC 2520
Bethesda, MD 20892-2520
Phone: 301-496-5717
http://www.niaid.nih.gov/ (April 30, 2001)

North American Vegetarian Society
P.O. Box 72
Dolgeville, NY 13329
Phone: 518-568-7970
http://navs-online.org/ (June 4, 2001)

The Vegetarian Resource Group
P.O. Box 1463
Baltimore, MD 21203
Phone: 410-366-8343
http://www.vrg.org/ (May 10, 2001)

9

Large Doses of Vitamins

Whether large doses of vitamins are helpful or harmful is not entirely clear. Some doctors and nutritionists claim that we are able to obtain all the vitamins we require simply by eating a balanced diet. Others suggest varying levels of supplementation. The amount of supplementation seems to differ from one expert to another, and "the studies that have been carried out frequently contradict each other" (Boyce: 18–19). There are many who advise large or even megadoses of vitamins—"the health equivalent of buying a fancy alarm system and a pit bull to protect your property" (Han and Walker: 28).

Vitamin supplements are an enormously lucrative business. It has been estimated that about 100 million Americans annually spend about $6.5 billion on different forms of vitamin supplements (Brody: Page A1). Do these supplements make a difference? According to Rima D. Apple in *Vitamania: Vitamins in American Culture*, "Manufacturers spend millions of dollars promoting the benefits of their products; consumers spend billions of dollars buying hundreds of different vitamin pills. Vitamin capsules are 'magic pills.' We take vitamins if we are under stress or tired. Vitamins promise sexual potency; they cure colds. Many take vitamin pills 'just in case.' Athletes take vitamin pills to maximize their achievements. We tell our children to 'eat your vitamins.' We buy vitamin-enriched beauty soaps and skin lotions. Vitamins are sold as candy. . . . Clearly vitamins are essential nutrients; people fall seriously ill when vitamins are missing from their diets. But do well-fed, middle-class Americans need to take vitamins?" (Apple: 1).

Writing in the *Baltimore Sun*, Nancy Menefee Jackson is even more emphatic. She claims that taking large doses of vitamins is not the same "as throwing money down the drain." Rather, it is more like "flushing money down the toilet." It will simply be eliminated by the body (Jackson: Page 1M). In an article in the *Sunday Telegraph*, Alasdair Palmer maintains that consuming large doses of vitamins is based on the notion that if something is good for you in small amounts it is even better for you in larger quantities. While that belief may work well with money and love, it does not have a similar effect with food and drinks (Palmer: 37).

On the other hand, Michael Janson, a doctor who has been using dietary supplements in clinical practice since 1976, is a vocal advocate of vitamins. He states that without supplementation, people are unable to achieve their optimum levels of health. Instead, they suffer from such medical problems as frequent colds, poor sleep, obesity, and accelerated aging (Jansen: 21–22). Similarly, John M. Ellis, who has conducted research on vitamin B6 since the early 1960s, contends that much of the food that is sold is devoid of nutrients. As a result, millions of Americans fail to consume even the minimum amount of vitamin B6 (Ellis and Pamplin: 2, 10).

According to Abram Hoffer, much of our food is devoid of nutritional value. Processed foods provide empty calories and inadequate amounts of vitamins and minerals. He cites soft drinks, white-flour bread, and white sugar as examples of foods that promote malnutrition (Hoffer and Walker: 16–17).

Some statistics seem to indicate otherwise. In 1997, a newspaper article in the *Times-Picayune* reported on a 13-year study of 10,758 Americans. It noted that "vitamin takers do not live longer or suffer fewer cancer deaths than those who do not take vitamins" (Brody: Page A1).

While the importance of certain nutrients in the diet now receives enormous media attention, it is not a new concept. "In 1747, Scottish surgeon James Lind discovered that feeding oranges and lemons to sailors not only cured those with scurvy, it prevented sailors without scurvy from getting sick." More than half a century passed before the British Navy realized the significance of the finding and decided to "add lemon juice to the men's diets" (Kirkey: Page B6, front). In 1906, Sir Frederick Hopkins, a British biochemist, found that foods had "accessory factors" or "compounds that appeared to act as catalysts and regulators for the transformation of food into cells and energy." In other words, Hopkins discovered how vitamins function. "Unlike the other essential constituents of food—proteins, carbohydrates and fats—they do not provide energy, or material that can be converted into tissue. Rather, vitamins help to speed up the reactions that ensure that food is converted into energy or tissue" (Thornton, Court, and Palmer: 21).

More of the general public soon concluded that certain dietary supplements could strongly impact physical and mental health. Supplements were not only for the seriously ill; they could resolve milder problems and even enable the healthy to retain their well-being.

ORTHOMOLECULAR MEDICINE

In the late 1960s, Linus Pauling, a chemist and Nobel laureate, "coined the word 'Orthomolecular' to denote the use of naturally occurring substances, particularly nutrients, in maintaining health and treating disease" (International Society for Orthomolecular Medicine Web site). The field of orthomolecular medicine was born. The goal was to use the proper molecules to restore or sustain health. *Ortho* is Greek for "right." The goal of orthomolecular medicine is to pick the "right molecule" (Barrett and Herbert: 331). Rather than focusing on the control of symptoms, emphasis is placed on resolving the biochemical causes of illness and preventing disease. "The object of orthomolecular medicine is to achieve a balanced metabolism by having the appropriate nutrient or biochemical molecule in the appropriate location at the appropriate time" (Haas: 87). Orthomlecular treatments may "include dietary manipulation, nutrition supplementation, herbal remedies, homeopathic treatments, detoxification . . . [as well as] safe forms of megavitamin therapy" (International Society for Orthomolecular Medicine Web site). Orthomolecular medicine practitioners commonly prescribe very large doses of vitamins. Pauling is believed to have "stirred 18 grams [of vitamin C] into his daily orange juice," and "he lived to the ripe old age of 93" (Boyce: 18–19). It should be noted that there are different definitions for supplement megadoses. "Some people use the word to define large doses or doses that exceed recommendations. In scientific terms, it has been defined as a dose that is 10 times the RDA [Recommended Dietary Allowance] or more" (Hay: 93).

According to the International Society for Orthomolecular Medicine, the following are the cardinal rules of the field:

1. Nutrition comes first in medical diagnosis and treatment.
2. Drug treatment is used only for specific indications and always with an eye to the potential dangers and adverse effects.
3. Environmental pollution and food adulteration are an inescapable fact of modern life and are a medical priority.
4. Biochemical individuality is the norm in medical practice; therefore stereotyped RDA values are unreliable nutrient guides.
5. Blood tests do not necessarily reflect tissue levels of nutrients.
6. Nutrient diagnosis is always defensible because nutrient-related disorders are usually treatment responsive or curable.
7. Hope is an indispensable ally of the physicians and an absolute right of the patient. (International Society for Orthomolecular Medicine Web site)

The International Society for Orthomolecular Medicine Web site includes a number of case studies that it claims demonstrate the effectiveness of this type of intervention, including a 45-year-old executive with depression, a 14-year-old boy who suffered from panic attacks, and a 4-year-old boy with mood swings. In each case, an orthomolecular program tailored to the person's specific circumstances allegedly led to significant improvements (International Society for Molecular Medicine Web site).

Orthomolecular medicine is probably best known for addressing a number of serious psychiatric problems such as schizophrenia. "It is a disease that causes enormous pain to individuals and families, carries a terrible stigma and can be associated with violent behavior" (Steed: Page F1). Moreover, "schizophrenia is an important factor in social aid and welfare costs, health care costs, employment inefficiency, impaired learning ability, alcoholism, broken homes and suicide. The average person with schizophrenia will cost one to two million dollars to society, directly and indirectly, in his/her lifetime" (International Society for Molecular Medicine Web site).

Years ago, Pauling wrote, "The functioning of the brain is dependent on its composition and structure; that is, on the molecular environment of the mind. . . . The proper functioning of the mind is known to require the presence in the brain of molecules of many different substances. . . . There is evidence that mental function and behavior are also affected by changes in the concentration in the brain of any of a number of other substances that are normally present" (International Society for Orthomolecular Medicine Web site).

The International Society for Orthomolecular Medicine maintains that about 35% of people with untreated schizophrenia recover on their own, but many seek professional help. A large number of these people could benefit from orthomolecular treatment. "Orthomoldcular treatment is reported to be effective in 80 percent or more of the cases and is the best treatment developed so far. This treatment usually includes a special diet, vitamins and minerals in accordance with the individual needs of the patient, and other therapeutic aids such as tranquilizers, supportive psychotherapy, and other treatments which the doctor thinks will be useful. Many persons with schizophrenia have low blood sugar (hypoglycemia) and allergies which are treated" (International Society for Orthomolecular Medicine Web site).

In *The Way Up from Down*, Priscilla Slagle, a psychiatrist who specializes in low moods and depression, wrote that an inadequate amount of certain essential nutrients may "cause an aberration in brain function" (Slagle: 112). The following substances are most related to mood control:

- The amino acids tyrosine or phenylalanine and tryptophan
- The B vitamins, in particular, B6, folic acid, and biotin

- Vitamin C
- The minerals (or enzymes) magnesium, zinc, iron, copper, and manganese
- Pancreatic enzymes (Slagle: 113)

There are also other mood-affecting factors, such as consuming too much refined sugar. In her book, Slagle recalled a patient with a host of psychiatric issues, including "chronic anxiety interspersed with panic attacks, confusion, restlessness, difficulty concentrating, memory lapses, suicidal thoughts, dizziness, palpitations and tightness in her chest, muscle weakness, pain and cramps, and chronic fatigue." Slagle found her diet mainly consisted of such foods as chocolate chip cookies, American cheese, hamburgers, soda, French fries, donuts, and hot dogs and buns. She had been eating this way for a long time. Her diet lacked protein, vegetables and fruits and consistently contained only one of the five basic food groups—grains. After years of such poor eating, it would take at least six months to a year for this woman to improve.

In *Total Nutrition*, Victor Herbert and Genell J. Subak-Sharpe report that in 1973, the American Psychiatric Association formed a task force to study orthomolecular therapy. "This group found no evidence to support the practice of it, and characterized the underlying therapy as superficial, inconsistent, and contradictory." Orthomolecular therapists attacked the task force's report, and orthomolecular therapy continued. Herbert and Subak-Sharpe state that studies have failed to determine that psychiatric patients do better with orthomolecular treatment (Herbert and Subak-Sharpe: 645).

There are few controlled orthomolecular medicine studies in which some patients are treated with conventional medicine and orthomolecular medicine and other patients are treated only with conventional medicine. This is primarily because orthomolecular physicians believe that "it is the duty of the physician to give every one of his patients the treatment that is his best judgment will be of the greatest value" (International Society for Orthomolecular Medicine Web site). They consider it unethical to withhold care that may be useful.

The International Society for Orthomolecular Medicine Web site contains summaries of a number of studies that it claims show orthomolecular treatments to be medically beneficial. In a review of 1,312 patients, selenium was found to reduce the risk of "total and lung cancer mortality, total cancer incidence, colorectal cancer and prostate cancer incidence." Another investigation divided 129 young healthy adults into two groups. For one year, one group took 10 times the recommended daily dose of nine vitamins; during the same time, the members of the other group took placebos. "Males taking the vitamins differed from those taking the placebo in that they reported themselves as feeling more 'agreeable' after 12 months. After 12 months the mood of the females taking the vitamin supplement was significantly improved in that they felt more 'agreeable,' more composed and reported better mental health" (International Society for Orthomolecular Medicine Web site).

A study of 177 elderly people found that those with folate deficiency were more likely to have a deteriorated functional and mental capacity than those with adequate folate levels. When 49 people who suffered from recurrent migraines were given 400 mg of riboflavin each day, their "mean number of migraine attacks fell by 67% and mean migraine severity improved by 68%." Over a period of four weeks, 58 patients received kava extract, a relaxant, or a placebo. There was "a significant reduction [in anxiety] in the group receiving kava extract" (International Society for Orthomolecular Medicine Web site).

SAFETY OF LARGE DOSES OF VITAMINS

The International Society for Orthomolecular Medicine states that taking large doses of vitamins is quite safe. "A small percentage of people experience some discomfort when taking vitamins, but the doctor can prescribe other forms of these vitamins or adjust the dose" (International Society for Orthomolecular Medicine Web site). Others disagree. An article published in 2000 in *Family Health* notes, "It is mistaken to think that if one dose of a supplement is good for you, two will be better, and five will be terrific. Unfortunately taking extra large doses of any product can have side effects. Some of these such as stomach upsets or allergic reactions can be very serious. Some can even be deadly" (Chornell: 11–14).

Some vitamins have been found to be potentially problematic in high doses. While vitamin B6, which is in foods such as cereals, potatoes, milk, meat, and beer, is believed to be useful for carpal tunnel syndrome, in larger amounts—more than 200 milligrams a day—it may cause nerve damage (Haukebo: Page 01C). This may lead to "numbness, clumsiness and tingling" (Laurance: 3). There are even reports of deaths (Philipps: 47). "People who are undergoing levodopa therapy for Parkinson's disease should avoid vitamin B6 supplements altogether. It has been found to reduce the drug's effectiveness" (Feinstein: 39).

Larger amounts of vitamin A seem to be risky for pregnant women. Boston University School of Medicine researchers interviewed 22,000 pregnant women. "Research showed that women who were taking large amounts of vitamin A were more likely to give birth to babies with serious birth defects, such as cleft palate and heart abnormalities" (Mermilliod: Page 24H2). Some women were taking 10,000 international units (IUs), which is twice the U.S. Recommended Daily Allowance. And, in

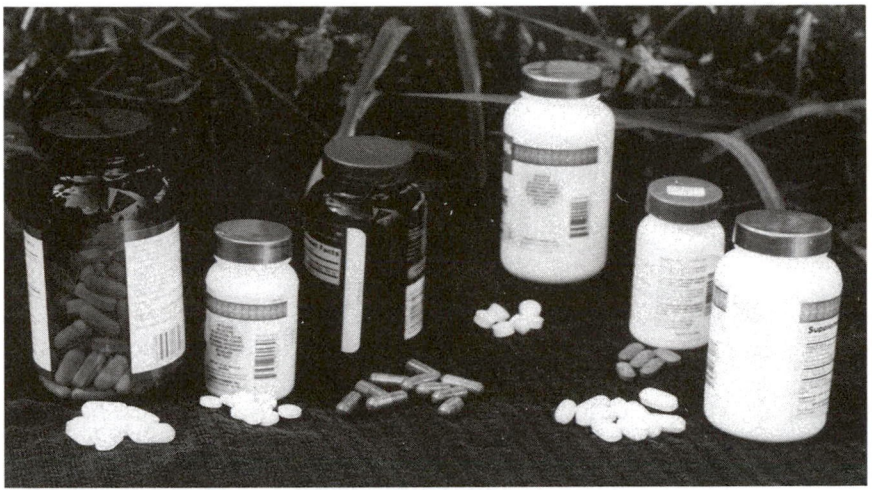

Large doses of vitamins are not necessarily healthful. Photo by Mark A. Goldstein.

Vitamin A, Thomas Moore, who was the Deputy Director of the Dunn Nutritional Laboratory in Cambridge, England in the 1950s, commented that Arctic explorers reported side effects from consuming large amounts of polar-bear liver, which is very high in vitamin A. These include "distress, nausea and peeling of the skin" (Moore: 445).

Large quantities of other vitamins and minerals have also been linked to medical concerns. Excessive amounts of potassium may be dangerous, particularly to those who have kidney problems. Too much vitamin K may affect clotting. "Women who are on the pill and taking megadoses of K could be at risk for blood clots" (Jackson: Page 1M). While extra vitamin D may be required by some, it is toxic for others. "Shut-ins and people with some types of intestinal or kidney disease need large doses of vitamin D because they're deficient in the nutrient, and their bodies can handle megadoses. In people who aren't deficient, the same large doses can cause serious, even deadly, side effects" (Cahill: Page Z15).

In an article published in the spring of 2000 in the *Proceedings of the National Academy of Sciences*, researchers at the University of Chicago reported a link between a mother's intake of high amounts of bioflavonoids, chemical compounds from plants, and the incidence of leukemia in infants and young children. Apparently, 10 out of the 20 bioflavonoids that were tested triggered breaks in the myeloid-lymphoid leukemia (MLL) area of the gene. That section of the gene is key to the development of the majority of infant leukemias (Strick et al.: 4790–4795).

A 1997 article by Jane E. Brody listed even more possible reasons to worry. "High doses of vitamin E can interfere with the action of vitamin

K, which promotes clotting. Large amounts of calcium can limit the absorption of iron and perhaps other trace elements. Zinc can reduce the level of copper in the body, impair immune responses and decrease the level of protective high-density lipoproteins in the blood, often called the 'good' cholesterol. Folic acid can react badly with anticonvulsant medications and mask signs of a B12 deficiency. Iron supplements can be deadly to small children. In fact, the most common cause of poisoning deaths among children is not caustic cleaning agents or aspirin, but iron supplements intended for adult use" (Brody: Page A1).

VITAMIN C

While almost any discussion of large doses of vitamins seems to generate heated rhetoric, perhaps the most controversy has centered around vitamin C (ascorbic acid). The clear catalyst for much of this debate was Pauling. "In 1970, Pauling announced in *Vitamin C and the Common Cold* that taking 1,000 mg of vitamin C daily will reduce the incidence of colds by 45 percent for most people but that some people need much larger amounts. . . . The 1976 revision of the book, retitled *Vitamin C, the Common Cold and Flu*, suggested even higher doses. A third book, *Vitamin C and Cancer* (1976) claims that higher doses of vitamin C may be effective against cancer" (Barrett and Herbert: 331).

Over the years, there have been many other proponents of vitamin C. In *Vitamin C*, Jennifer Hay notes that "in addition to vitamin C's known bodily functions—helping us to produce collagen, metabolize amino acids, cholesterol and nutrients, and maintain a healthy immune system—it has also been credited with" other positive roles. These include the following:

- Protecting against heart disease and stroke
- Improving immune response (including the response to viruses that cause colds)
- Protecting against cancer
- Protecting the lungs
- Protecting against cataracts
- Protecting the skin
- Speeding wound healing
- Decreasing diabetic complications
- Slowing the progression of osteoarthritis
- Improving fertility (Hay: 23)

Is vitamin C really that useful? Hay notes that although "many of the claims made for vitamin C have some substance," even well-designed research studies on the same subject have generated conflicting results. "Until a consensus emerges, vitamin C's various health benefits remain a matter of speculation" (Hay: 24).

In 1999, P. Samuel Campbell, a professor of biological sciences at the University of Alabama in Huntsville, reported at a meeting of the American Chemical Society that large doses of vitamin C boost the immune system. It appears that vitamin C lowers the "production of glucocorticoids—hormones released by the adrenal gland, including cortisol and cortisone—during times of stress." These hormones interfere with the body's ability to "fight off disease and infection." As a result, Campbell suggested that megadoses of vitamin C "may be especially important in protecting against the weakened immune system associated with chronic diseases such as AIDS, cancer, and diabetes, or for person who are under chronic or long-term stress" ("Cancer Tumors," 1999).

Meanwhile, other researchers have studied the effect of vitamin C on lead levels in the body. An investigation published in the *American Journal of Epidemiology* noted that Harvard researchers found that older men who consumed at least 339 mg of vitamin C each day had lower levels of lead in their blood than men who consumed less than 109 mg of vitamin C each day (Cheng et al.: 1162–1174). Similar results were obtained by researchers at the University of California at San Francisco. They concluded that "high serum levels of ascorbic acid are independently associated with a decreased prevalence of elevated blood lead levels." They further added that "if these associations are related casually, ascorbic acid intake may have public health implications for control of lead toxicity" (Simon and Hudes, June 1999: 2289–2293). In a separate analysis, these same researchers observed a relationship between vitamin C and cataracts. They determined that "ascorbic acid, a water-soluble antioxidant found in high concentrations in the lens, may be of importance for the prevention of cataract among older Americans" (Simon and Hudes, December 1999: 1207–1211).

Physicians in the Department of Traumatology at Kyorin University in Tokyo, Japan, have found that their patients with severe burns benefit from high doses of vitamin C. In the summary of their report, which appeared in the *Archives of Surgery*, the researchers noted that "adjuvant administration of high-dose ascorbic acid during the first 24 hours after thermal injury significantly reduces resuscitation fluid volume requirements, body weight gain, and wound edema. A reduction in the severity of respiratory dysfunction was also apparent in these patients" (Tanaka et al.: 326–331).

A 1999 article in the *Lancet* described a one-month study of people with mild to moderate hypertension (high blood pressure). Daily doses of 500 mg of vitamin C were found to lower blood pressure (Duffy et al.: 2048). During the same year, an article in *Circulation* found that daily consumption of 500 mg of vitamin C improved the dilation of blood vessels in people with coronary artery disease (Gokce et al.: 3234–3240).

With regard to cancer, the Linus Pauling Institute, which investigates the relationship between micronutrients, vitamins, and phytochemicals, states that it is wildly agreed that a greater consumption of fruits and vegetables reduces the risk of cancer. "In general, prospective studies in which the lowest group consumed more than 86 mg of vitamin C daily have not found differences in cancer risk, while studies finding significant cancer risk reductions found them in people consuming at least 80 to 110 mg of vitamin C daily."

The Linus Pauling Institute Web site acknowledges that Pauling and his associates believed that very large doses of vitamin C (10 grams daily or more) increased the length and quality of life of patients who were terminally ill with cancer. Nevertheless, two further studies by other researchers saw no difference between vitamin C and the placebo.

Then there is the age-old problem of the common cold. The Linus Pauling Institute Web site contends that vitamin C does not significantly affect the incidence of the common cold. "However, a few studies have indicated that certain susceptible groups (e.g. individuals with low dietary intake and marathoners) may be less susceptible to the common cold when taking supplemental vitamin C. Additionally, large doses of vitamin C have been found to decrease the duration and severity of colds, an effect which may be related to the antihistamine effects found to occur with large doses (2 grams) of vitamin C" (The Linus Pauling Institute Web site).

Several years ago, Finnish researchers reviewed three placebo-controlled studies that examined the role that vitamin C played for people under extreme physical stress. "In one study the subjects were schoolchildren at a skiing camp in the Swiss Alps, in another they were military troops training in Northern Canada, and in the third they were participants in a 90 km running race. In each of the three studies a considerable reduction in common cold incidence in the group supplemented with vitamin C . . . was found" (Hemila: 379–383).

In *The Vitamin Pushers*, Barrett and Herbert maintain that much of what has been written about vitamin C exaggerates its benefits. For example, "the largest clinical trials, involving thousands of volunteers, were directed by Dr. Terence Anderson, professor of epidemiology at the University of Toronto. Taken together, his studies suggest that extra vitamin C may slightly reduce the severity of colds, but it is not necessary to take the high doses suggested by Pauling to achieve this result." They also say that at least some of the research on vitamin C is seriously flawed. One such study, which compared people who took vitamin C to those who took a placebo, was conducted at the National Institutes of Health and reported in 1975. "Although the experiment was supposed to be double-blind, half of the subjects were able to guess which pill they were getting. When the results were tabulated with all subjects lumped together, the vitamin group reported fewer colds per person over a nine-month period. But among the half who hadn't guessed which pill they had been taking, no difference in the incidence of severity was found. This illustrates how people who think they are doing something effective (such as taking a vitamin) can report a favorable result even when none exists" (Barrett and Herbert: 331–332).

There is also a cautionary note for people who use the over-the-counter medication acetaminophen (commonly sold as Tylenol). In a small study, five people took 3,000 mg of vitamins 1½ hours after taking 1,000 mg of acetaminophen. Apparently, the high dose of vitamin C increased the level of acetaminophen in the blood, a condition that may be harmful to the liver (Harkness: Page E7). Further, "diarrhea can occur in people who take one gram of vitamin C a day or more," and "in lower doses . . . it can cause nausea, vomiting, abdominal cramps and fatigue" (Kirkey: Page B6, front).

Only a few studies have found large doses of vitamin C to be truly harmful. One of these, published in *Nature* in 1998, entitled "Vitamin C Exhibits Pro-Oxidant Properties," concluded that daily doses of 500 mg of vitamin C had both healthful antioxidant and damaging pro-oxidant properties. Following a great deal of controversy, many researchers concluded that the study was "hopelessly flawed" ("Can Vitamin C": 1–2). A study presented to the March 2000 meeting of the American Heart Association reported that daily doses of 500 mg of vitamin C increased the rate at which the carotid arteries thickened (Thornton, Court, and Palmer: 21). Responding to this study, Balz Frei, a professor of biochemistry and biophysics at Oregon State University and director of the Linus Pauling Institute, said that "the results from that study . . . are in direct conflict with a study published in 1995 in the American Heart Association journal *Circulation*. That research found a significant reduction in carotid artery wall thickness in people over 55 who consumed about 1,000 milligrams or more of vitamin C a day, compared to those consuming less than 88 milligrams per day." Frei added that the study presented at the meeting had not undergone peer review or been published. "The known health benefits of vitamin C far outweigh these alleged, unconfirmed risks. I believe that people taking vitamin C supplements should continue to do so. Vitamin C supplements have been shown to normalize vasodilation and lower blood pressure, two major cardiovascular risk factors" (The Linus Pauling Institute Web site).

In 1999, an alarm was also sounded by researchers at the Memorial Sloan-Kettering Cancer Center in New York City. They found "that cancer tumors consume large amounts of vitamin C" ("Cancer Tumors," 1999). As a result, they worried that vitamin C supplementation "could derail the beneficial effects of chemotherapy or even radiation" (Gottlieb: 2073–2075). In short, they questioned whether vitamin C could protect the cancer cells from chemotherapy and radiation, making them resistant to treatment.

At the same time, however, researchers at the University of Colorado Health Sciences Center said that high doses of vitamin C and other antioxidants "may not only protect normal cells during cancer treatment, but may actually help fight tumors" (Gottlieb: 2073–2075). Similar sentiments were expressed by the Linus Pauling Institute: "There is no clinical evidence that supplemental antioxidant vitamins, including vitamin C, harm cancer patients." Rather, "much of the recent cell culture and clinical research suggests that a *combination* of antioxidant vitamins and minerals as an adjunct to conventional therapy may have benefit" (The Linus Pauling Institute Web site).

In the midst of all this confusion and after nearly 60 years of adhering to the same RDAs, in the spring of 2000, the Food and Nutrition Board of the National Academy of Science's Institute of Medicine changed a few of its recommendations. Moreover, in addition to RDAs, the board noted amounts of acceptable upper intake levels (ULs). In the past, the Institute of Medicine had recommended daily vitamin C doses of 60 mg for men and women. That was increased to 75 mg for women and 90 mg for men. Those who smoke should add an extra 35 mg. The daily UL for vitamin C is 2,000 mg. RDAs and ULs for vitamin E and selenium were also noted: for vitamin E, an RDA of 15 mg/day and a UL of 1,000 mg/day ("This is equivalent to 22 IUs from natural-source vitamin E or 33 IUs of the synthetic form" [Wansbrough: 30–31]); for selenium, an RDA of 55 mcg (micrograms)/day and a UL of 400 mcg/day (Wansbrough: 30–31).

Dietary supplements were deemed unnecessary; vitamins should be obtained through food. Anything above UL amounts could place people at risk for health problems (Thornton, Court, and Palmer: 21). For example, higher amounts of vitamin C "can cause diarrhea and amounts above the RDA are likely to be excreted by the body unused." Similarly, a high amount of vitamin E "heightens the risk of bleeding," and high levels of selenium may cause selenosis, with hair and nail brittleness (Wansbrough: 30–31).

CONCLUSION

At this point, the consumer may well feel perplexed. Rima D. Apple writes in *Vitamania: Vitamins in American Culture* that science is unlikely to provide unambiguous answers to the vitamin controversy. Researchers, health-care professionals, advertisers, manufacturers, and government officials all use science for their own ends. Consumers must be aware of their motives as they try to make informed decisions (Apple: 196–197).

Although the use of large doses of vitamins is still very controversial, there are a few guidelines that teens and young adults may wish to follow. If generally healthy teens and young adults decide to include vitamin supplementation in their diets, they should consume only moderate amounts. Teens and young adults who would like to take larger amounts of vitamins for a medical problem should always discuss their wishes with a medical provider. As has been noted, in some instances, larger amounts of vitamins have the potential to harm.

TOPICS FOR DISCUSSION

1. Do you take vitamins? Why or why not?
2. Have you ever taken a large dose of a vitamin? Did you notice any positive or negative effects?
3. Do you agree that much of our food lacks nutritional value? Why or why not?
4. Do you believe that you eat a well-balanced diet? Are there ways you could improve your diet?
5. How do you interpret the varying opinions on the topic discussed in this chapter? How do you determine whom to believe?

REFERENCES AND RESOUCES

Books

Apple, Rima D. *Vitamania: Vitamins in American Culture.* New Brunswick, New Jersey: Rutgers University Press, 1996.

Barrett, Stephen, and Victor Herbert. *The Vitamin Pushers.* Amherst, New York: Prometheus Books, 1994.

Ellis, John M., and Jean Pamplin. *Vitamin B6 Therapy.* Garden City Park, New York: Avery Publishing, 1999.

Feinstein, Alice, managing editor. *Healing with Vitamins.* Emmaus, Pennsylvania: Rodale Press, 1996.

Haas, Elson M. *Staying Healthy with Nutrition.* Berkeley, California: Celestial Arts, 1992.

Hay, Jennifer. *Vitamin C.* Allentown, Pennsylvania: People's Medical Society, 1998.

Herbert, Victor, and Genell J. Subak-Sharpe, editors. *Total Nutrition.* New York: St. Martin's Griffin, 1995.

Hoffer, Abram, and Morton Walker. *Orthomolecular Nutrition*. New Canaan, Connecticut: Keats Publishing, 1978.

Janson, Michael. *The Vitamin Revolution in Health Care*. Greenville, New Hampshire: Arcadia Press, 1996.

Moore, Thomas. *Vitamin A*. Amsterdam: Elsevier Publishing Company, 1957.

Moyad, Mark A. *The ABC's of Nutrition and Supplements for Prostate Cancer*. Chelsea, Michigan: Sleeping Bear Press, 2000.

Slagle, Priscilla. *The Way Up from Down*. New York: St. Martin's Paperbacks, 1992.

Magazines, Journals, and Newspapers

Boyce, Nell. "Unknown Quantity: Megadoses of Vitamins Can Seriously Damage Your Health, But Nobody Knows How High You Can Safely Go." *New Scientist*, February 27, 1999: 18–19.

Brody, Jane E. "Vitamin Users Taking Gamble on Their Health." *Times-Picayune*, October 26, 1997: Page A1.

Cahill, Susan. "Getting By without Sun? Housebound Seniors May Need More Vitamin D." *Washington Post*, July 23, 1996: Page Z15.

"Cancer Tumors Consume Large Amounts of Vitamin C." *Cancer Weekly Plus*, September 27, 1999.

"Can Vitamin C Cause Harm in Large Doses?" *Tufts University Health and Nutrition Letter*, June 1998, 16(4): 1–2.

Cheng, Y., W.C. Willett, J. Schwartz, D. Sparrow, S. Weiss, and H. Hu. "Relation of Nutrition to Bone Lead and Blood Lead Levels in Middle-Aged to Elderly Men." *American Journal of Epidemiology*, June 15, 1998, 147(12): 1162–1174.

Chornell, J. Gary. "Healthy Eyes: The Key Is Good Food, Not Expensive 'Natural' Supplements." *Family Health*, March 2000, 16 (1): 11–14.

Duffy, Stephen J., Noyan Gokce, Monika Holbrook, Annong Huang, Balz Frei, John F. Keaney, Jr., and Joseph A. Vita. "Treatment of Hypertension with Ascorbic Acid." *Lancet*, December 11, 1999, 354(9195): 2048.

Gokce, N., J.F. Keaney, Jr., B. Frei, M. Holbrook, M. Olesiak, B.J. Zachariah, C. Leeuwenburgh, J.W. Heinecke, and J.A. Vita. "Long-term Ascorbic Acid Administration Reverses Endothelial Vasomotor Dysfunction in Patients with Coronary Artery Disease." *Circulation*, June 29, 1999, 99(25): 3234–3240.

Gottlieb, Nicole. "Cancer Treatment and Vitamin C: The Debate Lingers." *Journal of the National Cancer Institute*, December 15, 1999, 91(24): 2073–2075.

Han, Sallie, and Whitney Walker. "Swallowing a Dubious Claim: Vitamin-Loading Is Popular, But Evidence Is Slim." *New York Daily News*, October 13, 1997: Page 28.

Harkness, Richard. "Tylenol, Vitamin C May Not Be Safe Mix." *Times-Picayune*, September 19, 1999: Page E7.

Haukebo, Kirsten. "Take Your Vitamins?" *Courier-Journal*, September 21, 1998: Page 01C.

Hemila, H. "Vitamin C and Common Cold Incidence: A Review of Studies with

Subjects under Heavy Physical Stress." *International Journal of Sports Medicine*, July 1996, 17(5): 379–383.

Jackson, Nancy Menefee. "Megagood or Megawaste? Vitamins: Taking Huge Doses of Supplements, Experts Warn, May Be a Waste of Money—or Worse." *Baltimore Sun*, May 9, 1999: Page 1M.

Kirkey, Sharon. "C Is for Confusion: Is Vitamin C the Cure-all Some Claim, or Is It a Silent Killer?" *Ottawa Citizen*, March 28, 2000: Page, B6, front.

"Large Doses of Vitamin C Endorsed by Researcher." *Immunotherapy Weekly*, September 6, 1999.

Laurance, Jeremy. "Nerve Damage Warning over Vitamin Pills." *London Independent*, July 5, 1997: Page 3.

Maynard, Cindy. "Vitamins: How Much Is Enough?" *Current Health 2*, January 1999, 25(5): 16.

Mermilliod, Iris. "Birth Defects Linked to Large Doses of A." *Times-Picayune*, June 23, 1996: Page 24H2.

Palmer, Alasdair. "Vitamins We Can Do Without." *Sunday Telegraph*, July 26, 1998: Page 37.

Philipps, Rachel. "Science: Put a Lid On It; You Can Have Too Much of a Good Thing, Even Vitamins." *London Independent*, January 31, 1999: Page 47.

Podmore, Ian D., Helen R. Griffiths, Karl E. Herbert, Nalini Mistry, Pratibha Mistry, and Joseph Lunec. "Vitamin C Exhibits Pro-Oxidant Properties." *Nature*, April 9, 1998, 392(6676): 559.

Reynolds, Tom. "Antioxidants and Cancer: What Is the Evidence?" *Journal of the National Cancer Institute*, July 5, 2000, 92(13): 1033–1034.

Simon, J.A., and E.S. Hudes. "Relationship of Ascorbic Acid to Blood Lead Levels." *JAMA: The Journal of the American Medical Association*, June 23–30, 1999, 281(24): 2289–2293.

Simon, J.A., and E.S. Hudes. "Serum Ascorbic Acid and Other Correlates of Self-Reported Cataract among Older Americans." *Journal of Clinical Epidemiology*, December 1999, 52(12): 1207–1211.

Steed, Judy. " 'Scientific Battle' Way of Life for MD." *Toronto Star*, June 26, 1998: Page F1.

Strick, Reiner, Pamela L. Strissel, Susanne Borgers, Steve L. Smith, and Janet D. Rowley. "Dietary Bioflavonoids Induce Cleavage in the MLL gene and May Contribute to Infant Leukemia." *Proceedings of the National Academy of Sciences*, April 25, 2000, 97(9): 4790–4795.

Tanaka, H., T. Matsuda, Y. Miyagantani, T. Yukioka, H. Matsuda, and S. Shimazaki. "Reduction of Resuscitation Fluid Volumes in Several Burned Patients Using Ascorbic Acid Administration: A Randomised, Prospective Study." *Archives of Surgery*, March 2000, 135(3): 326–331.

Thornton, Jacqui, Mark Court, and Alasdair Palmer. "Vitamins Are Good for You . . . Aren't They?" *London Sunday Telegraph*, April 16, 2000: Page 21.

Wansbrough, Gillian. "How Much Is Too Much? A Joint Study between Canada and the U.S. Has Taken a New Look at the Intake of Antioxidants, This Time with Upper Limits, to Prevent Overdoses." *Medical Post*, May 16, 2000, 36(19): 30–31.

Organizations to Contact

Council for Responsible Nutrition
1875 Eye Street NW, Suite 400
Washington, DC 20006-5194
Phone: 202-872-1488
http://www.crnusa.org/ (August 17, 2000)

International Society for Orthomolecular Medicine
16 Florence Avenue
Toronto, Ontario, Canada M2N 1E9
Phone: 416-733-2117
http://www.orthomed.org/ (July 29, 2000)

The Linus Pauling Institute
Oregon State University
571 Weniger Hall
Corvallis, OR 97331-6512
Phone: 541-737-5075
http://www.orst.edu/dept/lpi/ (August 13, 2000)

United Nations University Headquarters
53-70, Jingumae, 5-chome
Shibuya-ku, Tokyo 150-8925, Japan
Phone: +81-3/3499-2811
http://www.unu.edu/ (July 28, 2000)

The Vitamin C Foundation
P.O. Box 73172
Houston, TX 77273
Phone: 1-888-443-3634, 1-281-443-3634
http://www.vitamincfoundation.org/ (August 26, 2000)

10

Fast Foods

With our busy lives, it is very tempting and convenient to eat fast food on a regular basis. Fast food is literally everywhere. In an interview published in 1998, Kelly Brownell, a national expert on weight control, commented that "fast food is infiltrating our culture. There are fast food restaurants inside some schools. Malls have food courts. Fast foods are showing up on airline flights and in airports" (Brownell and Liebman: 3–5). A January 2000 article in *Body Bulletin*, noted that every day about 25% of Americans eat in a fast-food restaurant ("About 25%": 2). But fast food tends to be high in calories and salt. An article from the *Nutrition Action Healthletter* said, "It's tough to walk out of a fast food restaurant without blowing at least half a day's artery clogging fat. A large fries will do it. So will a Big Mac, a Whopper, a Burger King Chicken Sandwich, or nine Chicken McNuggets." The meals keep getting bigger. "Fast food chains are tripping over each other to build bigger burgers. Fries have swollen to 'super sizes' that have as many calories as a Big Mac" (Hurley and Liebman: 13–15).

It seems only natural for teens to gravitate toward fast food. Since fast food may be eaten on the go, it fits into their busy schedules. Also, teens work at fast-food establishments, and eating fast food with their peers is a way to socialize.

Fast food commonly has a number of problems that were outlined in *Fast Food Facts* by registered dietician Marion J. Franz. A typical meal may contain half of the body's daily caloric requirement as well as the entire daily sodium intake—no more than 2,400 milligrams, according to the American Heart Association. "For example, if you have a fried fish sandwich, a milk shake, and large French fries, you've eaten 1100 calories, 45 grams of fat, and 1170 milligrams of sodium. This is over half the calories and sodium most adults need in a day." Similarly, "a quarter-pound burger with cheese, large fries, and a shake contain about 1200 calories and 52 grams of fat. A 1200-calorie meal might be okay for an active teenage boy, but it provides about 50% of the daily calories needed to maintain the weight of a 165-pound man, and 70% of the calories needed by a 128-pound woman. In fact, for someone on a diet, 1200 calories is practically the whole day's allotment" (Franz: 2).

The source of much of these calories is fat. Typically, about 40% to 60% of the calories in fast foods are derived from fat. The three major sources of fat in fast food are mayonnaise, cheese, and anything fried. Even chicken and fish, which are naturally lower in fat, may become sources of high fat content when they are coated with batter and deep fried. Eliminating or reducing these foods can transform a fast-food meal into a far healthier alternative. Mustard, ketchup, salsa, or low-fat dressings are good alternatives to mayonnaise. Low-fat cheese is better than regular cheese, and baked, grilled, broiled, and steamed foods are preferable to those fried in fat.

Salt and sugar levels are also high. "Several fast-food sandwiches contain 1500 to 2000 milligrams of sodium (⅔ to ¾ teaspoon of salt), more than half the daily recommended maximum sodium intake [of 2,400 milligrams]. . . . The greatest sources of sugar are soft drinks and shakes. A typical small (10-ounce) shake contains about 9 to 11 teaspoons of sugar, as much as a 12-ounce can of regular soda pop" (Franz: 3).

In a lunch from Boston Market, consisting of a soup, salad, and sandwich, one cup of tomato bisque soup contains 280 calories, 200 calories from fat, 1,280 mg of sodium, and 12 g of carbohydrate sugars. Four ounces of Caesar side salad contain 200 calories, 159 calories from fat, 450 mg of sodium, and 2 g of carbohydrate sugars. One chicken sandwich with cheese and sauce contains 750 calories, 300 calories from fat, 1,860 mg of sodium, and 13 g of carbohydrate sugars (Boston Market Web site). Add up the separate figures. This meal has a total of 1,230 calories. Of these calories, 659, more than half come from fat. There are also 3,590 grams of sodium. On top of all that are 27 grams of carbohydrate sugars.

At Wendy's, in comparison, one breaded chicken sandwich contains 440 calories, 160 calories from fat, 840 mg of sodium, and 6 of sugars. Eight ounces of cola soft drink contain 90 calories, 0 calories from fat, 10 mg of sodium, and 24 g of sugars. A medium, Frosty Dairy Dessert (16 ounces) contains 440 calories, 100 calories from fat, 260 mg of sodium, and 56 g of sugars (Wendy's Web site). This is not a big meal, but it has 970 calories, with 260 of these from fat. There are 1,100 mgs of sodium and 86 grams of sugar. While the calories/fat ratio is better than the Boston Market meal, there are too many calories, too much sodium, and far too much sugar.

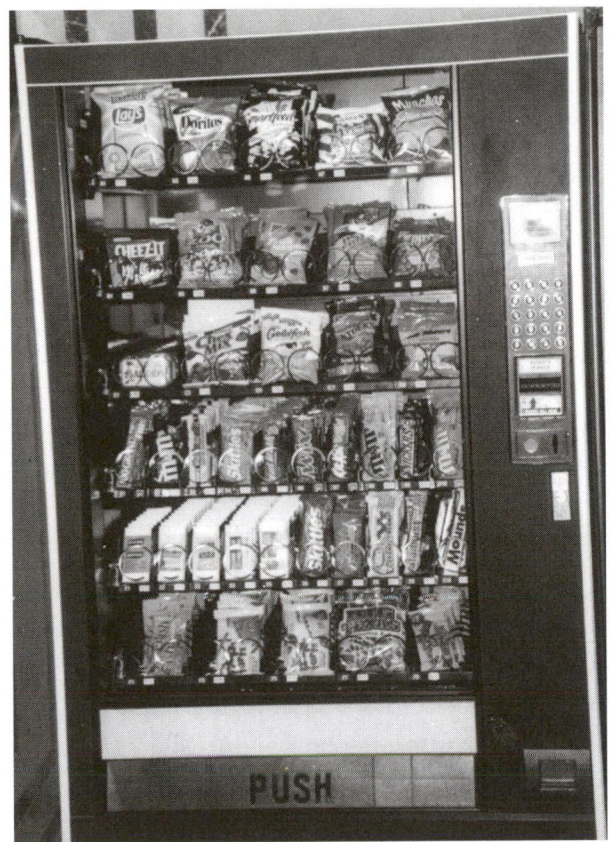

Fast food may have excessive calories, salt, sugar, and fats. Photo by Mark A. Goldstein.

Compare a pizza restaurant such as Domino's: Two slices of a Classic Hand Tossed Pizza (cheese only), 14-inch large, have 515.82 calories, 15.42 g of total fat, 6.72 g of saturated fat, 1080.21 mg of sodium, and 6.44 g of sugars. One breadstick has 116.14 calories, 4.05 g of total fat, 0.79 g of saturated fat, 152.19 mg of sodium, and 0.66 g of sugars. One barbecue Buffalo Wing has 50.08 calories, 2.43 g of total fat, 0.65 g of saturated fat, 175.3 mg and of sodium, and 1.26 g of sugars (Domino's Web site). While the values are a little better than those of some of the other foods, the amounts of fat and sodium remain on the high side.

One is able to eat healthier fast food. For example, a regular-sized grilled hamburger on a bun that may be purchased at many fast-food restaurants most likely has a more reasonable amount of fat and sodium if it is ordered without any mayonnaise or cheese. Wendy's is well known for having several healthier choices such as a wide variety of salads, baked potatoes, and low-fat sandwiches. Arby's highlights low-fat alternatives on a menu board ("Healthy in a Hurry": 1, 3–4).

The following are some additional suggestions for selecting healthier choices in fast-food restaurants:

- Plain baked potatoes, without sour cream, butter, and bacon bits, are wonderful offerings.
- Stay away from salads that appear to be filled with mayonnaise. Tuna salad is a common culprit. Croutons are generally high in fat and salt.
- Order a basic pizza. Added pepperoni, extra cheese, and sausage greatly increase the amount of fat.
- Try sushi, a low-fat Japanese food that is now sold in many restaurants and supermarkets.
- All too often, portions of food in fast-food restaurants are ridiculously large. Share a meal with a friend or save the extra food for another meal.
- Select steamed, baked, or roasted foods over those that are fried or deep fried.
- At salad bars, fill your plate with vegetables, peas, beans, pasta salads, and breads. Avoid the regular dressings. Use the lite ones.
- Low-fat yogurt is a tasty dessert.

In her book *Dining Lean*, Joanne A. Lichten shows how "deli sandwiches can be healthy or disastrous" (Lichten: 90). Here is a leaner choice:

	Calories	Fat (g)
3 oz. bagel	240	3
2 oz. turkey	60	1
Mustard, 1 T.	15	1
Baked potato chips, 12	110	1
Total	425	6

Here is Lichten's example of a "disaster" (90):

	Calories	Fat (g)
Tuna salad, ½ cup	380	20
Croissant, 3 oz.	360	20
Mayonnaise, 1 T.	100	11
Cheese, 1 oz.	100	8
Potato chips, 1 oz.	150	10
Total	1,090	69

In *Smart Fast Food Meals*, Peggy Reinhardt presents 48 lower-fat combo meals from 12 different fast-food chains. They all contain 700 calories or less and have no more than 30% of the calories from fat. For example, at Burger King, one broiler chicken sandwich and one small regular soft drink (16 ounces) contain 650 calories, 16.5 g of total fat, 4.5 g of saturated fat, 23% of calories from fat, and 750 mg of sodium. At KFC, one tender roast chicken breast, one order of mashed potatoes and gravy, one order of corn on the cob, and one small regular soft drink (16 ounces) contain 670 calories, 18.5 g of total fat, 4 g of saturated fat, 25% of calories from fat, and 1,305 mg of sodium. At Subway, one deli-style turkey breast sandwich with onions, lettuce, tomatoes, pickles, green peppers, and olives (no mayonnaise), one chocolate chip or chunk cookie, and one diet soft drink (16 ounces) contains 445 calories, 14 g of total fat, 5 g of saturated fat, 28% of calories from fat, and 1,125 mg sodium (Reinhardt: 29, 37, 91).

It is useful to note that the definition of "fast foods" can be extended to include some very basic healthy alternatives. Fruits, which are filled with fiber, contain a host of different vitamins and nutrients. Other healthy fast-food choices are low salt pretzels, pitas, raisins, and dried fruit. One can add more of these types of fast foods to the diet and reduce the alternatives that are filled with higher amounts of fat and salt.

CONCLUSION

With people leading such busy lives, it is very easy to save time on food preparation by eating a diet that includes lots of fast foods. Unfortunately, the majority of fast foods are high in calories and salt. But, there are fast food options that are lower in calories and salt. When you are making your fast food choices, try to select those.

TOPICS FOR DISCUSSION

1. What are the advantages and disadvantages of fast foods? How often is it reasonable to eat a meal at such a restaurant?
2. Do you have a fast-food restaurant in your school? Do you think that schools should have such restaurants? Why or why not? Should they have regulations?
3. What foods should these restaurants offer to balance diets?
4. Should fast-food restaurants be required to offer other healthier food choices? Why or why not?
5. Do you think that fast food contributes significantly to obesity in teens or in adults? Why or why not?

REFERENCE AND RESOURCES

Books

Brown, Amy C. *The Fast Food Freeway Guide*. San Diego, California: Mountain Top Productions, 1998.

Clark, Nancy. *Nancy Clark's Sports Nutrition Guidebook*. Champaign, Illinois: Human Kinetics, 1997.

Franz, Marion J. *Fast Food Facts*. Minneapolis: Chronimed Publishing, 1994.

Klein, Keith. *Weight Control for a Young America*. Wilsonville, Oregon: Book-Partners, 1999.

Lichten, Joanne V. *Dining Lean*. Houston, Texas: Nutrifit Publishing, 1998.

Mazel, Judy, and John E. Monaco. *Slim and Fit Kids*. Deerfield Beach, Florida: Health Communications, 1999.

Reinhardt, Peggy. *Smart Fast Food Meals*. New York: John Wiley and Sons, 1999.

Smith, J. Clinton. *Understanding Childhood Obesity*. Jackson: University Press of Mississippi, 1999.

Magazines, Journals, and Newspapers

"About 25% of Americans Eat in a Fast Food Restaurant Every Day." *Body Bulletin*, January 2000, 1(1): 2.

Brownell, Kelly, and Bonnie Liebman. "The Pressure to Eat: Why We're Getting Fatter." *Nutrition Action Healthletter*, July–August 1998, 25(6): 3–5.

Clark, Nancy. "Fast Food Best Bets." *Palaestra*, Fall 1998, 14(4): 51.

"Healthy in a Hurry." *Consumer Reports on Health*, October 1999, 11(10): 1, 3–4.

Hill, James O., and Frederick L. Trowbridge. "Childhood Obesity: Future Directions and Research Priorities." *Pediatrics*, March 1998, 101(3, part 2): 570–574.

Hodgkin, Georgia E. "Fantastic Fruits: Fast Food Alternatives for Health Meals at Home." *Vibrant Life*, May–June 1998, 14(3): 26–29.

Hurley, Jayne, and Leila Corcoran. "Meals to Go." *Nutrition Action Healthletter*, January 1998, 25(1): 12.

Hurley, Jayne, and Bonnie Liebman. "Fast Food Follow-Up: What's Left to Eat?" *Nutrition Action Healthletter*, November 1997, 24(9): 13–15.

Marquis, Julie. "Eating Habits Put Teens at Risk, Study Says." *Los Angeles Times*, September 26, 2000: Part A, part 1, page 1.

Maynard, Cindy. "Can You Live on Junk Food Alone?" *Current Health 2*, September 1997, 24(1): 18–20.

Maynard, Cindy. "How Does Your Diet Rate?" *Current Health 2*, March 1999, 25(7): 6.

Muha, Laura. "Too Fat?" *Parenting*, September 1998, 12(7): 128–133.

Platzman, Andrea D. "Eating Out Fast, But Healthfully: Is It Possible? EN Finds Out." *Environmental Nutrition*, July 1998, 21(7): 1–2.

"Quick Bites." *Consumer Reports*, March 2001, 66(3): 44–47.

Strauss, Richard S. "Childhood Obesity and Self-Esteem." *Pediatrics*, January 2000, 105(1): 15.

Styne, Dennis Michael. "Childhood Obesity: Time for Action, Not Complacency." *American Family Physician*, February 15, 1999, 59(4): 758, 761–762.

Organizations to Contact

Boston Market
14103 Denver West Parkway
P.O. Box 4086
Golden, CO 80401-4086
Phone: 800-365-7000
http://www.boston-market.com/ (December 6, 2000)

Center for Research on Human Nutrition and Chronic Disease Prevention
Wake Forest University Baptist Medical Center
Medical Center Boulevard
Winston-Salem, NC 27157
Phone: 336-716-2011
http://www.bgsm.edu/nutrition/ (December 3, 2000)

Center for Science in the Public Interest
1875 Connecticut Ave. NW, Suite 300
Washington, DC 20009
Phone: 202-332-9110
http://www.cspinet.org/ (December 15, 2000)

Domino's Pizza LLC
Attn: Customer Care Center
30 Frank Lloyd Wright Dr.
P.O. Box 997
Ann Arbor, MI 48106
Phone: 888-DOMINOS
http://www.dominos.com/ (December 3, 2000)

Food and Nutrition Information Center
USDA/ARS/National Agricultural Library, Room 304
10301 Baltimore Avenue
Beltsville, MD 20705-2351
Phone: 301-504-5719
http://www.nal.usda.gov/fnic/ (December 3, 2000)

McDonald's Nutrition Information Center
McDonald's Corporation
Oak Brook, IL 60523
Phone: 630-623-FOOD
http://mcdonalds.com/ (December 3, 2000)

Wendy's Customer Service
Wendy's International, Inc.
4288 W. Dublin-Granville Rd.
Dublin, OH 43017
Phone: 614-764-3100
http://www.wendys.com/index0.html/ (December 4, 2000)

11

Antioxidants

Antioxidants are in the news all the time. From the advertising, they appear to have a seemingly limitless number of benefits. But how much is media promotion and how much is reality?

The last time you left a half-eaten apple on the kitchen counter, it turned brown. The apple was literally attacked by free radicals—highly reactive oxygen molecules that are a by-product of normal metabolism.

Free radicals are not only out to decay apples. They destroy living cells. "Free radicals are vicious molecules missing an electron in their outer shell. Most are toxic forms of oxygen molecules. These unstable gangsters steal electrons from healthy cells, rendering them 'biologically rusted,' damaged, or destroyed" (Bushkin and Bushkin: 66–70). As a result, free radicals have been associated with a number of illnesses and medical problems. Most degenerative diseases, like arthritis, cataracts, or diabetes, are linked to free-radical damage. Free radicals also attack the brain and central nervous system and have been linked to heart disease and all types of cancer. They also weaken the immune system in various ways (Balch: 13).

Free radicals are able to harm a wide variety of tissues in the body. Most frequently, they hurt body fats, which are particularly at risk. They injure the nucleic acid bases that form DNA and prevent the DNA from correctly duplicating itself. "Damaged, or mutated, DNA leads to the replication of incorrect biological information—such as cancer cells." Free radicals may also impair proteins such as the collagen proteins in the skin. This causes the skin to toughen. "Damaged enzymes (which are proteins) will not work as efficiently to drive biochemical reactions. Nor will the repaired enzymes be able to repair as much free-radical damage, and a downward spiral causes a snowballing effect leading to faster aging and possibly cancer" (Passwater: 23, 24).

As dismal as this scenario may sound, the body is not helpless. It produces enzymes that neutralize free radicals. "In addition, the body uses antioxidant vitamins, minerals, and substances found in food and herbs to counteract the damaging effect" (Balch: 17).

Clearly, antioxidants are faced with a daunting task. "Antioxidants labor tirelessly to slow down and terminate this oxidation process. These kamikaze life-saver molecules continually seek and destroy free radicals, sacrificing themselves and self-destructing, to save other healthy cells from certain death" (Bushkin and Bushkin: 66–70).

The number of antioxidants keeps growing, but careful research studies have not been conducted on all of them. There is some disagreement about correct dosages. The Food and Drug Administration (FDA) considers antioxidants to be dietary supplements or nutrient additions to the diet. As such, they are not subject to presale analysis by the FDA. Nevertheless, it is useful to review current beliefs on some of the well-known antioxidants.

VITAMIN C

Perhaps the most acknowledged antioxidant is vitamin C (ascorbic acid). Although most animals synthesize their own vitamin C, primates do not. Therefore, all of our vitamin C must be obtained from our diet. Some good sources of vitamin C include citrus fruits, cauliflower, paprika, cabbage, turnip greens, broccoli, green peppers, tomatoes, and new potatoes (Williamson and Wyandt: 120+).

As was noted in chapter 9, in the early 1970s, Linus Pauling, who won a Nobel Prize in chemistry and a second one for peace, began to champion megadoses (1 to 4 g per day) of vitamin C. Pauling believed that such large quantities of this antioxidant could prevent and cure colds. The medical community greeted Pauling's beliefs with skepticism. "Dr. Pauling's thesis elicited a strong response by much of the medical community that contended (without much evidence) that megadoses of C were dangerous and would result in an epidemic of serious health problems including kidney stones, vitamin B deficiency, and even 'rebound scurvy,' which might occur if people suddenly stopped taking high doses of vitamin C" (Packer and Colman: 82–83).

In spite of the warnings, many people have placed themselves on high doses of vitamin C. As a rule, there have been few negative effects. Since vitamin C is a water-soluble vitamin, any excess intake is eliminated in the urine. "The only negative effects from too much vitamin C are abdominal cramping and diarrhea, which are uncomfortable but not particularly hazardous to your health. In very rare cases, people with a defect in iron or folic metabolism may experience an adverse reaction to megadoses of vitamin C, but there have been few reported cases" (Packer and Colman: 83).

A report presented to a March 2000 meeting of the American Heart Association (discussed in chapter 9) may cause some to rethink what they have said. James H. Dwyer, professor of preventive medicine at the Keck School of Medicine at the University of Southern California, studied 573 men and women between the ages of 40 and 60 who worked for an electric utility in Los Angeles. About 30% of the participants, who appeared to be relatively healthy, took vitamin C. Not only was there no evidence that the participants who took vitamin C benefited, but "those who consumed the most vitamin C from pills over a year and a half had more evidence of possible future arteriosclerosis." When researchers conducted ultrasound measurements on the participants' carotid arteries, they found that those who consumed at least 500 mg of supplemental vitamin C each day had "an inner artery wall layer 2.5 times thicker than that of people who did not take supplements. Among smokers, the supplement takers' inner artery layer was five times thicker. Such thickening precedes arteriosclerosis" (Monmaney: Part A, page 3). This study should be of particular concern to smokers, who are often told to take supplemental vitamin C to protect themselves from some of the negative effects of smoking.

The usefulness of high doses of supplemental vitamin C continues to be debated. Is vitamin C really a useful antioxidant? There is some evidence that a low intake of vitamin C is correlated with a higher risk of cancer, "especially cancers of the esophagus, mouth, pancreas, and stomach" (Williamson and Wyandt: 120+). Ralph W. Moss has written that vitamin C substantially reduces the risk of cancer by protecting genetic material from free-radical damage, strengthening the immune system, and increasing resistance to harmful chemicals. It also boosts other antioxidants, particularly vitamin E (Moss: 40). Further, while clinical studies have not found that vitamin C prevents or cures the common cold, "it may decrease the severity and duration of the virus" (Williamson and Wyandt: 120+). There is also some evidence that vitamin C supplements play a role in reducing heart disease. A study conducted at the School of Public Health at UCLA found that "men who took 300 milligrams of vitamin C daily had a 45 percent lower risk of heart disease than men who took less than 49 milligrams daily" (Packer and Colman: 90). Vitamin C may be effective in lowering the risk of cataracts. Research conducted at the USDA Human Nutrition Research Center at Tufts University determined that "women who took vitamin C for at least ten years were only 23 percent as likely to develop cataracts as women who did not" (Packer and Colman: 91). According to Lester Packer and Carol Colman, "It seems obvious that people who consume the lowest levels of vitamin C are not giving their bodies the tools they need to protect themselves against free radicals" (Packer and Colman: 90).

How much vitamin C should people take? The federal government says that the recommended daily allowance (RDA) for vitamin C is 75 mg for women and 90 mg for men. Smokers need to add an extra 35 mg. Packer contends that this amount is far too small and advises 250 mg twice a day. In his book *Eating Well for Optimum Health*, Andrew Weil, the director of the Program in Integrative Medicine at the University of Arizona, writes that he takes about 100 mg twice daily. In *Antioxidants against Cancer*, Ralph W. Moss says, "At a minimum, I suggest that you get at least 250 milligrams of vitamin C per day, in divided doses. 500 milligrams per day would be even better" (Moss: 50).

VITAMIN E

Fat-soluble vitamin E is also a frequently discussed and studied antioxidant. While it may be obtained from a variety of foods such as vegetables oils, whole grains, wheat germ, and nuts, it is usually believed that supplementation is necessary. "Disease due to deficiency of vitamin E is rare, but many people might not be getting enough of it to enjoy optimum health and protection from degenerative disease" (Weil: 130). Numerous benefits have been claimed for vitamin E. In *The Vitamin E Factor*, Andreas Papas states that "reducing heart disease is just the beginning" (Papas: 3). Studies of vitamin E have found that in addition to improving heart health, it may be useful for delaying aging; improving immunity; aiding in the prevention of Alzheimer's disease, cancer, Parkinson's disease, AIDS, male infertility, cataracts, macular degeneration, diabetes, asthma, and allergies; alleviating the effects of pollution; promoting skin health and wound healing; and delaying menopause (Papas: 3–4). A study conducted in Switzerland determined that "older people who took vitamin E supplements daily were 41 percent less likely to die of cancer, and 40 percent less likely to die of heart disease, than people who did not take vitamin E" (Moss: 53).

Apart from enhancing the quality of life, vitamin E may save money. At present, "the cost of treating cataracts is the biggest item in the Medicare budget," and "worldwide it ranks as the number one cause of blindness." Macular degeneration, which is the primary reason for blindness in Americans over the age of 65, is triggered, in part, by "oxidative damage." Since the retina has very high concentrations of oxygen, it is "particularly susceptible to such damage" (Golub: 1). It should be noted that other antioxidants have also been linked with eye health. These include lutein and zeaxanthin, which are found in dark green leafy vegetables such as kale, collards, and spinach.

Papas cautions that not all vitamin Es are alike. Vitamin E is actually composed of eight different compounds, four tocopherols and four tocotrienols. Some supplements may contain only one of these eight compounds. People who take these forms of vitamin E lose the potential benefits the other compounds may bring to their diets. Weil believes that for other vitamins, more expensive natural forms are a waste of money, no matter what the manufacturers claim, but that natural vitamin E contains compounds not found in synthetic vitamin E (Weil: 130). However, in a March 2000 story in the *Washington Post*, Robert Russell, a professor of medicine and nutrition at Tufts University and associate director of the U.S. Department of Agriculture's Human Nutrition Research Center, allegedly said the exact opposite: "This is one case where the synthetic form is actually better absorbed and is more bio available than the natural d form." "It goes against the common lore that the natural form is somehow better" (Squires: Page Z14).

The recommendations for adequate vitamin E intake seem to keep changing, but all the values tend to be low—around 30 IU. Many medical providers suggest that people consume higher amounts. Papas says that "100 IU plus 100 milligrams of mixed tocopherols and tocotrienols" is an "adequate level," but a "high, yet very safe dose" is "400 IU plus 400 milligrams of mixed tocopherols and tocotrienols" (Papas: 302). Weil has noted that "most experts on nutritional medicine agree that daily doses of 400 to 800 IU are necessary for maximum antioxidant effect, optimum health, and surest disease prevention" (Weil: 130). A 1999 article in the *American Journal of Clinical Nutrition* reported that daily doses of 2,000 IU were safely administered to elderly people for a period of two years (Vatassery, Bauer, and Dysken: 793–801).

While the vast majority of studies on vitamin E supplementation have concluded that it is beneficial, a brief article published in early 2000 in the *Lancet* raised at least a minor caution. One investigation of 2,545 women and 6,996 men, aged 55 or older, who were at high risk for cardiovascular problems found that those "who took vitamin E for a mean of 4.5 years fared no better than controls in terms of cardiovascular outcome" (Senior: 383).

Another study that was presented to a meeting of the American Society for Cell Biology at the end of 1999 described the work of Rudolf I. Salganik and his associates at the University of North Carolina. They divided a strain of mice that develops brain tumors into two groups. One was fed a regular diet; the second was fed a diet devoid of vitamins A and E. The tumors in the mice who ate the food without vitamins A and E were half the size of the tumors in the other mice. "Moreover, 20 percent of the tumor cells in the antioxidant-deprived mice were undergoing a type of cell death called apoptosis, which is driven by free radicals. The body ordinarily uses this programmed suicide to rid itself of old or wounded cells. In the mice on the normal diet, just three percent of cancer cells were undergoing apoptosis" (Raloff, January 1, 2000: 11). In this case, at least, it appears that the antioxidants aided the growth of cancer cells (Salganik: 909–914).

As a result of these findings, some doctors are advising patients undergoing chemotherapy to either eliminate antioxidant supplements or consume only modest amounts. That is exactly what appears to be happening with a number of physicians at the Memorial Sloan-Kettering Cancer Center in New York, where researchers founds that "large doses of vitamin C [were] interfering with cell kill in people with prostate cancer, breast cancer and leukemia" (Stahl: 510).

People who are taking blood-thinning medications need to take lower dosages of vitamin E. "Patients receiving warfarin (Coumadin) therapy should limit vitamin E intake to 200 IU per day and should avoid vitamin E if they are at high risk for bleeding" (Adams, Wermuth, and McBride: 895–902).

In September 1999, a study published in *Lancet* noted that the combination of vitamins C and E appears to prevent pre-eclampsia in pregnant women who are at increased risk. Pre-eclampsia, a toxic condition characterized by weight gain and a dangerous rise in blood pressure, "is an important cause of maternal morbidity and mortality and accounts for more than 40% of the iatrogenic [physician-induced] premature deliveries." At 16 to 22 weeks of gestation, a total of 283 high-risk women were either given 1,000 mg/day of vitamin C and 400 IU/day of vitamin E or a placebo. "Those who were taking the supplements had less than half the incidence of pre-eclampsia than those in the placebo group" (Chappell et al.: 810–816).

COENZYME Q10

Another well-publicized antioxidant is coenzyme Q10. Although its name is a bit unusual, according to Stephen T. Sinatra, author of *The Coenzyme Q10 Phenomenon*, coenzyme Q10 (also known as ubiquinone) "is a naturally occurring substance that is found in virtually all cells of the human body." It is also contained in a number of foods such as "beef heart, pork, sardines, anchovies, mackerel, salmon, broccoli, spinach and nuts." On average, people take in about 10 mg/day. "However, the amount received from dietary sources is insufficient to produce any substantial clinical effects, especially in those with pathological situations such as periodontal disease, high blood pressure, heart disease, impaired immunity and so on" (Sinatra, 1998: 15). As of June 1998, Sinatra suggested the following doses: 90 to 120 mg daily as a preventive in cardiovascular or periodontal disease and for patients taking HMG-CoA reductase inhibitors (cholesterol-lowering drugs); 120 to 240 mg daily for the treatment of angina pectoris, cardiac arrhythmia, high blood pressure, and moderate gingival disease; and 240 to 450 mg daily for congestive heart failure and dilated cardiomyopathy. He recommended even higher doses of coenzyme Q10 for a severely impaired immune system, as in cancer (Sinatra, 1998: 29).

The literature contains numerous reports of positive outcomes facilitated by coenzyme Q10. An article in *RN* summarized a double-blind clinical trial in which "people who had suffered an acute MI [heart attack] were given either 100 mg a day of oral CoQ or a placebo for 28 days. Those on CoQ experienced less angina pectoris, fewer arrhythmias, and better left ventricular function. Even more impressive was the fact that the coenzyme was linked to fewer cardiac deaths and nonfatal MIs" (Cerrato: 61–62). An article in *Better Nutrition* listed a series of studies showing the remarkable health gains from coenzyme Q10 (Scheer and Guest: 52). The number of positive accounts seems endless.

Not everyone is convinced. A 1999 *Harvard Heart Letter* described "a small but careful and rigorous trial that evaluated coenzyme Q10 in 30 patients enrolled in a heart-failure and transplant program" in Australia ("Coenzyme Q10 Disappoints": ITEM99221005). The researchers found no positive outcome from coenzyme Q10, but they also observed no negative consequences.

Another investigation published in 2000 in the *Annals of Internal Medicine* examined the results of treating patients with congestive heart failure with coenzyme Q10 versus giving them placebos. As might be expected, the patients who took coenzyme Q10 had higher amounts of the antioxidant in their blood, but "the compound had no positive effect on the heart compared to the placebo. It also had no effect on exercise duration or oxygen consumption during exercise" (Khatta et al.: 636).

OTHER ANTIOXIDANTS

While vitamins C and E and coenzyme Q10 are the antioxidants that appear to generate the most publicity, there are a host of others that are now being investigated. Many are in the foods you may already eat. Some are in foods that you may wish to try. A smaller number are most readily obtained through supplementation.

For example, during the past few years, scientists have determined that the flavonoids (plant pigments that act as antioxidants) in blueberries fight aging. At the U.S. Department of Agriculture (USDA) Human Nutrition Research Center on Aging at Tufts University, researchers studied older rats who had lost their ability to traverse a maze, an activity they had previously mastered. After two months of supplementation with blueberry extract, that skill returned. Moreover, "the rats' balance, coordination, and running speed also improved" (McCord, June 1999: 122). Studies have also found blueberries useful for preventing urinary-tract infections and for relieving eye problems such as night blindness and eyestrain. Apparently, the healthy benefits of blueberries are a direct result of anthocyanins, the pigments that give them their deep blue color. Ronald Prior, one of the Tufts scientists who studied blueberries, has suggested that people add half a cup of blueberries to their daily diets. In a 1999 article in *Prevention* magazine, he was quoted as saying, "With ½ cup of blueberries, you can just about double the amount of antioxidants most Americans get in one day. If you want to slow down the free radical aging process, blueberries are the leader of the pack" (McCord, June 1999: 122–127).

Then there is the antioxidant tea. Tea is the second most consumed drink in the world. Only water is more common. It now appears that green tea contains polyphenols, powerful antioxidants that offer "protection against cancer, heart disease, and high cholesterol." A study published at the end of 1999 found that Chinese green tea lowered the cholesterol of laboratory rats. Another report, published in early 2000, determined that green tea reduced the risk of coronary heart disease (McCommons: 24). "One [study] showed that both men and women who drank 10 or more cups of green tea daily developed cancer several years later than non-drinkers" (Saltus: Pages E1, E5).

Meanwhile, a 1999 article published in the *Archives of Internal Medicine* noted an inverse relationship between drinking black tea and advanced stages of aortic atherosclerosis. In other words, the more black tea one drinks, the less likely one will develop hardening of the arteries. This association is especially strong in women. It is theorized that the flavonoids in black tea serve as protective antioxidants (Geleijnse et al.: 2170–2174).

An interesting study published early in 2000 in the *Journal of the National Cancer Institute* found a relationship between the intake of quercetin (found in onions and apples) and naringin (found in white grapefruit), two flavonoids, and lung cancer. "An inverse association with lung cancer that approached statistical significance was observed for quercetin. Although not statistically significant, the risk estimates for naringin were also consistent with the reduction in risk seen for white grapefruit. The inverse associations with onions, apples, and white grapefruit were present in both sexes and in almost all ethnic groups" (Marchand et al.: 154–160).

Fat- and water-soluble alpha lipoic acid, or thioctic acid, which is found in "spinach, meats (especially liver), and brewer's yeast" (Kalyn: 234), has been said to be "useful against everything from aging and heart disease to Parkinson's disease and lupus" (Webb: 69–70). At present, there is no proof for most of these claims. However, there is some evidence that alpha lipoic acid may prevent "bad" (LDL) cholesterol. In *Alpha Lipoic Acid*, Allan E. Sosin and Beth M. Ley Jacobs write that there are numerous studies that show that antioxidants protect low-density lipoprotein (LDL), the bad type of cholesterol, from oxidation. "In addition to providing powerful antioxidant properties itself, alpha lipoic acid recycles other antioxidants in the body such as vitamin C and E. Together they act synergistically as crucial components to warding off free radical damage and maintaining healthy circulation to the heart and throughout the body. In one study, blood samples of 36 African Americans, ages 16 to 37, showed an inverse correlation between LDL, alpha-tocopherol content, and LDL oxidation rates. LDL samples with higher alpha-tocopherol content exhibit slower LDL oxidation lag rates, demonstrating the ability of vitamin E to increase LDL resistance to oxidation" (Sosin and Jacobs: 123–124).

Alpha lipoic acid is already being viewed as a means to relieve diabetic neuropathy, a complication of high sugar levels in people with diabetes, in which damaged nerve endings trigger "stabbing, tingling, and burning in the legs, feet, and hands, especially at night" (Webb: 69–70). In *The Healing Power of Vitamins, Minerals, and Herbs*, it is noted that "in a trial at multiple medical centers, 328 people with diabetic nerve damage were given 100 mg, 600 mg, or 1200 mg of alpha-lipoic acid a day over a three-week period. Patients receiving 600 mg reported the most significant reduction in pain and numbness, compared with other groups." Further, "Alpha-lipoic acid may also benefit the 25% of diabetes sufferers who are at risk of sudden death from nerve-related heart damage. After four months of taking 800 mg of alpha-lipoic acid a day, these patients showed a notable improvement in their heart function tests." It may also help memory. "A study of aged mice indicated that alpha-lipoic acid improved long-term memory, possibly by preventing free-radical damage to brain cells" (Kalyn: 235).

While no one is saying that alpha lipoic acid is a cure for HIV/AIDS, it might have possible value to those who are dealing with this serious medical problem. In *Encyclopedia of Natural Medicine*, Michael Murray and Joseph Pizzorno describe a study on the effect alpha lipoic acid has on HIV-positive patients. The study demonstrated that supplementation with alpha lipoic acid "led to significant beneficial changes in the blood of HIV infected patients. Perhaps the most significant of these effects was the increase in the glutathione content, since the level of glutathione is directly linked to preventing the progression to AIDS" (Murray and Pizzorno: 206).

In *The Alpha Lipoic Acid Breakthrough*, Burt Berkson writes that he has found alpha lipoic acid useful for almost all of his patients. Many have witnessed significant improvements in medical conditions ranging from cardiovascular problems to complications of diabetes. He offered a detailed description of 50-year-old Mr. Green, who was skeletally thin because he found it extremely painful to eat. Several doctors had told him that this was a complication of his adult-onset diabetes, and that he just had to live with it. A neurosurgeon suggested severing the nerve to his digestive tract. "Mr. Green came to me looking for an alternative. . . . In addition to his regular diabetes medication, I put Mr. Green on a good, healthy diet with nutritional supplementation, prescribed moderate exercise, and started him on an oral dose of ALA [alpha lipoic acid]. Within three weeks most of his pain subsided and he rapidly put on weight. As a bonus, his blood sugar fell to close to normal. Also, as a result of the treatment and exercise, Mr. Green's muscle mass and energy levels increased" (Berkson: xiv–xv).

Foods contain only very small amounts of alpha lipoic acid. "For example, it takes seven pounds of spinach to produce just 1 mg" (Webb: 69–70). Anyone interested in taking this antioxidant must turn to a supplement. Some medical providers recommend doses as low as 20 to 50 mg/day. Others say that the doses need to be significantly higher— 300 to 600 mg/day or twice that amount. Those considering a higher dose should discuss their plans with a medical provider. Moss cautions against high doses. "When the dose is increased, there may be some low toxicity, such as over-alertness or insomnia. Stomach upset is a possibility at higher amounts. In doses over 500 milligrams per day or more, a slight blood glucose lowering effect is observed. Some allergic skin reactions have also been reported in a few people at these high doses. However, there is no evidence that lipoic acid promotes mutations, birth defects, or cancer" (Moss: 68).

Another less recognized antioxidant is grape seed extract, which "used to be considered a worthless by-product of wine production." According to Varro Tyler, a well-known expert on herbs, "Weight for weight, its antioxidant activity is some 50 times greater than that of vitamin E and 20 times greater than vitamin C" (Tyler: 105).

Grape seed extract is said to be useful for a number of medical problems, including inadequate blood flow in the veins, eye stress, and macular degeneration. It is believed to be at least partially responsible for "the French paradox," the fact that the French, who tend to eat a diet that is high in fat, have a relatively low incidence of heart-related diseases. "The answer appears to be in their choice of beverage: red wine. Following the harvest of the grapes, along with their stems and leaves, the grapes are pressed and the entire crush is placed in fermentation vats. During the process, the alcohol with the juice extracts the most soluble antioxidants from the grape seeds and skin into red wine. . . . It is healthier to drink the red wine because this wine contains antioxidants that have been leached from the grape skins and seeds during the fermentation process" (Balch: 113–114).

"The French paradox" should not be used as an excuse for someone to drink excessively. While a study in France found that "those who drank two to three glasses of wine a day had 35 percent fewer heart attacks, 24 percent fewer cancers, and 30 percent fewer deaths from all causes . . . , at four glasses of wine per day, there is a major reversal of the statistics and the death rates and cancer rates rise! At that point, the oxidative effects of the alcohol itself surpass the benefits of the antioxidants" (Balch: 119).

Those who are not of drinking age or who prefer not to consume alcohol may obtain comparable benefits by drinking grape juice, particularly purple grape juice. When researchers at the University of Wisconsin Medical School studied 15 men and women with coronary artery disease, they found that they improved with daily doses of purple grape juice. "Their vasodilation (ability of arteries to open to allow better blood flow) improved almost three-fold (from 2.2 percent to 6.4 percent)" (Orr: 18). Another study at the same medical school determined that drinking purple grape juice inhibited the formation of artery-clogging platelets in dogs and monkeys (Osman et al.: 2307–2312). A 1999 article in *Vegetarian Times* concluded that "preliminary studies show that purple grape juice has the same salutary effects as the daily glass of red wine we've heard so much about" (Marandino: 14).

Supplementation is also an option. As with other antioxidants, dosage recommendations vary. Generally, a grape seed extract maintenance dose is 50 to 100 mg/day. For the therapeutic treatment of a problem, a dose as high as 300 mg/day may be warranted.

Selenium is found in seafood, kidney, liver, and other meats as well as protein-rich plant foods such as seeds and nuts. Brazil nuts are an especially good source. Two such nuts a day provide all the selenium the body requires. At present, the suggested dosage is 55 micrograms (mcg) a day for women and 70 mcg a day for men. Some, such as Moss, advise higher levels. "Selenium is so important that I believe that practically every adult should take a 200 microgram selenium supplement every day" (Moss: 81). Still, a warning should be noted. "Selenium can be toxic in amounts above 1,000 micrograms a day; the early signs of toxicity are peeling of fingernails and brittleness of hair" (Weil: 135).

A 1999 article in the *Journal of the American Dietetic Association* underscores the point that true selenium deficiency is rare. "The primary group of people who have developed selenium deficiency have been those receiving total parenteral nutrition without selenium for extended periods." Still, a selenium deficiency "may exacerbate damage from other disease-causing factors" (Holben and Smith: 836–843).

In *Formula for Life*, Eberhard Kronhausen and Phyllis Kronhausen state that selenium serves a variety of important functions. "For one thing, a vital enzyme system—glutathione peroxidase—is selenium-dependent, and even marginal selenium deficiency may prevent its proper functioning. Furthermore, selenium protects against several common degenerative diseases, such as coronary artery disease, cerebrovascular disease (strokes), and degenerative joint disease (arthritis and rheumatoid arthritis). Most important to us, however, after a couple of cancer scares, is its role in boosting cellular immunity. . . . Recently, it has been shown that the AIDS virus slowly depletes the body of selenium—just as it does with glutathione. When the virus has used up all the selenium in an immune system cell, it breaks out in search of more, spreading the infection to other cells" (Kronhausen and Kronhausen: 54). Further, a short article in the January/February 2000 issue of *Men's Health* reported that during a study of the effect of selenium on skin cancer, researchers at the University of Arizona found that it lowered the incidence of prostate cancer, apparently by increasing the levels of the antioxidant glutathione peroxidase (Spiker: 32).

The antioxidant ginkgo has often been featured in scientific journals and in all forms of the written and televised media. Ginkgo, which is derived from the leaves of the ginkgo tree, has ancient roots. Some researchers believe that the species is more than 200 million years old. It has been part of Chinese medicine for 5,000 years. "Traditionally, ginkgo has been used in the elderly for age-related memory loss and diminished mental functioning. In this capacity it works as an antioxidant and as a blood thinner. By thinning the blood, ginkgo assists in guaranteeing a good supply of blood to the tiny vessels of the brain" (Starbuck, 1999: 48). A study published in the *Journal of the American Medical Association* investigated 202 patients with dementia. "Patients who took 120 mg of ginkgo biloba extract a day were more likely to stabilize or improve their mental and social functions, compared with those given a placebo. The effects were modest and of limited duration" (Kalyn: 299).

Ginkgo is also said to be beneficial for depression, memory loss, Alzheimer's disease, vertigo/dizziness, peripheral arterial disease, PMS, ringing in the ears, moodiness, and anxiety. Some data are striking. For instance, "when 40 patients with senile dementia of the Alzheimer's type received 80 milligrams of Ginkgo biloba [ginkgo] extract three times a day, their memory and attention span were observed to significantly improve after only one month" (Craig: 14). Similarly, daily doses of ginkgo ranging from 120 mg to 240 mg were given to 31 healthy people between the ages of 30 and 59. "Researchers noted a slight increase in memory among those that took the ginkgo, but the effect was most highly pronounced in subjects 50 to 59 years old" ("Ginkgo": 46). Another double-blind study of 165 women found "that ginkgo was effective in significantly reducing breast tenderness prior to the menses. The women were given either a placebo, or 80 mg of ginkgo, twice a day, from day 16 of their cycle through day 5 of the next cycle. The ginkgo group fared far better in terms of breast symptoms than did the placebo group" (Starbuck, 2000: 72).

In *Miracle Cures*, Jean Carper, a medical writer and author of books on health and nutrition, describes the case of an elderly woman with Alzheimer's disease who was treated unsuccessfully with a variety of medications. Finally, her son, a scientist, turned to ginkgo. He "began giving her ginkgo biloba in standardized doses of 240 milligrams daily, which is used in Germany to treat Alzheimer's." While she did not recover her lost memory, the progression of the disease stopped. "Her son is convinced it has helped his mother, now age eighty-eight, function with dignity in an assisted-living center far better and longer than would have been expected otherwise" (Carper: 60–61).

In *Ginkgo Biloba*, Glenn S. Rothfeld and Suzanne LeVert reviewed several studies of ginkgo. One found that ginkgo was effective in reducing loss of concentration, memory loss, and symptoms of senility. Another indicated a significant improvement in reaction time of healthy young women performing a memory test after ginkgo was administered. A third study showed that ginkgo inhibits the activity of monoamine oxidase, an enzyme involved in depression. Other studies found that ginkgo benefited patients with tinnitus, macular degeneration or vertigo (Rothfeld and LeVert: 39, 41).

Different people recommend varying amounts of ginkgo. Commonly, dosages are around 160 mg/day. In clinical trials, doses have been higher. However, a warning needs to be noted. People who are taking blood-thinning medications such as warfarin or high-dose aspirin should avoid it; otherwise, they are at risk for developing bleeding problems. Other possible side effects of ginkgo include nausea, diarrhea, leg pain, and dizziness. Unprocessed ginkgo leaves should not be used in any form. "They contain potent chemical (allergens) that can trigger allergic reactions" (Kalyn: 298). During processing, these are removed.

Until 1996, beta-carotene foods and supplements were thought to contain some of the best antioxidants, and the supplements were believed to be effective against a number of medical problems such as cancer and macular degeneration. A yellowish compound, beta-carotene consists of numerous pigments known as carotenoids and is found in a number of fruits and vegetables such as cantaloupes and carrot juice. A precursor of vitamin A, beta-carotene converts into vitamin A in the body.

However, in that year, a study published by *JAMA: The Journal of the American Medical Association* reported that two large clinical trials had found that high doses of supplemental beta-carotene and vitamin A offered no protection for people at high risk of lung cancer—former smokers and asbestos workers. Moreover, in one of the studies, "there was even evidence of the opposite effect—a lung cancer rate that was higher in at-risk patients who took high-dose supplements of beta carotene and vitamin A than in at-risk patients who took a placebo" (Marwick: 422–423).

Since then, other studies have found that beta-carotene supplements have neither a positive nor a negative effect on cancer, cardiovascular disease, and type 2 diabetes. Weil cautions that people should learn from the experience with beta-carotene. "To recommend the use of one, isolated element of a complex family of protective compounds in plants is to fall under the spell of reductionism, the belief that the part equals the whole. Unfortunately, that way of thinking now dominates Western medicine and science" (Weil: 139).

While beta-carotene supplementation seems to have lost its glow, no one talks against the value of eating foods containing beta-carotene. All diets should have generous amounts of fruits and vegetables with beta-carotene.

While many high-antioxidant foods are vegetables and fruits, such as kale, spinach, broccoli, prunes, raisins, and various berries, one surprising antioxidant is chocolate. Chocolate is not marketed as a health food, but it is obtained from beans that have large amounts of flavonoids. "A 40-gram serving of milk chocolate typically contains around 400 milligrams of antioxidants, about the same quantity as a glass of red wine." A serving of dark chocolate "contains more than twice that quantity— roughly the same amount as a cup of black tea" (Raloff, March 18, 2000: 188–189). "A small candy bar (1 to 2 ounces) has the same amount of these antioxidants, called phenols, as you'd get in a five-ounce glass of red wine. Even a cup of hot chocolate made with 2 tablespoons of coca powder contains 146 milligrams of phenols. Dark chocolate has the most phenolics, while white chocolate has none. Better yet, the antioxidants in chocolate appear more potent than those in wine" (Somer: 83). Turning to chocolate to improve health is not a new phenomenon. Those who are well versed in nutritional history know that several centuries ago chocolate and cocoa treatments were used for a variety of medical problems such as anemia and gastrointestinal complaints.

CONCLUSION

It is a little unsettling to close this chapter with so many unexplained findings. Why does one study find this or that antioxidant useful when another concludes that it may be detrimental to one's health? In a 1999 article in the *American Family Physician*, Robert Kiningham speculates that antioxidants may require certain other antioxidants and nutrients in order to work effectively. When these other antioxidants and nutrients are absent, the antioxidants may fail to function at optimum capacity. The overall nutritional state of the individual may also be a factor in their effectiveness (Kiningham: 742).

Michael T. Murray, an authority on natural medicine, author, and lecturer, agrees. "In addition to consuming a diet rich in plant foods . . . , I recommend using a combination of antioxidant nutrients rather than high dosages of any single antioxidant. Mixtures of antioxidant nutrients appear to work together harmoniously to produce the phenomena of synergy—in other words, $1 + 1 = 3$" (Murray: 16).

However, Victor Herbert, professor of medicine at Mount Sinai School of Medicine in New York, notes that he advises against using antioxidant supplements. "Vitamins and other nutrition in food are balanced nutrition. In supplement pills they are unbalanced nutrition. . . . No pill, be it a single vitamin and/or mineral and/or omega-3 (or other) fatty acid, or a multivitamin/mineral pill, ever comes close to the balance of ingredients (including various kinds of fiber), per unit volume, bulk, and weight, achieved by nature in food" (Herbert and Subak-Sharpe: 118).

While the issues surrounding antioxidants remain controversial, it is obvious that many people could increase their intake simply by adding more fruits and vegetables to their daily diet. That is probably the easiest and most effective lifestyle modification the average person should do. Foods such as blueberries, raisins, prunes, spinach and kale appear to be particularly useful. Healthy teens and young adults normally do not require antioxidant supplementation. But, those faced with medical problems may wish to consult with a doctor or nutritionist to see whether antioxidant supplementation is advisable.

TOPICS FOR DISCUSSION

1. Do you or any members of your family regularly take any antioxidant supplements? Which ones do you take? Have you noticed any positive or negative changes?

2. Do you think that it is best to have food as your primary source of antioxidants, or do you believe that supplementation may be needed? Why?

3. One researcher says that you should take vitamin E in the natural form. Another says that the synthetic variety is better. Whom do you agree with and why?

4. What antioxidant foods do you incorporate into your diet? Why?

5. Has reading this chapter changed how you feel about antioxidants? Why or why not?

REFERENCES AND RESOURCES

Books

Balch, James F. *The Super Antioxidants*. New York: M. Evans and Company, 1998.
Berkson, Burt. *The Alpha Lipoic Acid Breakthrough*. Rocklin, California: Prima Publishing, 1998.

Carper, Jean. *Miracle Cures*. New York: HarperCollins, 1997.

Herbert, Victor, and Genell J. Subak-Sharpe, editors. *Total Nutrition*. New York: St. Martin's Griffin, 1995.

Kalyn, Wayne, editor. *The Healing Power of Vitamins, Minerals, and Herbs*. Pleasantville, New York: Reader's Digest, 1999.

Kronhausen, Eberhard, and Phyllis Kronhausen. *Formula for Life*. New York: Quill, 1999.

Moss, Ralph W. *Antioxidants against Cancer*. Brooklyn, New York: Equinox Press, 2000.

Murray, Michael T., and Joseph E. Pizzorno. *Encyclopedia of Natural Medicine*. Rocklin, California: Prima Health, 1998.

Packer, Lester, and Carol Colman. *The Antioxidant Miracle*. New York: John Wiley and Sons, 1999.

Papas, Andreas. *The Vitamin E Factor*. New York: HarperPerennial, 1999.

Passwater, Richard A. *All about Antioxidants*. Garden City Park, New York: Avery Publishing Group, 1998.

Rothfeld, Glenn S., and Suzanne LeVert. *Ginkgo Biloba*. New York: Dell Publishing, 1998.

Sinatra, Stephen T. *The Coenzyme Q10 Phenomenon*. New Canaan, Connecticut: Keats Publishing, 1998.

Sinatra, Stephen T. *Optimum Health*. New York: Bantam Books, 1997.

Somer, Elizabeth. *Food and Mood*. New York: Henry Holt and Company, 1999.

Sosin, Allan E., and Beth M. Ley Jacobs. *Alpha Lipoic Acid*. New York: Kensington Books, 1998.

Taylor, Nadine. *Green Tea*. New York: Kensington Books, 1998.

Weil, Andrew. *Eating Well for Optimum Health*. New York: Alfred Knopf, 2000.

Magazines, Journals, and Newspapers

Adams, Alexandria K., Ellen O. Wermuth, and Patrick E. McBride. "Antioxidant Vitamins and the Prevention of Coronary Heart Disease." *American Family Physician*, September 1, 1999, 60(3): 895–902.

Adderly, Brenda. "New Hope for Chronic Fatigue Sufferers." *Better Nutrition*, April 2000, 62(4): 48–52.

Bushkin, Estitta, and Gary Bushkin. "Anti-Aging with Antioxidants." *Better Nutrition*, February 2000, 6(2): 66–70.

Cerrato, Paul L. "Coenzyme Q and Heart Disease." *RN*, June 1999, 62(6): 61–62.

Chappell, Lucy C., Paul T. Seed, Annette L. Briley, Frank J. Kelly, Rosalind Lee, Beverley J. Hunt, Kiran Parmar, Susan J. Bewley, Andrew H. Shennan, Philip J. Steer, and Lucilla Poston. "Effect of Antioxidants on the Occurrence of Pre-Eclampsia in Women at Increased Risk: A Randomised Trial." *Lancet*, September 4, 1999, 354(918): 810–816.

"Coenzyme Q10 Disappoints in Rigorous Study." *Harvard Heart Letter*, August 1999, 9: ITEM99221005.

Craig, Winston J. "Going with Ginkgo to Enhance Immune Function." *Vibrant Life*, January 2000, 16(1): 14.

Geleijnse, Johanna G., Lenore J. Launer, Albert Hofman, Huibert A.P. Pols, and

Jacqueline C.M. Witteman. "Tea Flavonoids May Protect against Athero-sclerosis: The Rotterdam Study." *Archives of Internal Medicine*, October 11, 1999, 159(18): 2170–2174.

"Ginkgo: The End of Alzheimer's Disease?" *Psychology Today*, March 2000, 33(2): 46.

Golub, Catherine. "Fending Off Vision Loss: Produce May Have the Power to Protect Your Eyes." *Environmental Nutrition*, September 1999, 22(9): 1.

Henderson, Charles W. "Antioxidants and Progression of Human Immunodeficiency Virus (HIV) Disease." *AIDS Weekly Plus*, August 16, 1999.

Holben, David H., and Anne M. Smith. "The Diverse Role of Selenium within Selenoproteins: A Review." *Journal of the American Dietetic Association*, July 1999, 99(7): 836–843.

Jancin, Bruce. "Ginkgo Plus Anticoagulation Can Lead to Hemorrhage." *Family Practice News*, February 15, 2000, 30(4): 65.

Khatta, Meenakshi, Barbara S. Alexander, Cathy M. Krichten, Michael L. Fisher, Ronald Freudenberger, Shawn W. Robinson, and Stephen S. Gottlieb. "The Effects of Coenzyme Q(10) in Patients with Congestive Heart Failure." *Annals of Internal Medicine*, April 18, 2000, 132(8): 636–640.

Kiningham, Robert. "The Value of Antioxidant Vitamin Supplements." *American Family Physician*, September 1, 1999, 60(3): 742.

LoBuono, Charlotte, and Mary Desmond Pinkowish. "Purple Grape Juice: A Liter a Day Keeps the Doctor Away." *Patient Care*, November 15, 1999, 33(18): 229.

Marandino, Cristin. "Heart Copy." *Vegetarian Times*, February 1999, 258: 14.

Marchand, Loic Le, Suzanne P. Murphy, Jean H. Hankin, Lynne R. Wilkens, and Laurence N. Kolonel. "Intake of Flavonoids and Lung Cancer." *Journal of the National Cancer Institute*, January 19, 2000, 92(2) 154–160.

Marwick, Charles. "Trials Reveal No Benefit, Possible Harm of Beta Carotene and Vitamin A for Lung Cancer Prevention." *JAMA: The Journal of the American Medical Association*, February 14, 1996, 275(6): 422–423.

McCommons, James. "Tea Helps Hearts Stay Healthy." *Organic Gardening*, May/June 2000, 47(3): 24.

McCord, Holly. "The Miracle Berry." *Prevention*, June 1999, 51(6): 122–127.

McCord, Holly, and Sherry Weiss Kiser. "Grape Juice with the Most Punch." *Prevention*, October 1999, 51(10): 58.

Monmaney, Terence. "Heart Not Protected by Vitamin C, Study Finds." *Los Angeles Times*, March 3, 2000: Part A1, page 3.

Murray, Michael T. "Power in Numbers—'Team Up' Antioxidants for Best Results." *Better Nutrition*, November 1999, 61(11): 16.

Orr, Tamara B. "4 Ways to Keep Cholesterol Levels in Balance, Naturally." *Better Nutrition*, February 2000, 62(2): 18.

Osman, Hashim, Nabil Maalej, Dhanansayan Shanmuganayagam, and John D. Folts. "Grape Juice But Not Orange or Grapefruit Juice Inhibits Platelet Activity in Dogs and Monkeys." *Journal of Nutrition*, December 1998, 128(12): 2307–2312.

Raloff, Janet. "Antioxidants May Help Cancers Thrive." *Science News*, January 1, 2000, 157(1): 11.

Raloff, Janet. "Berry Good Protection for Aging Brains." *Science News*, September 18, 1999, 156(12): 180.

Raloff, Janet. "Chocolate Hearts." *Science News*, March 18, 2000, 157(12): 188–189.

Roan, Shari. "No Verdict Yet on Vitamin C." *Los Angeles Times*, April 17, 2000: Page 1.

Salganik, Rudolf I., Craig D. Albright, Jerilyn Rodgers, John Kim, Steven H. Zeisel, Mikhail S. Sivashinskiy, and Terry A. Van Dyke. "Dietary Antioxidant Depletion: Enhancement of Tumor Apoptosis and Inhibition of Brain Tumor Growth in Transgenic Mice." *Carcinogensis*, May 2000, 21(5): 909–914.

Saltus, Richard. "The Tao of Tea." *Boston Globe*, June 13, 2000: Pages E1, E5.

Saunders, Carol S. "The Final Say on Beta Carotene?" *Patient Care*, February 29, 2000, 34(4): 14.

Scheer, James F., and Donna K. Guest. "Getting to the Heart of the Matter with CoQ10." *Better Nutrition*, June 1999, 61(6): 52.

Senior, Kathryn. "Setback for Vitamin E as Preventive Therapy for Cardiovascular Disease." *Lancet*, January 29, 2000, 355(9201): 383.

Spiker, Ted. "Prostate Protector." *Men's Health*, January/February 2000, 15(1): 32.

Squires, Sally. "High Irony: New Supplement Labels Are Short on Facts." *Washington Post*, March 7, 2000: Page 14.

Stahl, Patricia. "The Antioxidant Conundrum: Two Recent Studies Point in Different Directions." *Journal of the American Dietetic Association*, May 2000, 100(5): 510.

Starbuck, J. Jamison. "Beyond Brainboosting." *Better Nutrition*, April 2000, 62(4): 72.

Starbuck, J. Jamison. "Why You Need Ginkgo." *Better Nutrition*, April 1999, 61(4): 48.

Tyler, Varro. "The Miracle of Anti-Aging Herbs." *Prevention*, November 1999, 51(11): 105.

Vatassery, Govind T., Timothy Bauer, and Maurice Dysken. "High Doses of Vitamin E in the Treatment of Disorders of the Central Nervous System in the Aged" *American Journal of Clinical Nutrition*, November 1999, 70(5): 793–801.

Webb, Denise. "For Diabetes Nerve Pain, Try Alpha-Lipoic Acid." *Prevention*, May 2000, 52(5): 69–70.

Williamson, John S., and Christy M. Wyandt. "What to Tell Your Patients about Antioxidants." *Drug Topics*, December 6, 1999, 143(23): 120+.

Organizations to Contact

Center for Research on Human Nutrition and Chronic Disease Prevention
Wake Forest University Baptist Medical Center
Medical Center Boulevard
Winston-Salem, NC 27157
Phone: 336-716-2011
http://www.bgsm.edu/nutrition/ (May 27, 2002)

Human Nutrition Research Center on Aging
711 Washington Street
Boston, MA 02111-1524
Phone: 617-556-3000
http://www.hnrc.tufts.edu/ (June 25, 2000)

United States Department of Agriculture
14th & Independence Ave. SW
Washington, DC 20250
Phone: 202-720-2791
http://www.usda.gov/ (June 25, 2000)

12

Organic Foods

Advertising tries to persuade consumers that organic food is healthier and worth the extra price. Whether organic foods indeed provide the benefits claimed for them is a matter of controversy. In the supermarket, there is a large display of apples that sell for 99 cents per pound. There is also a similar arrangement of organic apples. However, these retail for $1.49 per pound. Are the organic apples worth the extra 50 cents per pound? Are they better than the regular apples?

Until the 1970s, there were few commercially available organic foods, most found only at small co-ops. That has all changed. Now organic foods are available at regular suburban grocery stores as well as specialty shops and are purchased by consumers from all ethnic backgrounds and economic classes. Organic foods are at least a six-billion-dollar business that keeps growing. "Sales of organic food in North America have been increasing 20 to 30 percent annually over the past decade, and organic food is now the fastest-growing segment of the natural-foods market" (Kett: 11).

Who is buying organic foods? Read what the Organic Trade Association as to say:

- A study conducted in March 2001 found that, at some point, 63% of Americans buy organic foods and beverages.
- Organic users tend to be 31% more concerned about the environment and pollution than the general population.
- More than 40% of the people who use organic food are between the ages of 36 and 55. People who use organic products are 25% more likely to have a bachelor's or graduate degree. (Organic Trade Association Web site)

STANDARDS FOR ORGANIC FOODS

What makes a food organic has little to do with the food; instead, it is primarily a function of how the soil was prepared and how the food was produced. "In fact, to understand what you're getting when you buy organic, you have to forget fruits and vegetables for a moment and think about dirt" (Shapiro: 54). According to a 1998 article in *Consumer Reports*, the techniques organic farmers use to control weeds and insects have existed since the beginning of agriculture: crop rotation, cultivation, mulching, soil enrichment, and the encouragement of natural predators and microorganisms that keep pests in check. The report added that farmers who produce organic products "are allowed to use only natural pesticides: insecticidal compounds extracted from plants, bacteria that attack crop pests, soaps, and a few types of metals and minerals. (Some of these can be just as toxic as synthetic pesticides, which is why organic farmers are supposed to use them only as a last resort)" ("Greener Greens": 12–18).

A September 2000 article in the *Baltimore Sun* stated that in order to be considered organic, "crops must be grown without chemical or biological interference, without genetic modifications, on land that is free of contaminants. For animal products, it means animals raised for food must be treated in a humane manner, not confined, not genetically altered, and not given hormones or antibiotics that might show up in meat or dairy products" (Menzie: Page 1F). This type of farming increases labor costs and makes organic foods more expensive (Shapiro: 54).

According to Ronald F. Schmid, a naturopath, "Organic agriculture truly lives and breathes. The soil teems with microorganisms that give vigor and resistance to plants, with worms to aerate the soil and insect predators to control pests. High in humus and nurtured with natural fertilizers, a living soil provides plants with strength to resist disease and insects, as well as superior taste and nutritional value" (Schmid: 170–171). Organic growers manage their farms as whole systems. They focus on improving soil health and use farming methods that prevent problems, such as rotating crops from field to field to manage pests and weeds and to improve soil health and fertility, using animal manures and vegetative matter as fertilizers, monitoring fields regularly to determine when pest or weed control should be done, and recycling and composting organic wastes (Organic Alliance Web site).

For many years, certification of organic farmers was conducted by more than 40 state and private organizations. In December 2000, the USDA issued a universal standard. The new standard, which required more than 10 years to develop and did not become fully effective until mid-2002, prohibited "the use of irradiation, biotechnology and sewer-sludge fertilizer for any food labeled organic." It also forbade "synthetic

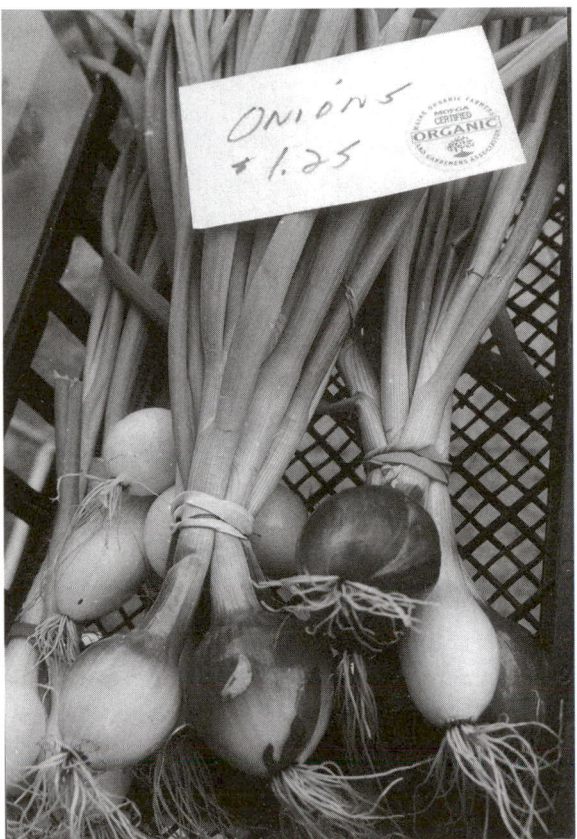

Should consumers pay extra for organic foods? Photo by Samantha A. Goldstein.

pesticides and fertilizers in the growing of organic food, and antibiotics in meat labeled organic" (Burros: Page A20). Further, dairy cattle must "have access to pasture" (Brasher: Page A3). Foods that meet the standard's criteria are labeled "USDA Organic." A USDA news release noted that "all agricultural products labeled organic must originate from farms or handling operations certified by a state or private agency accredited by the USDA. Farms and handling operations that sell less than $5,000 worth per year of organic agricultural products are exempt from certification" (USDA Web site).

The standard also established four categories for labeling. Foods that are labeled "100 percent organic" must contain only organic ingredients. Ninety-five percent of the ingredients of any food labeled "organic" must be organic. Foods that contain at least 70% organic ingredients may contain a label that says, "Made with Organic Ingredients." Three of the ingredients may be noted on the front of the package. Finally, "Processed products with less than 70 percent organic ingredients may list organic ingredients on the information panel but may not carry the term 'organic' anywhere on the front of the package" (Burros: Page A20).

When the standard was announced, Dan Glickman, then the secretary of Agriculture, noted, "Let me be clear about one thing. The organic label is a marketing tool. It is not a statement about food safety. Nor is 'organic' a value judgment about nutrition or quality. USDA is not in the business of choosing sides, of stating preferences for one kind of food, one set of ingredients or one means of production over any other. As long as rigorous government safety standards are being met, we stand ready to do what we can to help support any farmer and help market any kind of food" (National Organic Program Web site).

More than a decade ago, the Organic Foods Protection Act (OFPA) of 1990 was passed. It mandated that the USDA create national standards for organically produced agricultural products. To be sold as organic, products needed to adhere to these standards. "The OFPA and the National Organic Program (NOP) require that agricultural products labeled organic originate from farms or handling operations certified by a State or private agency that has been accredited by the U.S. Department of Agriculture (USDA). The OFPA and proposed regulations do not address food safety or nutrition. The USDA Agricultural Marketing Service, the part of the USDA that set marketing standards, is charged with implementing the NOP" (National Organic Program Web site).

In December 1997, Glickman "proposed federal organic standards for U.S. food crops [that] included . . . genetic engineering, the use of sewage sludge as fertilizer, irradiation and livestock confinement practices" (Rembert: 16–19). The National Organic Program Web site noted that the USDA "received 275,603 public comments, explaining why and how the rule should be rewritten." It is believed that the proposed standards were created following much lobbying from the giant businesses. How else, for example, could one explain the addition of sludge? "Sewage sludge contains some 60,000 toxic chemicals, a mix of residential, industrial and commercial discharge that includes hospital wastes, street runoff, heavy metals, PCBs, dioxin, solvents, asbestos and radioactive wastes" (Rembert: 16–19). New standards that prohibited the use of genetic engineering and addressed the other contested issues were proposed in March 2000. All products labeled "USDA Certified Organic" must "be produced without toxic pesticides or toxic 'inert ingredients'; . . . antibiotics, growth hormones, and rendered animal protein cannot be administered or fed to animals; . . . intensive confinement of livestock will not be allowed; and . . . no synthetics or chemicals will be allowed in organic production without the approval of the NOSB [National Organic Standards

Board]" (Cummins: 12). The standards were further modified and, as noted, presented in their final form in December 2000.

PESTICIDES

Organic farmers use no synthetic pesticides. The previously mentioned *Consumer Reports* story stated that pesticides are poisonous compounds that are designed to kill elements of nature that damage crops, including insects and fungal pests. As such, they have the potential to cause a variety of medical problems. Information about the effects of pesticides has primarily been obtained from studies of pesticide applicators and farmworkers. Common reactions to pesticides include nausea, lung and eye irritation, and temporary nerve damage. Long-term and chronic medical problems have been harder to verify, but farmers using more pesticides seem to be at greater risk than nonfarmers for some forms of cancer and amyotropic lateral sclerosis (Lou Gehrig's disease), and tests on animals indicate that some pesticides may cause birth and immune-system defects. It is suspected that many pesticides may interfere with hormone systems that regulate functions like reproduction. "For consumers in general, the unsettling truth is that no one really knows what a lifetime of consuming the tiny quantities of pesticides found on foods might do to a person. The effect, if any, is likely to be small for most individuals—but may be significant for the population at large" ("Greener Greens": 12–18).

In *The Organic Gourmet: Feast of Fields*, Tracy Kett, a writer, caterer, and promoter of organic agriculture, noted, "Several studies have found that the possible short- and long-term human health effects of agricultural chemicals are numerous and range from respiratory problems in field workers (despite hazardous working conditions, farmers and their employees often work without any kind of safety clothing or respiratory protection) to severe allergic and asthmatic reactions, reproductive disorders, cancer and degenerative diseases in both consumers and farm workers." Most of these chemicals have no purpose. "According to research done at Cornell University, 500 million kilograms (1.1 billion pounds) of pesticide chemicals are applied in North America every year. Of that amount, 99.9 percent miss the target organism" (Kett: 13–14).

In *Eating with the Seasons*, Paula Bartimeus, a professional nutritionist and regular writer for health magazines, said that "although the Government states that the levels of pesticides used are well within the safety margins, random testing has proved otherwise. Many farmers mix chemicals before spraying, and the combined and cumulative effects of such concoctions are still uncertain" (Bartimeus: 7–8). The author of *Designer Poisons*, Marion Moses, lists some precautionary statements from pesticide labels: "Avoid inhalation or contact with eyes or skin. Harmful if swallowed. May cause eye irritation." "Avoid eye contact. Wash thoroughly after handling." "Corrosive to eyes. Causes eye damage. Do not get in eyes. Harmful if swallowed. Avoid contact with skin or clothing." "Do not apply to excessively sunburned or damaged skin. May cause skin reaction in rare cases." "Do not get in eyes, on skin, or clothing. Harmful if swallowed, inhaled or absorbed through skin" (Moses: 21).

The Environmental Protection Agency (EPA) regulates pesticides, but there is concern that the regulation is inadequate. A 1998 article in *Country Living* magazine noted that a number of groups concerned about the use of pesticides believe that the EPA "has not tested all the ingredients in these chemicals and does not require companies to disclose or label their so-called inert ingredients." Moreover, the EPA fails to "take into consideration the effects of combinations of pesticides (only the effects of individual pesticides have been studied)." Further, there is no acknowledgment that almost all pesticides "drift from their point of application" (Howe: 44–45). The *Consumer Reports* article noted, "The legal limits for pesticide residues on foods—all 9700 of them—are based mainly on animal toxicity tests, with an additional 'uncertainty factor' as a theoretical safety margin for human exposure. If a pesticide, applied according to the package label, doesn't result in residues higher than a safe level, that safe level becomes the legal limit. But the legal limit can sometimes exceed the level that safety alone would require if the government decides the benefit to farmers outweighs the risk to consumers" ("Greener Greens": 12–18).

Another concern is that "because government standards for pesticide levels are based on the height and weight of an adult man, it's unclear whether pesticide consumption at those levels might be harmful to a child" (Gallagher: 81–82). A five-year study completed by the National Academy of Sciences found that children were more vulnerable to pesticides than adults (Cheney: 90–93). Nutritionist Susan M. Kleiner offered several reasons. "Children eat more food in proportion to their body weight than do adults, so their exposure to pesticides in greater. Children eat more fruit . . . compared with adults. Children will often eat a lot of one or two specific foods. If that food has pesticide residues, it will increase their exposure to pesticides" (Kleiner: 15–16).

The Environmental Working Group (EWG), a leading content provider for public interest groups with a special interest in the effect pesticides have on children, arranged for laboratory evaluations of baby foods produced by Gerber, Heinz, and Beech-Nut. The testers "found 16 different pesticides in eight baby food products tested. Of those 16 pesticides, three are probably human carcinogens, five are possible human carcinogens, eight are neurotoxins, five are endocrine disruptors, and five are categorized as oral toxicity 1 chemical, the most toxic designation. More than half of all samples (53 percent) contained detectable levels of pesticides, 18 percent of samples had two or more pesticides in them, and one sample contained three different pesticides" (Environmental Working Group Web site).

The EWG obtained data from the U.S. Food and Drug Administration on the pesticide content of 42 fruits and vegetables. "More than half of the total dietary risk from pesticides in these foods was concentrated in just 12 crops. The pesticides that were found in these foods are classified by the Environmental Protection Agency (EPA) as probable human carcinogens, nervous system poisons and endocrine system disrupters." The 12 most contaminated foods, in order of levels of contamination, were strawberries, bell peppers (green and red) and spinach (tied), cherries (U.S.), peaches, cantaloupe (Mexican), celery, apples, apricots, green beans, grapes (Chilean), and cucumbers (Environmental Working Group Web site).

It should not be surprising that there has been a boom in the sale of organic baby food. "According to a study conducted by the U.S. Department of Agriculture's (USDA) Economic Research Service, sales of organic baby food increased a whopping 2,200% between 1989 and 1995." Additionally, "supermarkets posted a sales gain of nearly 25% for organic and natural baby food during the 12-month period [that] ended [in] April 1999" (Donegan: 51–54).

At least one school system—Berkeley, California—is offering pesticide-, herbicide-, and hormone-free foods to its students. "For now, schools are buying their goods from Berkeley's twice-a-week farmers' market, from where organic farmers and vendors are regularly invited to visit with students to explain their natural farming techniques. Educators hope to integrate gardening know-how with classroom education, and, in the future, individual schools plan to start up organic gardens of their own" (Wright: 13).

One cannot just wash off the pesticides before preparing the food, because some pesticides are not water soluble. Also, "Many chemicals routinely used in farming can penetrate the fruit or vegetable skin and therefore can't be washed off. Peeling helps remove them but eliminates valuable nutrients in the process. And . . . a wax coating . . . not only seals in pesticides, but the wax itself may contain fungicides, coloring agents and other potentially unhealthy substances" (Cheney: 90–93).

LIMITATIONS OF ORGANIC FOODS

Organic foods, however, are not necessarily healthful or safe. A high-fat food that is made from organic products remains high in fat. "You can buy organic chocolate bars, ice cream and cookies—all made with ingredients that are pesticide-, chemical-, antibiotic- and hormone-free— but they'll be laden with fat, sugar and calories" (Gallagher: 81–82).

Moreover, the manure that organic farmers may use could contain bacteria. "The only real difference between organic and nonorganic food is in the growing—and that's not a big enough difference to protect your health from bacteria." An article in *Newsweek* noted that a food scientist and director of research at an organic food distributor said, "There really isn't any difference between organic and nonorganic as far as the risks for, say, cyclospora or E. coli" (Rogers: 31).

Commenting on the manure used by organic farmers, the Organic Trade Association Web site noted, "Conventional and organic agriculture both use manure as a part of regular farm soil fertilization programs. Certified organic farmers, however, must maintain a strict farm plan detailing the methods used to build soil fertility, including the application of manure as mandated by the Organic Foods Production Act of 1990. No other agricultural regulation in the United States imposes such strict control on the use of manure" (Organic Trade Association Web site).

Like other forms of food production, there may be compromises in the healthfulness of the organic food environment. In a January 1999 issue of the *Humanist*, Lisa Hamilton wrote that the major producers "may dump obscene amounts of quick-to-leach chicken manure on poor soil, carrying hazardous nitrates directly to groundwater, or blast crops with the nonexclusive, plant-based pesticide Pyrethrum, killing most (if not all) insects in range, including beneficial ladybugs and lacewings" (Hamilton: 41).

Nevertheless, a May 2000 survey of 1,029 men and women commissioned by the National Center for Public Policy Research, a Washington, DC, nonprofit education foundation, found that the majority of the public believe that products labeled "USDA Certified Organic" would be "safer," "better," and "healthier for consumers" than nonorganic foods. Responding to the results of this study, John Carlisle, director of the Environmental Policy Task Force at the National Center for Public Policy Research, said that misperceptions about the benefits and risks of organically certified products would be heightened by this USDA proposed label. "Clearly, consumers want the USDA to amend this rule to include specific language on the USDA proposed seal to inform consumers that organic certification is based on production methods and conveys no assurance of food safety, nutrition or other quality" (National Center for Public Policy Research Web site).

As a result of this study, the National Center for Public Policy Research advised against the creation of a USDA organic seal that would only impart misinformation and create confusion. A letter from John E. Frydenlund, the director of the taxpayer watchdog group Citizens against Government Waste, to the program manager of the federal government's National Organic Program stated that "there is no scientific evidence that organic food is safer, healthier, or, in any way, better than non-organic food." Moreover, Frydenlund continued, there are "inadequate safeguards to protect consumers from the health dangers caused by composted and raw manure used in organic production. This inadequacy is exacerbated by a failure to provide adequate information informing consumers of the particular health dangers that exist in the consumption of organic foods" (Citizens against Government Waste Web site). Nevertheless, a USDA organic seal was designed and made available when the December 2000 organic standard was issued.

According to the National Center for Public Policy Research, there are some additional limitations to organic farming. "Because organic farmers eschew pesticides and herbicides used by conventional farmers, they cannot use modern conservation tillage techniques that have been extraordinarily successful in reducing soil erosion. As a result, compared to conventional farming, organic farming is woefully inadequate in controlling soil erosion. . . . But the most glaring environmental disadvantage of organic farming is its exorbitant need for land. Organic farming is only about half as productive as conventional farming, which means organic farming requires far more land to feed the world than modern methods" (National Center for Public Policy Research Web site). In an interview published in the April 2000 issue of *Reason*, Nobel Peace Prize winner Norman Borlaug, an agronomist, noted, "Even if you could use all the organic material that you have—the animal manures, the human waste, the plant residues—and get them back on the soil, you couldn't feed more than four billion people. In addition, if all agriculture were organic, you would have to increase cropland area dramatically, spreading out into marginal areas and cutting down millions of acres of forests" (Bailey: 30).

These are essentially the beliefs of Dennis T. Avery, an expert in international agriculture, in *Saving the Planet with Pesticides and Plastic*. "With present knowledge levels, no responsible authority or organization should recommend either organic farming or traditional low-yield farming systems as a broad-gauge alternative to high-yield agriculture. In fact, slashing farm chemical usage is likely to produce more soil erosion, more human cancer, and less wildlife habitat. At present, organic farming could not even sustain the fertility of our existing cropland, or protect it effectively from erosion" (Avery: 167).

Regardless, the previously noted *Consumer Reports* article concluded by advising people to incorporate organic food into their diets. "Organic food guarantees you a diet as low in pesticide residues as possible. On a public scale, organic agriculture practices are much less harmful to the environment than conventional chemical agriculture" ("Greener Greens": 12–18).

CONCLUSION

Is organic food worth the extra cost? That depends on how you feel about production of the food that you eat. If you believe, as the federal government contends, that the pesticides used are generally safe, then you will most likely be comfortable with regular commercially prepared foods. On the other hand, if you worry about the long-term consequences of ingesting pesticides, then you should probably pay extra for organic products. But remember not to assume that the organic seal indicates that a food is safe, superior, or healthful. The organic seal only denotes how the product was produced.

TOPICS FOR DISCUSSION

1. Why do you think the organic food market is growing at such a fast pace?
2. Does your family buy organic foods? Why or why not?
3. Has your family ever had an organic garden? If so, was it successful? How would you rate the food that was grown?
4. Do you think that the USDA was correct in issuing a universal organic standard? Why or why not?
5. Do you think that pesticides are as harmful as some people contend?Why or why not?

REFERENCES AND RESOURCES

Books

Avery, Dennis T. *Saving the Planet with Pesticides and Plastic*. Indianapolis: Hudson Institute, 1995.

Bartimeus, Paula. *Eating with the Seasons*. Boston: Element Books, 1998.

Chandler, Gary, and Kevin Graham. *Natural Foods and Products*. New York: Twenty-First Century Books, 1996.

Dominé, André, editor. *Organic and Wholefoods*. Cologne, Germany: Könemann, 1997.

Haas, Elson M. *The Staying Healthy Shopper's Guide*. Berkeley, California: Celestial Arts, 1999.

Harrison, John Bede. *Growing Food Organically*. Seattle: Waterwheel Press, 1993.

Jack, Alex. *Let Food Be Thy Medicine*. Becket, Massachusetts: One Peaceful World Press, 1999.

Kett, Tracy. *The Organic Gourmet: Feast of Fields*. Toronto, Ontario, Canada: Robert Rose, 1998.

Moses, Marion. *Designer Poisons*. San Francisco: Pesticide Education Center, 1995.

Peavy, William S., and Warren Peary. *Super Nutrition Gardening*. Garden City Park, New York: Avery Publishing Group, 1993.

Richard, David, and Dorie Byers, editors. *Taste Life!* Bloomingdale, Illinois: Vital Health Publishing, 1998.

Schmid, Ronald F. *Traditional Foods Are Your Best Medicine*. Rochester, Vermont: Healing Arts Press, 1997.

Magazines, Journals, and Newspapers

Bailey, Ronald. "Billions Served." *Reason*, April 2000, 31(11): 30.

Brasher, Philip. "Standards for Food Labeled Organic." *Boston Globe*, December 21, 2000: Page A3.

Burros, Marian. "U.S. Imposes Standards for Organic-Food Labeling." *New York Times*, December 21, 2000: Page A20.

Cheney, Susan Jane. "Organics: Are They Worth the $$?" *Vegetarian Times*, November 1999, 267: 90–93.

Cummins, Ronnie. "USDA Surrenders on Organic Standards." *Animals' Agenda*, May–June 2000, 20(3): 12.

Donegan, Priscilla. "Whole Health Hits the Baby Aisle." *Grocery Headquarters*, August 1999, 65(8): 51–54.

Fulmer, Melinda. "USDA Finally Sets Down Rules for Organic Food." *Los Angeles Times*, December 21, 2000: Part C, page 1.

Gallagher, Stephanie. "Organic Foods: Pricier, But Safer?" *Kiplinger's Personal Finance Magazine*, July 1997, 51(7): 81–82.

"Greener Greens." *Consumer Reports*, January 1998, 63(1): 12–18.

Hamilton, Lisa. "Diamonds in the Dirt?" *Humanist*, January 1999, 59(1): 41.

Howe, Maggy. "Pesticides in Our Produce: What Goes into the Fresh Fruits and Vegetables You Buy?" *Country Living*, March 1998, 21(3): 44–45.

Howell, Debbie. "Popularity Growing for Organics." *DSN Retailing Today*, May 22, 2000, 39(10): 4.

Kleiner, Susan M. "Should You Opt for Organic?" *Physician and Sportsmedicine*, December 1995, 23(12): 15–16.

Loftus, Margaret, and Mary Brophy Marcus. "Hold the Chemicals: Chefs and Grocers Sell More Organic Food; Defining It Is Tricky." *U.S. News and World Report*, May 18, 1998, 124(19): 74–76.

Lunna, Rebecca. "Eat Organic." *MPLS–St. Paul Magazine*, April 2000, 28(4): 150.

Menzie, Karol V. "U.S. Poised to Define Organic Foods for National Standards." *Baltimore Sun*, September 27, 2000: Page 1F.

Rembert, Tracey C. "Food Porn: Organic Foods May Be Grown with Sewage Sludge and Drugs." *E*, May/June 1998, 9(3): 16–19.

Rogers, Adam. "Trendy—But Is It Safe?" *Newsweek*, September 1, 1997, 130(9): 31.

Shapiro, Laura. "Is Organic Better?" *Newsweek*, June 1, 1998, 131(22): 54.

Wright, Fred W., Jr. "Small Soldiers and Better Food." *Mother Earth News*, February 2000: Page 13.

Organizations to Contact

Center for Global Food Issues
P.O. Box 202
Churchville, VA 24421-0202
Phone: 540-337-6354
http://www.cgfi.com/ (December 29, 2000)

Citizens against Government Waste
1301 Connecticut Avenue NW, Suite 400
Washington, DC 20036
Phone: 202-467-5300
http://www.cagw.org/ (December 29, 2000)

Environmental Working Group
1718 Connecticut Ave NW, Suite 600
Washington, DC 20009
Phone: 202-667-6982
http://www.ewg.org/ (November 11, 2000)

The National Center for Public Policy Research
777 N. Capitol St. NE, Suite 803
Washington, DC 20002
Phone: 202-371-1400
http://www.nationalcenter.org/ (November 20, 2000)

National Organic Program
USDA-AMS-TMP-NOP
Room 4008-South Building
14th and Independence Ave. SW, Ag Stop 0268
Washington, DC 20250-0020
Phone: 202-720-3252
http://www.ams.usda.gov/ (November 19, 2000)

Organic Alliance
400 Selby Avenue, Suite T
St. Paul, MN 55102
Phone: 651-265-3678
http://www.organic.org/ (November 16, 2000)

Organic Trade Association
P.O. Box 547
Greenfield, MA 01301
Phone: 413-774-7511
http://www.ota.com/

United States Department of Agriculture
14th and Independence Ave. SW
Washington, DC 20250
Phone: 202-720-2791
http://www.usda.gov/ (December 20, 2000)

13

High-Protein Diets

Millions of Americans are trying to lose weight. Only a small number accomplish their goal. Some contend that a high-protein diet is the best way to achieve this.

An estimated 54 million Americans are on a diet (International Food Information Council Web site). There are some people who believe that the solution to weight loss lies in high-protein diets or diets that include a higher proportion of protein than most people consume. They argue that this is how humans are genetically programmed to eat.

Clearly, protein is a vital component of everyone's diet. "Second only to water, it makes up the greatest percentage of our body weight. This key nutrient provides the building blocks kids and adults need for growing, maintaining, and repairing worn-out cells. Without protein, our bodies couldn't regulate fluids and our immune systems would shut down. In fact, if it weren't for protein there would be no hormones or enzymes—the protein compounds that take part in every single physical function" (Albertson: 118). Protein builds skin, bones, and muscle. Our bodies are formed from the protein we obtain from foods.

In *Charles Hunt's Diet Evolution*, Charles Hunt, who developed his own fitness program, notes that Stone Age anthropologists have found that "wherever grains became the mainstay of human diets, there was a universal drop in height, muscularity, and even cranial capacity" (Hunt: 14). Further, Hunt adds, people do not overeat high-protein foods. "Nobody binges on roast, fish or steak. Nobody binges on sticks of butter or lard by themselves. They are naturally self-limiting. When you've had enough to satisfy your nutritional needs, you stop. No problem. Try that with sugar-grain combinations (like cake and cookies), sugar-fat combinations (like ice cream and icing), and grain-fat combinations (like potato

chips, corn chips and bread)! We become 'bottomless pits' with no natural shut-off valve" (Hunt: 13–14).

High-protein diets are not new. Some doctors have advocated them
for decades. There have been a number of different varieties. All are
controversial. Every high-protein diet increases protein intake while
sharply reducing carbohydrate consumption. A 1997 article in the *Harvard Health Letter* notes that "these diets generally urge people to eat a
lot of protein-rich foods—such as steak and cheese—and to avoid rice,
pasta, grains, and many fruits and vegetables." While the specifics of the
diets vary, "the underlying theory is the same: carbohydrates—not just
in pasta and bread but also in fruit—are to blame for most weight problems" (Norris: 1–3). They maintain that eating carbohydrates stimulates
the release of excess insulin, "causing carbohydrates to be taken to the
cells and stored as fat instead of being used for energy" (Heart Information Network Web site). To lose weight, dieters must decrease starchy
carbohydrates and sweets and instead focus on eating meats and vegetables. A 2000 article in *Prevention* that lists a number of positive elements
in high-protein diets says that "for most people, that means trading in
nutrient-empty white flour and sugar for nutrient-laden protein and produce" (Pierre and Robertson: 134).

As might be expected, high-protein diets have generated heated debate. In fact, some contend that high-protein diets have the potential to
be quite dangerous. The American Dietetic Association, the American
College of Sports Medicine, and the Women's Sports Foundation have
denounced them (International Food Information Council Web site). The
Heart Information Network notes that "all the major professional health
organizations, including the American Heart Association, the National
Cholesterol Education Program, and the American Cancer Society, endorse a diet that is composed of 10% to 15% protein, 55% to 60% carbohydrates, and 25% to 30% fat" (Heart Information Network Web site).
While the percentages of protein, carbohydrates, and fat advocated by
the high-protein diets vary from diet to diet, they generally call for at
least twice this amount of protein, at least half the amount of carbohydrates, and about the same amount of fat.

According to the Heart Information Network, high-protein diets are
based on faulty science. Carbohydrates are not the only source of weight
gain. Rather, calories from all foods "are converted into glucose to be
stored for energy. Glucose is stored as fat only when you have consumed
excess calories. So it's your overall calorie intake and not carbohydrates
that cause fat storage and weight gain. Besides, foods high in protein,
such as meats and cheeses, are also high in saturated fat. These foods
are known to increase cholesterol levels when eaten in excess" (Heart
Information Network Web site).

SPECIFIC ELEMENTS OF SOME HIGH-PROTEIN DIETS

The most popular of all high-protein diets is the Atkins Diet introduced by Robert C. Atkins, a New York City cardiologist, in his 1970s best-seller *Dr. Atkins' Diet Revolution*. Since that first book on his diet, Atkins has written several more. His works have sold millions of copies.

Atkins contends that the majority of people follow the wrong route to weight loss. They eliminate red meat from their diets and prepare their scrambled egg whites with little or no oil; they remove the skin from their chicken and use no butter on their potatoes and pasta. Oatmeal and skim milk become preferred breakfast foods, and desserts may consist of frozen yogurt or fruit sorbet. But the weight does not drop.

Atkins says that most doctors believe that the only way to lose weight is to reduce calories. To Atkins, that is incorrect. "Different kinds of diets can have different effects on the amount of calories a person's body consumes daily, and, by taking different metabolic pathways, can cause the body to *require* different amounts of energy to do its work. On a low-carbohydrate diet, there are metabolic advantages that will allow you to *eat as many or more calories as you were eating before starting the diet and still begin losing pounds and inches*. And if you eat fewer calories—most people do on this diet—you'll lose weight very fast" (Atkins: 10).

There are negative aspects that Atkins does not address. High amounts of dietary cholesterol—especially over an extended period of time—are dangerous. Foods high in cholesterol contribute to an elevated cholesterol level and other cardiovascular problems. While rapid weight loss may be psychologically desirable, it is not necessarily good for the body. It is far healthier to lose weight continuously over a longer period of time.

Atkins says that Americans historically ate very little sugar. In 1828, the average American consumed only 12 pounds a year. In 1990, it was found that the typical American annually ate 137.5 pounds of sugar (Atkins: 44). "Since the average person eats 425 grams of carbohydrates a day, 105 grams of protein, and 168 grams of fat, sugar constitutes 40% of the carbohydrate total and nearly one fourth of our daily food by weight. Sugar has no nutritional value and is directly harmful to your health" (Atkins: 45).

Atkins says that earlier Americans were carnivores whose diets included beef, fish, fowl, pork, and eggs. But, he maintains, hardly anyone died from heart attacks. As a result, Atkins claims that the human body was designed to eat those types of foods. He says that the host of medical problems facing Americans today is largely caused by the contemporary diet. Still, the lifestyle of the average earlier American required a good deal of hard labor, and they probably burned off much of the fat that they ate. The Atkins diet does not focus on exercise. Yet,

Atkins does advise it and calls it an "essential part of the program" (Atkins: 202).

Atkins says that the amount of insulin in the blood is a function of the level of carbohydrates. Diets that are high in carbohydrates encourage the production of insulin. When there is too much sugar in the blood for the available insulin to handle, the excess is converted to fat. When fewer carbohydrates are consumed, the body will burn its own fat for energy.

During the first 14 days of the Atkins diet, known as the "Induction Diet," dieters are able to eat all the high-protein foods they wish. Carbohydrates are limited to 20 grams per day—"about one hot-dog bun's worth." The goal is to "trigger ketosis," the burning of stored fat for energy. Then, until the ideal weight is achieved, between 25 and 75 grams of carbohydrates may be consumed each day. When maintenance is reached, there may be a little more flexibility (Jibrin: 78).

In *Dr. Atkins' New Diet Revolution*, Atkins describes people who have witnessed dramatic improvements on his diet. One example is an overweight man in his 60s who survived three heart attacks. The man also had arthritis and high cholesterol. Atkins eliminated ice cream and French fries from his diet and "urged him to eat a lot of meat, fish, fowl, and eggs when he wanted them, nuts, salads, vegetables, and a little cheese." The man's cholesterol went down from 228 to 157, and his weight dropped from 228 to 190, "a pretty good weight for a powerfully built six-footer." The man also experienced an improvement in his arthritis symptoms (Atkins: 10–11).

Another hugely popular high-protein diet, the Zone, was introduced by Barry Sears, a biochemist, in his mid-1990s best-seller *The Zone*. In the preface of this book, Sears explains his motivation to find a healthier lifestyle: he was a "walking genetic time bomb" (Sears, 1995: ix). Sears says that he was genetically programmed to die young of heart disease. Before they reached the age of 54, his grandfather, father, and three uncles died from heart attacks. Searching for a way to avoid this fate, Sears eventually came upon eicosanoids—hormones that "act as 'master switches' that control virtually all human body functions—including the cardiovascular system, the immune system, and the systems that govern how much fat we store (and therefore how much we weigh)." Sears believes that many diseases such as heart disease, diabetes, arthritis, and cancer are caused by imbalances among the eicosanoid hormones. He claims that maintaining and restoring the balance "might help prevent or even become the primary treatment for these diseases" (Sears, 1995: xiv).

Eicosanoids have the potential to do even more. They "might help maintain a state of nearly perpetual good health: a molecular definition of 'wellness' that would lead to a better quality of life. As an ultimate payoff, keeping eicosanoids in balance might help all of us reach that near-euphoric state of maximum physical, mental, and psychological performance that athletes call 'the Zone' " (Sears, 1995: xiv).

Sears says that his diet uses food "to manipulate [the] eicosanoid balance." This manipulation is a "passport to the Zone" (Sears, 1995: xv). In Sears's system, all calories are not created equal. "The hormonal effect of a calorie of carbohydrate is different than the hormonal effect of a calorie of protein, and is still different from the hormonal effect of a calorie of fat. Each of these three nutrients has its own unique effects on your body's hormones. In the proper balance, these three nutrients are exactly what your body needs to remain healthy by keeping insulin within the Zone." When the nutrients are imbalanced and insulin levels rise, the body's hormonal stability is altered, "resulting in weight gain, an increased likelihood of chronic disease, and acceleration of the aging process." However, "if insulin levels are too low, your cells begin to starve because a certain amount of insulin is required to drive life-sustaining nutrients into your cells" (Sears, 2000: 3–4).

Sears recommends a diet that is 40% carbohydrate, 30% protein and 30% fat; it has a daily intake of between 1,100 and 1,600 calories. Each meal should include a low-fat protein. In the Zone diet, protein is obtained from leaner sources such as turkey, fish, skinless chicken, egg whites, soy meat substitutes, tofu, and 1% cottage cheese. A tiny amount of good fat, such as that in nuts or olive oil, is advised. At least for the first two weeks, rather than eating pasta, bread, and potatoes, carbohydrates should be obtained from fruits and vegetables. According to Sears, people who follow his diet should lose between 1 and 1½ pounds per week without feeling hungry (Stedman: 73–74).

After *The Zone*, Sears wrote several more books. In *A Week in the Zone* he summarized the basic Zone rules:

1. Always eat a Zone meal within one hour after waking.
2. Try to eat five times per day: three Zone meals and two Zone snacks.
3. Never let more than five hours go by without eating a Zone meal or snack.
4. Eat more fruits and vegetables and less bread, grains, and other starches.
5. Drink at least eight eight-ounce glasses of water every day.
6. Don't worry about an occasional mistake at a meal; just be sure to make the next meal a Zone meal. (Sears, 2000: 5–6)

In the same book, Sears listed some of the long-term benefits of the Zone diet: permanent fat loss, reduced risk of heart disease, breast cancer, and type 2 diabetes, protection from arthritis and osteoporosis, and fewer infections (Sears, 2000: 19–20). He also disputed the generally accepted notion that his diet is high in protein, noting that it consists of more carbohydrates than protein (Sears, 2000: 16–17).

In *The Carbohydrate Addict's Lifespan Program*, Richard F. Heller and Rachael F. Heller maintain that some people are "addicted" to carbohydrates. They define this addiction as "a compelling, recurring or, at times, escalating craving for starches such as bread, pasta, rice, or potatoes, or for snack foods such as chips, popcorn, or pretzels, or for sweets such as cookies, cakes, pies, donuts, muffins, or chocolate." These people have "a tendency to gain weight easily or, over time, to regain weight that has been lost by dieting." The Hellers add that carbohydrate addicts do not necessarily eat more food than nonaddicts. Sometimes they eat less, but, "The carbohydrate addict's body . . . may be much more efficient at turning food energy into fat" (Heller and Heller: 21–22).

According to the Hellers, carbohydrate addiction is caused by an imbalance of insulin in the body. Some carbohydrate addicts produce too much insulin. Others have cells that resist insulin, and the excess insulin remains in the bloodstream. Some carbohydrate addicts have both problems (Heller and Heller: 24). Whatever the cause, there is too much insulin in the blood.

In essence, the Hellers advise an eating plan that has two high-protein/high-fiber vegetable meals per day and one meal that includes carbohydrates. The meal with carbohydrates should begin with two cups of fresh salad. The remaining foods should look like a plate divided into thirds. "Place the vegetables, the proteins, and the carbohydrates (including dessert) in each of the thirds" (Heller and Heller: 112). Second helpings are permitted, but they must be eaten in the same proportions— no seconds of carbohydrates without the vegetables and proteins. All the food should be consumed within an hour. A daily consumption of six to eight glasses of water is required.

In the hugely popular *Sugar Busters!* H. Leighton Steward, a writer and former business executive, and doctors Morrison C. Bethea, Samuel S. Andrews, and Luis A. Balart contend that the primary culprit for ill health and excess weight is sugar. In their diet, people need to avoid "foods or combinations of foods that require the secretion of large amounts of insulin." To these authors, "*refined* sugar in any significant quantity is toxic to many human bodies, and it certainly helps make many bodies fat" (Steward et al.: 2–3). They advise a diet of "natural unrefined sugars, whole unprocessed grains, vegetables, fruits, lean meats, fiber, and alcohol (in moderation)" and provide lists of acceptable foods (Steward et al.: 118, 123–126). Foods such as potatoes, beets, and carrots, which are "simply starch, a storage form of glucose," are eliminated because they are converted to pure sugar during digestion (Steward et al.: 120–121). *Sugar Busters!* advises drinking only a small amount

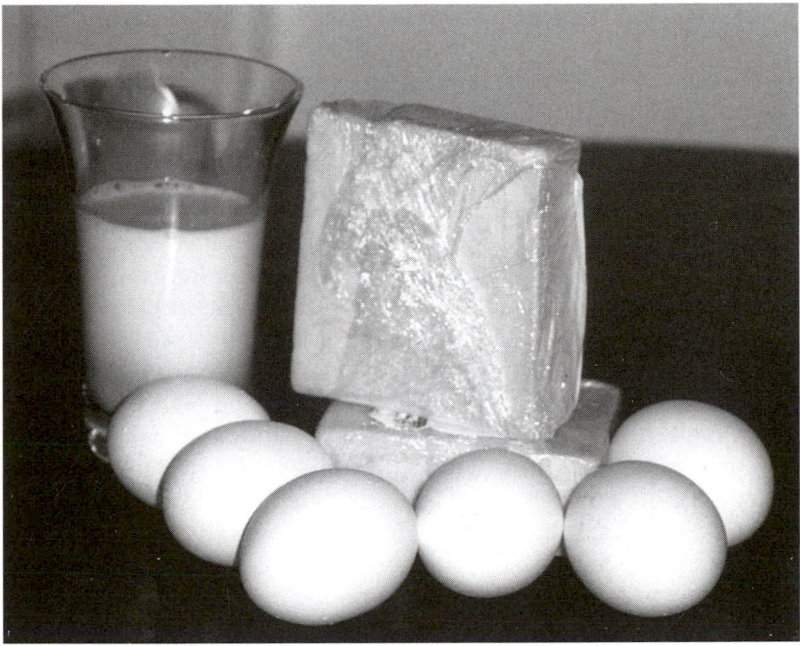

High protein diets may not necessarily be healthful. Photo by Mark A. Goldstein.

of fluids with meals. It contends that excess fluids impair digestion. On the other hand, additional fluids may be consumed between meals.

LIMITATIONS OF HIGH-PROTEIN DIETS

A 1997 article in the *Harvard Health Letter* raised a number of concerns about high-protein diets. While it is true that about 25% of Americans are insulin resistant, it is generally believed that this is not caused by eating too many carbohydrates. On the contrary, it is thought to be a direct result of excess weight and a sedentary lifestyle. Some people lose a considerable amount of weight on high-protein diets. When they do, this is assumed to be caused by eating fewer calories. The American Dietetic Association suggests that a 154-pound man eats about 2,600 calories per day. A man of that size on the Zone diet would eat about 900 calories a day. That is quite restrictive (Norris: 1–3).

The same article notes that Americans do not consume inadequate amounts of protein. On the contrary, Americans eat about 80 to 90 grams each day, almost twice what they need. In sharp contrast to the proponents of high-protein diets, this article emphasizes that these diets foster cardiovascular disease and high cholesterol levels and increase the risk of cancer. The article also criticizes Atkins's view of ketosis, or the burning of fat for energy. Because of the loss of water, sodium, and potassium, ketosis may trigger an uneasy feeling and lightheadedness. The lack of fiber may result in constipation. There may be a diminished appetite and nausea. If the uric acid level rises too high, it could set off an episode of gout (Norris: 1–3).

While acknowledging that people are losing weight on high-protein diets, a 1999 story in *Men's Health* mentioned some of the limitations. Like the previous article, it expressed concern about ketosis, which may also produce bad breath and heart irregularities. It further noted that there might be a reduced ability to exercise. The diet could also be dangerous for people with impaired kidney function (Jibrin: 78).

A 2000 article in the *Journal of the American Dietetic Association* said that books on high-protein diets are filled with anecdotal evidence, but there are few if any hard data to prove the theses. "Often the information communicated in the diet books is exaggerated or interpreted in such a way that cannot be proven" (Stein: 760). Additionally, the International Food Information Council Web site says, "There is a dire lack of scientific research to corroborate the theories expounded in the majority of diet books currently on the market. . . . Authors may simplify or expand upon biochemistry and physiology in an effort to help support their theories and provide a plethora of scientific jargon that people do not understand but that seems to make sense. And few, if any, offer solid scientific support for their claims in the form of published research studies. Instead, most evidence is based on anecdotal findings, theories, and testimonials of short-term results." This Web site also lists concerns specific to each of several high-protein diets, such as those of Atkins and Sears.

Writing in 1999 in *Prevention*, Elizabeth Somer, a registered dietician, says that high-protein diets may prompt depression. "Ironically, all that protein has the effect of lowering the level of the amino acid tryptophan in your brain, which is the building block for the mood-lifting brain chemical serotonin. High levels of serotonin boost your mood, but low levels can result in depression. No other nerve chemical is as strongly linked to your diet as is serotonin." In sharp contrast to the high-protein advocates, Somer advises people to "make sure that every meal contains some carbohydrate-rich foods, especially whole grain foods such as whole wheat bread, oatmeal, or brown rice. Carbohydrates trigger the release of insulin, which allows tryptophan to freely enter your brain, causing serotonin levels to rise" (Somer, December 1999: 124–129).

Two separate studies published in 1998 in the *American Journal of Clinical Nutrition* found that high-protein diets may predispose people to some nutritional deficiencies. One study found that a high-animal-protein diet was correlated with the loss of calcium in the urine (Itoh, Nishiyama, and Suyama: 438–444). The other study determined that young women on high-protein diets appear to have greater requirements for vitamin B6 (Huang et al.: 208–220).

A 2000 article in *Runner's World* advises runners not to follow a high-protein diet for a number of reasons. The diet does not contain a sufficient amount of carbohydrates to "fuel" running. Runners require a minimum of 400 grams per day of carbohydrates. "But possibly the worst part of the high-protein diets—for runners—is how tired you feel. . . . After a week or so on the diet, you must either give up running or agree that this low-carbohydrate thing is for the birds (or more accurately, cats, who survive best on a high-protein diet)" (Applegate: 30).

A 1997 article in *Prevention* magazine included input from Jay Kenny, a nutritionist with the Pritikin Longevity Center. According to the author, Colleen Pierre, Kenny wondered why the Japanese, who eat a high-carbohydrate diet, are "enviably slim." Insulin, he added, does not make people overweight. Instead, extra weight raises insulin levels. Losing weight generally reduces the amount of insulin in the blood (Pierre: 85–91).

A study published in 1998 in *Pediatrics* described the effects of a high-protein, very low-calorie diet on six morbidly obese adolescents. The adolescents, between the ages of 12 and 15, all weighed more than 200% of the ideal body weight. For the first eight weeks, "daily intake consisted of 650 to 725 calories, which was substantially in the form of protein (80–100g). The diet was very low in carbohydrates (25g)." During this phase, the patients lost an average of 15.4 kg, an amount that was statistically significant. Then, for an additional 12 weeks, two carbohydrates (30g) were added at each meal. While on this phase of the diet, one subject regained the weight. The remaining five lost an average of 4.9kg, a figure that was not statistically significant. As a result, the researchers concluded that the very low-calorie, high-protein diet "can be used effectively for rapid weight loss in adolescents with morbid obesity. Loss in lean body mass is blunted, blood chemistries remain normal and sleep abnormalities significantly decrease with weight loss." Nevertheless, there were a few words of caution. Although the subjects consumed large amounts of supplemental calcium, during the high-protein phase, "bone mineral density decreased significantly" (Willi et al.: 61–67).

Though it does not advocate high-protein diets, a 2000 article in *Prevention* lists some ways to make them healthier:

- Have your doctor test your kidney function before you start a high-protein diet to make sure that your kidneys are healthy.
- Choose a diet that maximizes intake of high-fiber, brightly colored vegetables and be sure to eat all the vegetables that are allowed.

- Select a diet that emphasizes low-saturated-fat meat and poultry. Trim fat. Don't char.
- Pick a diet that includes at least 50 grams of carbohydrates daily to prevent ketosis.
- Drink 8 cups of fluid daily to help the kidneys.
- Select whole-grain breads and cereals when possible.
- Choose soy-based foods, legumes, and fish to provide protein.
- Choose low-fat dairy foods and calcium supplements to reach 1,500 to 2,000 milligrams of calcium daily.
- Take a standard (not high-potency) multivitamin/mineral supplement daily. (Pierre and Robertson: 134–141)

CONCLUSION

For years, people have been losing weight on high-protein diets. However, from the beginning, there has been concern about their safety and their ability to create new medical problems, especially if followed over a longer period of time. Some highly regarded professional organizations, such as the American Dietetic Association, have opposed them. Still, they have many followers and their advocates continue to sell millions of books. When considering diets, it is always better to think in moderation and to check with a medical provider you trust.

TOPICS FOR DISCUSSION

1. The Atkins diet tells people to eat high-protein, high-calorie foods such as steak and cheese, yet some people lose weight. How does that happen?
2. Do you think that the Atkins diet is healthful and safe? Why or why not?
3. Compare and contrast the different high-protein diets. What do they have in common? What are their differences?
4. Do you think that any aspects of the diets are dangerous? Should people be concerned?
5. What are the most healthful components of the diets? Why?

REFERENCES AND RESOURCES

Books

Atkins, Robert C. *Dr. Atkins' New Diet Revolution*. New York: Avon Books, 1992.

Daoust, Joyce, and Gene Daoust. *40-30-30 Fat Burning Nutrition*. Del Mar, California: Wharton Publishing, 1996.

Eades, Michael R., and Mary Dan Eades. *Protein Power*. New York: Bantam Books, 1996.

Eades, Michael R., and Mary Dan Eades. *The Protein Power Lifeplan*. New York: Warner Books, 2000.

Heller, Richard F., and Rachael F. Heller. *The Carbohydrate Addict's Lifespan Program*. New York: Plume, 1998.

Hunt, Charles. *Charles Hunt's Diet Evolution*. Beverly Hills, California: Maximum Human Potential Productions, 1999.

McCullough, Fran. *Living Low-Carb*. Boston: Little, Brown and Company, 2000.

Sears, Barry. *The Top 100 Zone Foods*. New York: Regan Books, 2001.

Sears, Barry. *A Week in the Zone*. New York: Regan Books, 2000.

Sears, Barry. *The Zone*. New York: Regan Books, 1995.

Somer, Elizabeth. *Food and Mood*. New York: Henry Holt and Company, 1999.

Steward, H. Leighton, Morrison C. Bethea, Samuel S. Andrews, and Luis A. Balart. *Sugar Busters!* New York: Ballantine Books, 1998.

Magazines and Journals

Albertson, Ellen. "Walking the Protein Tightrope." *Better Homes and Gardens*, April 1999, 77(4): 118.

Applegate, Liz. "Just the Facts." *Runner's World*, April 2000, 35(4): 30.

Huang, Yi-Chai, Wei Chen, Marc A. Evans, Madeleine E. Mitchell, and Terry D. Shultz. "Vitamin B-6 Requirement and Status Assessment of Young Women Fed a High-Protein Diet with Various Levels of Vitamin B-6." *American Journal of Clinical Nutrition*, February 1998, 67(2): 208–220.

Itoh, Roichi, Noriko Nishiyama, and Yasuo Suyama. "Dietary Protein Intake and Urinary Excretion of Calcium: A Cross-Sectional Study of a Healthy Japanese Population." *American Journal of Clinical Nutrition*, March 1998, 67(3): 438–444.

Jibrin, Janis. "Don't Have a Cow, Man."*Men's Health*, December 1999, 14(16): 78.

McGinn, Paul. "The Skinny on Sugar." *American Medical News*, April 20, 1998, 41(15): 13–16.

Norris, Eileen. "High-Protein Diets: Where's the Beef?" *Harvard Health Letter*, January 1997, 22(3): 1–3.

Pierre, Colleen. "The Secret of High-Protein Diets." *Prevention*, June 1997, 49(6): 85–91.

Pierre, Colleen, and Sarah Robertson. "Good News about Those High-Protein Diets." *Prevention*, March 2000, 52(3): 134–141.

Somer, Elizabeth. "Make Your Own 'Happy Food.' " *Prevention*, December 1999, 51(12): 124–129.

Stedman, Nancy. "The Best Secrets of 'Zone' Dieting." *Redbook*, November 1997, 190(1): 73–74.

Stein, Karen. "High-Protein, Low-Carbohydrate Diets: Do They Work?" *Journal of the American Dietetic Association*, July 2000, 100(7): 760.

Thomas, David. "Dangerous Dieting: Weight-Loss Fads Can Be Hazardous to the Health." *Maclean's*, February 10, 1997, 110(6): 54–55.

Willi, Steven M., Mary Joan Oexmann, Nancy M. Wright, Nancy A. Collop, and L. Lyndon Key, Jr. "The Effects of a High-Protein, Low-Fat Ketogenic Diet on Adolescents with Morbid Obesity: Body Composition, Body Chemistries, and Sleep Abnormalities." *Pediatrics*, January 1998, 101(1): 61–67.

Organizations to Contact

American Dietetic Association
216 W. Jackson Blvd.
Chicago, IL 60606-6995
Phone: 312-899-0040, 800-877-1600
http://www.eatright.org/ (February 4, 2001)

Heartinfo.org
TriGenesis Communications Inc.
26 Main Street
Chatham, NJ 07928
Phone: 973-701-6035
http://www.heartinfo.org/ (January 26,2001)

International Food Information Council
1100 Connecticut Avenue NW, Suite 430
Washington, DC 20036
Phone: 202-296-6540
http://www.ific.org/ (February 1, 2001)

14

Popular Diets

Vast numbers of Americans are overweight. In many ways, obesity is a national epidemic. In response, there are many popular diets. Some seem to be effective, but their long-term effects are unclear.

According to the National Institute of Diabetes and Digestive and Kidney Diseases (NIDDK), more than half of all U.S. adults are overweight. Almost 25% are obese. A normal body-mass index (BMI) is between 18 and 24. People with a BMI of 25 are viewed as overweight; those with a BMI of 30 are obese. To calculate your BMI, multiply your weight in pounds by 703. That number should be divided by your height in inches. Finally, divide the number a second time by your height in inches.

The high rates of excess weight exact a terrible toll on individuals and society at large. Overweight and obese adults are at far greater risk for a host of medical problems such as heart disease, stroke, gallbladder disease, type 2 diabetes, osteoarthritis, high blood pressure, sleep apnea, hypertension, and certain types of cancer. These may require costly medical care and expensive medications, for which all of society pays dearly. It is believed that every year 300,000 Americans die prematurely from obesity (Diamond and Schnell: 34). Further, there are emotional issues. Society favors thinner people. Just look at the most sought-after movie and television stars. Think about the famous people and models on the covers of magazines. Almost without exception, the females are thin: the men are trim and muscular. There are a few who are overweight or obese. They gain notoriety in part because they stand out from the crowd.

The numbers of overweight and obese children and teens are also on the rise. In the United States today, obesity in children and teens is reaching epidemic proportions. "Depending on how overweight . . . is defined, at least 11% and possibly as many as 25% of US children and adolescents are overweight. These numbers may be much higher in some ethnic groups" (Hill and Trowbridge: 570–574). In *Understanding Childhood Obesity*, J. Clinton Smith noted, "Since the early 1960s, the number of American children, adolescents and adults who have become overweight or obese has increased dramatically. Of special concern is the evidence that African Americans and Mexican Americans are getting heavier at faster rates than white Americans. Why this is so is unknown, but what is suggested is that cultural factors may play a major role in the development of obesity. Other ethnic groups, such as some Pima, Navajo, and Cherokee Americans, also have high rates of excessive weight" (Smith: 30).

Funded by the California Endowment, a 1998 study of more than 1,200 California teens between the ages of 12 and 17 found that "nearly a third ... were overweight or on the verge of being so." These statistics are not unique to California. "Nationwide, particularly in the last decade, both children and adults are getting fatter. The percentage of children deemed overweight has doubled since the mid-1970's" (Marquis: Part A, part 1, page 1).

Overweight kids and teens are at greater risk for a number of medical problems. In the most obese children and adolescents, these include high blood pressure, abnormal blood fats, and non-insulin-dependent diabetes mellitus (NIDDK Web site). A 1998 article in *Parenting* magazine listed a host of different weight-related problems, including kidney disease, hip and ankle problems, high blood pressure, high cholesterol, sleep apnea, and inflammation of the pancreas. Further, obese children are almost twice as likely to become obese adults with medical problems. "By the time they're teens, many have the beginnings of heart disease or diabetes. . . . Early puberty—common among both overweight boys and girls—has been linked to breast cancer in women later in life" (Muha: 128–133).

They are also at greater risk for emotional issues. "Studies also show that overweight kids ages 6 and older tend to have fewer friends, are less involved with extracurricular activities, are more depressed, and have lower self-esteem than their thinner peers" (Muha: 128–133). A January 2000 article published in *Pediatrics* said that obese Hispanic females and obese white females demonstrated less self-esteem than Hispanic and white females who were not obese. Similar results were observed in boys (Strauss: Page e15). Do the emotional problems trigger overeating and weight gain, or does the excess weight result in emotional distress? Most likely, they both play a strong role.

There are many reasons for the escalating rates of obesity, including fewer mandated physical education programs in schools and the lack of safe areas where inner-city youth may exercise. In addition, people of all ages spend too much time in front of their television sets or at their computers. When people are not active, they do not burn higher amounts of calories. Hours of sitting—which may be accompanyied by snacking— lead to excess weight gain. A 1996 report by the surgeon general suggested that "children get at least 30 minutes of moderate physical activity almost every day, whether it's at once or spread out over several short sessions. And playtime isn't the only activity that counts—walking to school or helping to wash the car also qualifies" (Muha: 128–133). Like children and teens, to maintain their weight, adults also require exercise. Most experts suggest at least 30 minutes of a moderate aerobic exercise such as walking three or four times a week combined with some form of weight training several times a week, but this is a minimum.

Genetics and family eating patterns play a role in obesity. Children who are overweight usually have at least one parent who is overweight. Another key component is diet. In *Understanding Childhood Obesity*, Smith wrote, "As a matter of fact, not only dietary habits but also total calories and nutrient intake have been shown to 'cluster' in some families" (Smith: 68).

It is not surprising that the United States is a country obsessed with weight loss. If one types the word "diet" in one of the larger Internet bookstores, hundreds of selections will appear. Weight loss is a huge business. Annually, about $50 billion is spent on diet products and programs (Brandt: 37). It has been estimated that every year 80 million Americans go on some form of weight-loss diet. However, about 95% of the dieters gain back the weight (Diamond and Schnell: 29). While no chapter could cover all of the diet approaches that have gained prominence, it is useful to review a few of the most common. Since high-protein diets are discussed in chapter 13, they will not be reintroduced here.

DIETING WITH THE DUCHESS/WEIGHT WATCHERS

For most of her life, Sarah, the Duchess of York, the former Sarah Ferguson and ex-wife of Prince Andrew of England, battled excess weight. Over and over again, the duchess tried to lose pounds. After her marriage ended in the mid-1990s, Weight Watchers International approached the duchess and asked her to be a spokesperson. She was startled by the offer. "Here I was, a single working mother who certainly had her share of highs and lows, in life as well as with my weight. How could I motivate others to take control of their lives when I was still struggling with mine?" (Mountbatten-Windsor, 1998: 11).

Nevertheless, Sarah accepted the challenge and began the Weight Watchers 1-2-3 Success® Weight Loss Plan. The plan employs a point system that is based on calories, fat, and fiber. Each food has a specific point value. Though it varies from person to person, depending upon a person's weight, most people have a daily consumption of between 22 and 29 points. One keeps a careful tally of the point values of foods consumed. Obviously, foods with higher point values must be eaten in moderation, but nothing is off limits. If one balances the day with two lower-point meals, a larger meal is permitted. The diet tends to be low in calories (between 1,225 and 1,725 each day) and high in fiber.

A key component of the Weight Watchers strategy is support. Usually, people following the Weight Watchers diet attend regular meetings led by program graduates. Dieters share their experiences and frustrations with other dieters, and they learn hints that help them successfully lose weight. According to the Weight Watchers Web site, "Preliminary scientific research shows that people who regularly attend Weight Watchers meetings lose more weight than people who try to lose weight on their own." The meetings give them the incentive and support that they need to adhere to the diet, something that many may not be able to do without assistance.

It is not difficult to locate a meeting site. There are more than 20,000 in the United States (Weight Watchers Web site). When a number of employees want to follow the program at the same time, Weight Watchers will even set up meetings at work-site locations. There is a modest one-time registration fee, and weekly fees, between $10 and $15, are charged at the support-group meetings.

The Weight Watchers diet has been generally well received. It does require a good deal of vigilance and patience. Point values for food must be carefully tallied so it is not a good diet for people who are in a hurry to lose weight and who do not have the patience to keep track of the points. Still, there are no foods to weigh or calories to count. It is not necessary to scrutinize labels or to purchase Weight Watchers products.

Weight Watchers does not promise quick weight loss. Though some dieters lose up to two pounds a week, the Weight Watchers program is premised on slow, steady progress and lifestyle changes. Once weight loss is achieved, one remains on a maintenance program. Self-conscious men might think twice before joining. Weight Watchers meetings are comprised almost entirely of women. In order to be accepted into the program, a dieter must be at least five pounds overweight.

Commenting on the Weight Watchers diet, an article in *Town and Country* noted that it "is the most respected and least costly commercial diet program in the country" (Vreeland and Maroukian: 150–151). A Weight Watchers survey found that after two years about half of the lifetime members had maintained their weight loss. *The Diet Advisor*, written by the editors of *Health Magazine*, notes that while there is no detailed information about the survey methods, "Given Weight Watchers' sensible overall approach . . . such encouraging results seem entirely possible" (Editors of *Health Magazine*: 175).

EAT MORE, WEIGH LESS

More than two decades ago, Dean Ornish, a cardiologist who teaches at the School of Medicine, University of California at San Francisco, determined that even severe cases of heart disease could be reversed, if patients were willing to adhere to a very low-fat diet combined with moderate exercise, emotional support, smoking cessation, and stress management. In the process, patients also lost weight. Soon, Ornish concluded that he should share his program with the millions of people (who may or may not have heart problems) struggling to lose weight. That is why he wrote *Eat More, Weigh Less*. He claims that by following his diet, which he calls Life Choice, people are able to lose weight and improve their overall health.

According to Ornish, the diet of the average American consists of about 40% fat. Most diets reduce that amount to about 30%. People lose weight because they eat reduced portions. Quite naturally, they feel hungry and deprived.

Ornish states that all calories are not alike. There are twice as many calories in fat as there are in either proteins or carbohydrates. When the typical American diet is reduced from 40% of calories from fat to the 10% of calories from fat advised in Ornish's diet, people are able to eat one-third more food while consuming the same amount of calories (Ornish, 1993: 19–20).

Ornish says that people convert ingested fat into body fat. It requires only 2.5 calories to store 100 fat calories as body fat. On the other hand, the body needs 23 calories to convert 100 calories of dietary protein or carbohydrate into body fat. Just a tiny 1% of dietary protein and carbohydrate become body fat (Ornish, 1993: 20).

It is important to avoid diets that deprive the body of food. With these, the body believes that it is starving. In response, metabolism slows. As a result, fewer calories are burned, and weight loss slows or stops (Ornish, 1993: 23).

With Life Choice, one does not count calories. Instead, one eats a low-fat, high-carbohydrate, vegetarian diet with lots of beans and other legumes, fruits, grains, and vegetables. Small amounts of nonfat dairy products, nonfat mayonnaise, nonfat salad dressings, and other very low-fat commercial products such as whole-wheat breakfast cereal are permitted. Meats, poultry, fish, oil, sugar, alcohol, olives, low-fat dairy products, egg yolks, avocados, and commercial foods with more than two grams of fat per serving are eliminated.

In addition, Ornish advises some form of regular exercise such as walking and a "daily soul nourishment" such as meditation. "Among other benefits, this enables you to shift from fight-or-flight and eat-and-run to eating more peacefully, with joy and awareness. The ritual itself is comforting and provides both a sense of order and a sense of greater meaning" (Ornish, 1993: 73). To balance the diet and ensure proper nutrition, Ornish recommends various supplements.

Ornish's diet is difficult for most people to maintain. Since Americans commonly eat far higher quantities of fat and since most prepared foods are filled with fat, keeping one's intake of fat to 10% or lower is a herculean task. "Even highly motivated people can have a hard time eating less than 20% fat for long—and Ornish's regimen allows for only half of that" (Editors of *Health Magazine*: 95). However, people who adhere to this diet do lose weight and keep it off.

Nevertheless, in *Fad-Free Nutrition*, Frederick J. Stare and Elizabeth Whelan said that the diet is not realistic. Most people would not follow such a low-fat diet for an extended period of time. It may also result in an insufficient intake of essential fatty acids (Stare and Whelan: 202).

Others have noted that some of Ornish's claims are based on inaccurate information. Among these are Kevin Vigilante and Mary Flynn. In their book *Low-Fat Lies*, the authors say that when Ornish writes for other scientists, his works are scientifically sound. However, when he is addressing the lay public, his advice is sometimes incorrect. For example, unlike most diet researchers who applaud the inclusion of small amounts of olive oil in the diet, Ornish has indicated that olive oil is harmful. Vigilante and Flynn say that there is absolutely no proof that the consumption of olive oil negatively impacts the body.

People with diabetes may wish to steer clear of Ornish's approach. While consuming such a high amount of carbohydrates, they may have trouble controlling their glucose levels. It has been determined that diabetics generally do better eating lower amounts of carbohydrates.

EAT RIGHT 4 YOUR TYPE

As a result of years of clinical observation, Peter J. D'Adamo, a naturopathic physician, maintains that people should eat a diet based on their blood type. According to D'Adamo, people who eat the foods that their blood type craves are healthier. They age more slowly, and they naturally gravitate toward their ideal weight. Further, they have greater protection from infections, diabetes, cancer, and heart disease.

D'Adamo says that lectins or diverse proteins that are contained in foods are the key elements in this process. "They have agglutinating—gluing or sticking—properties that affect your blood. When you eat a food containing protein lectins that are incompatible with your blood type antigen, the lectins target an organ and begin to agglutinate blood cells in that area. In effect, lectins gum up the works, interfering with digestion, insulin production, food metabolism, and hormone balance" (D'Adamo, 1998: 9).

People with the type-O blood have genetic ancestors who were hunters and gatherers. Since their digestive tracts "retain the memory of ancient times," they do best on a diet that is higher in lean animal protein. They also require a good deal of exercise (D'Adamo, 1996: 52).

People with type-A blood had ancestors who were farmers. D'Adamo says that this is why they do best on a vegetarian diet with lots of soy protein, grains, and vegetables. Meats and dairy foods should be avoided. People with type-A blood store meat as fat. Whereas people with type O have high stomach acid, which easily digests meat, type As have low amounts of stomach acid (D'Adamo, 1996: 98). D'Adamo says that people with type-A blood do better with stress-reducing exercises. These include golf, swimming, and low-impact aerobics.

People with type-B blood have ancestors who were nomads. They should eat red meat, fish, and most dairy foods. However, they need to stay away from chicken, shellfish, and wheat. Eliminating wheat from the diet is especially important for those who want to lose weight. For type Bs, exercise should incorporate some of the more physical components that type Os require with some of the calmer ones that type As need.

Only 2 to 5% of the population has type-AB blood, which has been around for less than 1,000 years. Foods that are problematic for either type As or type Bs are generally off limits for type AB. To lose weight, people with type AB should limit their intakes of meat and wheat. They should follow the exercises recommended for people with type-A and type-B blood.

By adhering to this diet, people avoid the lectins that agglutinate their type of blood. D'Adamo claims that his diet is effective about 90% of the time. Further, "the more severe the problem, the faster it works" (D'Adamo, 1998: 3).

A 1997 story in *Good Housekeeping* magazine noted that there was essentially no scientific evidence to prove D'Adamo's theories. Although D'Adamo refers to his research, he "does not list a single study he has published in a scientific journal." It is possible to eat a reasonably nutritious diet on this plan, and since there are so many eliminated foods, weight loss may be achieved, but the article claims that it is not worth the bother. The combination of the diet's numerous restrictions and its inconvenience with the lack of proven benefits means that many people will have little inclination to follow its unusual regimen (Hammock, "Eat Right": 132).

In *Fad-Free Nutrition,* Stare and Whelan say, "This is not only one of the most preposterous books on the market, but also one of the most frightening. It contains just enough scientific-sounding nonsense, carefully woven into a complex theory, to actually seem convincing to the uninitiated." Stare and Whelan contend that the essential thesis of the book is simply erroneous. They maintain that D'Adamo bases his thesis on the presumption that components in food may cause red blood cells to agglutinize, or clump. In essence, D'Adamo says that the blood-type gene is the same gene that directs food and digestive capabilities. Such a contention is "arbitrary" and "irresponsible." To Stare and Whelan, D'Adamo "could just as easily have chosen to link food with eye color— and he would have been no farther off target" (Stare and Whelan: 209– 210).

SOMERSIZING, SUZANNE SOMERS'S DIET

During a 1992 trip to a medieval French village, Suzanne Somers ate a dinner of pâté, fish cooked in butter, fresh vegetables, cheese, and wine. As she was leaving, she picked a few cherries off a tree and quickly "popped them into her mouth." When her French host saw what she had done, he told her that eating fruit after a big meal would give her indigestion. Sure enough, it did. It also introduced Somers to the notion of food combining—foods that should or should not be eaten with other foods. "Somers eventually figured out that she could lose weight and still have many of the indulgent treats she loved—as long as she didn't eat certain foods with them" (Wolfson: 110). This program is called "Somersizing." By following this diet, Somers reduced her weight from 130 to 116 pounds. In *Suzanne Somers' Get Skinny on Fabulous Food*, Somers wrote, "And because I give my body real foods, my hunger is satisfied and I am meeting my body's nutritional needs. In the last six years my weight has not fluctuated by more than five pounds" (Somers, 1999: 8).

With Somersizing, proteins and fats may be eaten together, but not with carbohydrates. Fruits may only be consumed on an empty stomach. Vegetables, bread, cereal, and whole-grain pasta are also permitted, but not with fats and proteins. To Somers, the worst foods are those high in starch and sugars such as potatoes, white flour, and white rice. She terms these "funky foods." But this category also includes foods that others characterize as healthy such as carrots, bananas, and acorn squash.

Somers begins by categorizing foods. There are pro/fats, which are foods like meat and poultry and fats in their natural state like butter and cream. Veggies are low-starch, fresh vegetables such as peppers and zucchini. Whole-grain pasta, breads, and nonfat dairy foods are carbos. There are also fruits, which range from apples to tangerines, and the previously noted funky foods.

Then Somers lists the seven basic guidelines of her program. First, all funky foods must be eliminated. Next, fruit must not be eaten with any other food and must be consumed when the stomach is empty. Pro/fats and carbos may each be eaten with veggies. Pro/fats and carbos should be consumed separately. When switching from a pro/fats meal to a carbos meal or vice versa, people should wait three hours. Meals should not be skipped, and people should eat until they are comfortably full (Somers, 1999: 11).

Once weight loss has been achieved, dieters may transition to Level Two, the maintenance program. Although there is no portion control on the first part of the program, dieters on Level Two have more variety, but they must be careful when they created imbalanced eating. To prevent weight gain, they may wish to limit some portions. Somers maintains that Somersizing reprograms the metabolism and balances the hormones. According to Somers, it is hormone imbalance, not fat and calories, that causes people to gain weight.

In *Eat, Cheat, and Melt the Fat Away*, Somers explains why her diet is different from other diets, such as those that eliminate food groups. She says that her diet is balanced and has all the needed vitamins to maintain excellent health. Further, it is not a "crash" diet that may interfere with an individual's metabolism, and, she contends, it is easy to follow. "This program is also *backed up by sound medical studies* that will explain why sugar, not fat, is the real enemy" (Somers, 2001: 3). A few of these are briefly referenced. While Somers does not spend much time discussing exercise, she does advise people to make time for regular workouts.

Most people disagree with Somers's assertion that calories do not count. Whether calories come from proteins, fats, or carbohydrates, caloric intake is directly related to weight gain or loss. As for Somers's food-combining theories, there is no scientific proof supporting her beliefs. Her contention that people may eat as much fat as they wish—in the forms of butter, oil, sour cream, and other foods—may have serious negative health consequences. It is well known that high-fat diets have been linked to a number of problems such as cardiovascular disease and colon cancer.

On the other hand, Somers's advice on limiting refined sugars is praiseworthy. Refined sugars are simply empty calories. Americans eat far too much sugar, much of it hidden in processed foods.

Remaining on the Somers diet for an extended period of time may be quite challenging, especially with its somewhat rigid rules for food combining. Somersizing has the potential to be confusing. For example, in a carbos meal, only protein without fat may be eaten, so a carbos meal may include nonfat milk but not whole milk (Somers, 1999: 49).

In a discussion of Somersizing, an article in *Good Housekeeping* magazine noted that dieters are not guaranteed to lose weight, even when portions are fairly moderate. Moreover, the diet is "a mishmash of nonsensical rules that make healthy low-calorie eating a lot more difficult than it needs to be." Those who try this diet should "limit fat (and calories) by opting for more carb/veggie meals than protein/fat meals and include skim milk and other calcium-rich, low-fat, low-fat dairy products" (Hammock, "Suzanne Somers": 127–128).

THE BODY CODE

Jay Cooper, who authored *The Body Code* with Kathryn Lance, is wellness director of the Green Valley Spa in St. George, Utah. He is a marathon runner, triathlete, and fitness trainer. For more than two decades, he has been involved with weight-loss wellness programs.

Cooper contends that there is no one diet that works for everyone, because everyone is born with one of four different categories of body types—warrior, nurturer, communicator, and visionary. People should first determine their body type. After that, they need to combine a regular exercise program with a body-type-appropriate diet.

The warrior has a stronger upper body and a shorter neck. Excess body fat tends to be located in the upper portions of the body. Warriors are assertive, decisive, task oriented, orderly, and extroverted. Their exercise regimen should concentrate on cardiovascular training and flexibility. They are known to crave meat and fatty foods, which stimulate their dominant glands; they are healthiest when they consume a plant-based diet including whole grains, fruits, and vegetables.

The nurturer has a curvy, more ample lower body and a smaller upper body. Excess fat may be found in the buttocks, outer and inner thighs, triceps, and hamstrings. Nurturers tend to be friendly, extroverted, caring, service-oriented people. They should focus on cardiovascular training, with strength training only for the upper body. While they may crave creamy and/or spicy foods, they do better when they eat high-water-content foods, including lots of fruits and vegetables.

The communicator has a longer-looking physique and bony hands and feet. Excess fat is located in the spare-tire area, the top front of the legs, and the triceps. Communicators are creative, verbal, extroverted, spirited, moody perfectionists. They enjoy a variety of exercises that should include cardiovascular training, strength training, and flexibility exercises. Though they love sweets and carbohydrates, they do better eating high-quality, animal-based protein.

The visionary has a less developed physique and a youthful appearance. Hands and feet tend to be small. Excess weight looks like puffiness. Visionaries are either calm, introverted, and intellectual or childlike, witty, curious, and extroverted. While they are not natural exercisers, they do best on a strength and flexibility program, with a little cardiovascular exercise for overall health. Visionaries should eat light proteins and vegetables with few or no dairy products.

Cooper believes that each of these body types is driven by one of four glands—the warrior by the adrenal, the nurturer by the ovaries (therefore, only women are nurturers), the communicator by the thyroid, and the visionary by the pituitary. The adrenal gland regulates appetite and reactions to stress; the gonads control sexuality and reproduction; the thyroid directs metabolism; and the pituitary oversees all the other glands. The dominant gland causes the body to crave foods that stimulate it, but these are the very foods that should be avoided. In order to balance the body, Cooper advises people to eat foods that stimulate the other three glands.

In his book, Cooper outlines very detailed instructions for each body type. There is little emphasis on calories and no discussion of how much weight one may expect to lose. This is not an easy diet to follow. Dieters must avoid the foods that they most wish to eat. Very specific rules must be followed. For example, communicators may not eat any carbohydrates before noon, and nurturers must severely restrict their intake of red meat.

There are no scientific studies or data to prove or disprove Cooper's theories. Instead, they are based on his personal observations and years of experience. One cannot help but wonder if many of Cooper's clients lose weight not because they adhere to certain body-type diets, but rather because he advises a great deal of exercise and many of his food suggestions are low in calories. When followed for an extended period of time, such a diet may lead to nutritional deficiencies. Dieters may find that they are unable to incorporate so much exercise into their already pressed schedules. With so many inconveniences, it is all too easy to become discouraged and quit.

ESSENTIAL DIET PRINCIPLES

Which diet should people follow if they want to lose weight and keep it off? That is not always clear. In all probability, people who adhere to any of the previously discussed diets will initially lose weight. Between the food restrictions and the caloric limitations, the pounds are bound to fall. When people return to their prediet eating patterns and find excuses not to exercise, they will regain weight. That is why many doctors advise their patients to make long-term, healthy dietary changes that are combined with lifestyle modifications. While it is evident that there is no one diet that meets the needs of everyone, there are essential principles that will help most people maintain a healthier weight.

In *The American Dietetic Association's Complete Food and Nutrition Guide*, Roberta Larson Duyff lists a number of basic ADA dietary guidelines. The goal is to present a sensible, easy-to-follow diet that may readily fit into the average person's lifestyle, rather than a fad diet that one rigorously follows for a period of time, before quitting in abject frustration. People should eat a variety of foods and participate in some form of physical activity. Diets should contain lots of grain products, vegetables, and fruit. They should be low in fat, saturated fat, and cholesterol and modest in sugars and salt. If alcohol is consumed, it should be limited. "Food variety—along with balance and moderation—is the cornerstone of an eating style that's both healthful and enjoyable. These same qualities apply to daily food choices that almost all healthy people need, regardless of their age, food preferences, energy needs, and lifestyle" (Duyff: 8). People should cook with less fat and watch for hidden fats in processed foods. They should consume more foods with fiber. Insoluble fibers, such as wheat bran, aid in digestion; soluble fibers, such as oat bran, seem to help lower cholesterol and regulate the body's use of sugars. Additionally, since foods with fiber make the body feel fuller, people who eat them are able to eat less and better control their weight.

Edited by cardiologist Bernard J. Gersh, the second edition of the *Mayo Clinic Heart Book*, which has contributions from more than 125 specialists from the prestigious Mayo Clinic based in Rochester, Minnesota, notes that "a typical day's healthy diet" for a person over the age of two should include the following:

- Less than 10 percent of total calories from saturated fat
- About 30 percent of calories from all types of fat
- At least 55 percent of total calories from complex carbohydrates
- No more than 300 milligrams of cholesterol
- A maximum of 6,000 milligrams of salt per day (2,400 milligrams of sodium)
- Enough calories to maintain a healthy body weight

Additionally, the book recommends eating a wide variety of foods, most of which are derived from plant sources. The daily diet should consist of at least five servings of fruits and vegetables and six or more servings of bread, pasta, and cereal grains. Foods that are high in fat, especially animal fat, and simple sugars should be eaten sparingly (Gersh: 191).

The American Heart Association adds that many Americans could lose weight if they controlled their intake of calories and exercised more. "Exercise combined with cutting calories is more healthful for you than a severely restricted caloric intake. . . . If you eat less fat without increasing your caloric intake, you'll naturally lose weight because fat contains a high concentration of calories" (American Heart Association: 14). In *Safe Dieting for Teens*, Linda Ojeda, a certified nutritional consultant, contends that there is no mystery to weight loss. Weight loss is a function of a reduced intake of calories coupled with an increase in physical activity. Moreover, "the diet you follow to lose weight should be very close to the diet you are going to stay on for the rest of your life." Dieters must always remember that it takes time to drop the pounds. "It didn't take you two months to put the weight on, and it won't take just a few weeks to take it off" (Ojeda: 2–3).

CONCLUSION

The 1.3 million people who live in Okinawa, a chain of islands that stretches from Japan to Taiwan, have the longest life expectancy—81.2 years—of any place in the world. In their relatively small population, they have more than 400 centenarians, about 34 for every 100,000 residents. With all its sophisticated medical care, the United States has between 5 and 10 centenarians per every 100,000 (Willcox, Willcox, and Suzuki: 2). Not only do Okinawans live longer, they are far healthier, and they tend to be slim.

What about their lifestyle lends itself to good health and long life? About three-quarters of their diet is from plants. Every day, they eat between 9 and 17 servings of vegetables and between 7 and 13 servings of whole grains. There are ample amounts of foods with antioxidants and calcium and relatively low amounts of fat, refined sugars, and protein. Further, they practice a cultural habit called "hara hachi bu," in which they stop eating when they feel the first hint of fullness. Exercise is woven into everyday life. "Okinawans keep fit in all three components of fitness—anaerobic, flexibility, and aerobic—mainly through martial arts, which they have been practicing for centuries; traditional dance, which many Okinawan men and women learn from a very young age and continue to perform; and gardening and walking" (Willcox, Willcox, and Suzuki: 7). Perhaps, instead of gravitating to one of the popular diets, Americans might do better to model their diets and aspects of their lifestyle after the Okinawans, with moderation in both eating habits and exercise. By eating reasonable amounts of more plant-based foods and including regular exercise in their lifestyles, greater numbers of Americans could drop the pounds and improve their health in a safe and sensible way.

TOPICS FOR DISCUSSION

1. Are you overweight? If so, do you have any related medical problems? What are you doing about the situation?

2. Ornish recommends a diet that is extremely low in fat. Do you think that this is realistic for the average person? Why or why not?

3. Had you heard of D'Adamo's blood-type diet before you read this chapter? Do you think that his science is sound? Please explain.

4. Some diets recommend different types of food combining. Do you think that people really lose weight from specific foods combinations? Comment further.

5. Have you ever been on a diet? Did you lose weight? What do you think that people should do to maintain a healthy weight?

REFERENCES AND RESOURCES

Books

American Heart Association. *Low-Fat, Low-Cholesterol Cookbook*. 2nd ed. New York: Times Books, 1997.

Cooper, Jay, with Kathryn Lance. *The Body Code*. New York: Pocket Books, 1999.

D'Adamo, Peter J., with Catherine Whitney. *Cook Right 4 Your Type*. New York: G.P. Putnam's Sons, 1998.

D'Adamo, Peter J., with Catherine Whitney. *Eat Right 4 Your Type*. New York: G.P. Putnam's Sons, 1996.

Diamond, Marilyn, and Donald Burton Schnell. *Fitonics for Life*. New York: Avon Books: 1996.

Duyff, Roberta Larson. *The American Dietetic Association's Complete Food and Nutrition Guide*. Minneapolis: Chronimed, 1996.

Editors of *Health Magazine*. *The Diet Advisor*. Alexandria, Virginia: Time-Life Books, 2000.

Gersh, Bernard J., editor-in-chief. *Mayo Clinic Heart Book*. 2nd ed. New York: William Morrow, 2000.

Mazel, Judy, and John E. Monaco. *Slim and Fit Kids*. Deerfield Beach, Florida: Health Communications, 1999.

Mountbatten-Windsor, Sarah, Duchess of York, and Weight Watchers. *Dieting with the Duchess*. New York: Simon and Schuster, 1998.

Mountbatten-Windsor, Sarah, Duchess of York, and Weight Watchers. *Reinventing Yourself with the Duchess of York*. New York: Simon and Schuster, 2001.

Mountbatten-Windsor, Sarah, Duchess of York, and Weight Watchers. *Win the Weight Game*. New York: Simon and Schuster, 2000.

Ojeda, Linda. *Safe Dieting for Teens*. Alameda, California: Hunter House, 1993.

Ornish, Dean. *Eat More, Weigh Less*. New York: HarperCollins, 1993.

Ornish, Dean, with Janet Fletcher, Jean-Marc Fullsack, and Helen Roe. *Everyday Cooking with Dr. Dean Ornish*. New York: HarperCollins, 1996.

Rolls, Barbara, and Robert A. Barnett. *The Volumetrics Weight-Control Plan*. New York: Quill, 2000.

Smith, J. Clinton. *Understanding Childhood Obesity*. Jackson: University Press of Mississippi, 1999.

Somer, Elizabeth. *The Origin Diet*. New York: Henry Holt and Company, 2001.

Somers, Suzanne, *Suzanne Somers' Eat, Cheat, and Melt the Fat Away*. New York: Crown Publishing, 2001.

Somers, Suzanne, *Suzanne Somers' Get Skinny on Fabulous Food*. New York: Crown Publishing, 1999.

Stare, Frederick J., and Elizabeth Whelan. *Fad-Free Nutrition*. Alameda, California: Hunter House, 1998.

Vigilante, Kevin, and Mary Flynn. *Low-Fat Lies*. Washington, DC: LifeLine Press, 1999.

Weight Watchers International. *Weight Watchers Coach Approach*. New York: Macmillan, 1997.

Willcox, Bradley J., D. Craig Willcox, and Makoto Suzuki. *The Okinawa Program*. New York: Clarkson Potter, 2001.

Magazines, Journals, and Newspapers

Brandt, Laura A. "Desperately Seeking Satiety!" *Prepared Foods*, February 2001, 170(2): 37.

Brink, Susan. "The Low-Fat Life." *U.S. News and World Report*, July 12, 1999, 127(2): 56.

Brody, Jane E. "New Guide Puts Most Americans on Fat Side." *New York Times*, June 9, 1998: Section F, page 7, column 1.

Brody, Jane E. "Warning: The Wrong Nutritionist Can Be Dangerous to Your Health." *New York Times*, April 17, 1998: Section 6, part 2, page 36, column 1.

Chima, Cinda Williams. "Another Health Plan with More Questions Than Answers." *Plain Dealer*, August 25, 1997: Page 2E.

Crayhon, Robert. "Is the Stone Age Diet the Ideal for Humans?" *Total Health*, April–May 1999, 211(2): 46–49.

Eveld, Edward M. "Spreading the Word: New Book Stresses Enzymes and Mental Exercise." *Kansas City Star*, November 18, 1996: Page E3.

Foreman, Judy. "Evidence Shows Blood Types Have Evolved as Disease-Fighters." *Boston Globe*, November 6, 2001: Pages C1–C2.

Gavalas, Elaine. "The Great Diet Debate." *Better Nutrition*, May 2000, 62(5): 32.

Gerosa, Melina. "Sarah, Bright and Dark." *Ladies' Home Journal*, April 1999, 116(4): 136.

Hammock, Delia. "Eat Right 4 Your Type." *Good Housekeeping*, June 1997, 224(6): 132.

Hammock, Delia. "Suzanne Somers' *Eat Great, Lose Weight*." *Good Housekeeping*, June 1997, 224(6): 127–128.

Heinrich, Richard L. "Cave Woman Wisdom?" *Better Nutrition*, October 2000, 62(10): 26.

Hill, James O., and Frederick L. Trowbridge. "Childhood Obesity: Future Directions and Research Priorities." *Pediatrics*, March 1998, 101(3, part 2): 570–574.

Linder, Lawrence. "Eating Right: A New Contender in the Battle of the Bulge; Swimming against the Tide of Diet Hype, *Volumetrics* Weighs in with a Refreshingly Honest Approach." *Washington Post*, January 4, 2000: Page Z16.

Mandell, Terri. "The Living Laboratory." *American Fitness*, March–April 2000, 18(2): 37–38+.

Marquis, Julie. "Eating Habits Put Teens at Risk, Study Says." *Los Angeles Times*, September 26, 2000: Part A, part 1, page 1.

Melton, Lisa. "And Now for the Good News." *New Scientist*, September 22, 2001, 171(2309): 32.

Muha, Laura. "Too Fat?" *Parenting*, September 1998, 12(7): 128–133.

Powell, Joanna. "A Royal Survivor." *Good Housekeeping*, April 1998, 226(4): 94–98.

Puhn, Adele. "Diet Special: At Last! Cosmo's 1998 'No Willpower Required' Diet." *Cosmopolitan*, January 1998, 224(1): 188–191.

Rhodes, Maura. "American's Top Six Fad Diets." *Good Housekeeping*, July 1996, 223(1): 100–102.

Schwartz, Rosie. "Forget Diet Book Fads; Eat Well to Curb Cravings." *Ottawa Citizen*, November 6, 1996: Page E3.

Strauss, Richard S. "Childhood Obesity and Self-Esteem." *Pediatrics*, January 2000, 105(1): e15.

Styne, Dennis Michael. "Childhood Obesity: Time for Action, Not Complacency." *American Family Physician*, February 15, 1999, 59(4): 758, 761–762.

Vreeland, Leslie, and Francine Maroukian. "Losing It: A Guide to Weight-Management Programs." *Town and Country*, June 1996, 150(5193): 150–151.

Ward, Elizabeth M. "Winnowing Weight-Loss Programs to Find a Match for You." *Environmental Nutrition*, January 1998, 21(1): 1, 4+.

Wolfson, Nancy. "The Suzanne Somers Diet." *Good Housekeeping*, July 2000, 231(1): 110.

Organizations to Contact

Center for Science in the Public Interest
1875 Connecticut Ave. NW, Suite 300
Washington, DC 20009
Phone: 202-332-9110
http://www.cspinet.org/ (September 22, 2001)

National Institute of Diabetes and Digestive and Kidney Diseases
Office of Communications and Public Liaison
NIH
Building 31, Room 9A04
31 Center Drive, MSC 2560
Bethesda, MD 20892-2560
Phone: 301-496-3583
http://www.niddk.nih.gov/ (August 2, 2001)

Weight Watchers
175 Crossways Park West
Woodbury, NY 11797
Phone: 800-651-6000
http://weightwatchers.com/ (November 6, 2001)

15

Genetically Modified Foods

Increasingly, genetically modified foods are making their way to the marketplace. Since they are not labeled, consumers generally do not know that they are eating such products. Not everyone is comfortable with the present system.

A few years ago, one rarely heard about genetically modified organisms (GMOs). In fact, few people knew exactly what they were. That is no longer the case. GMOs, or plants, animals, or microorganisms that have been genetically altered or engineered for a specific purpose, are everywhere. It has been estimated that almost half of all American farmers grow some variety of genetically modified crops, also known as genetically engineered crops (BioScience Productions Web site).

According to the U.S. Department of Agriculture, in 1996, about 8 million U.S. acres were devoted to crops that had been genetically engineered. By 1998, that figure was up to 67 million acres (U.S. Department of Agriculture Web site). A March 2000 article in *Frozen Food Age* noted that in 1996 only 2% of all soybeans were genetically modified. By 2000, that figure was up to more than half. "About a third of corn (maize, or hard corn used for corn meal—not sweet cob corn) has also been genetically modified" (Thayer: 34–36).

The U.S. Food and Drug Administration (FDA) says that GMOs are filling the shelves of stores. "Tomatoes, potatoes, squash, corn, and soybeans have been genetically altered through the emerging science of biotechnology. So have ingredients in everything from ketchup and cola to hamburger buns and cake mixes" (FDA Web site). A 2000 article in *Better Homes and Gardens* said that "by one estimate, 70 percent of the processed foods sold in the United States contain some GM [genetically modified] ingredients" (Gower: 256). Meanwhile, a 2000 article in *Current Health 2* noted, "If you've gobbled down a crispy taco, a bowl of cornflakes, a

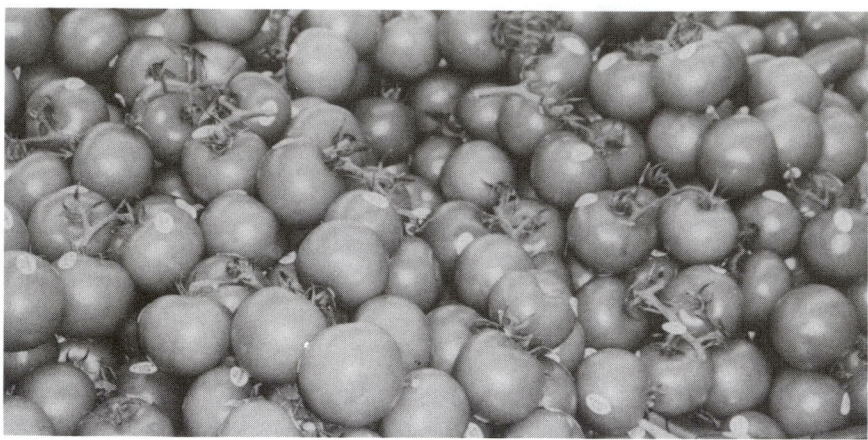

Large numbers of tomatoes are genetically modified. Photo by Mark A. Goldstein.

baked potato, or cheese pizza lately, chances are you've eaten genetically engineered foods" (Maynard: 22)

In *Genetically Engineered Food*, Martin Teitel, executive director of the Council for Responsible Genetics, and Kimberly A. Wilson, director of the council's program on Commercial Biotechnology and the Environment, describe the sweeping changes brought about by GMOs. "The genetic engineering of our food is the most radical transformation in our diet since the invention of agriculture 10,000 years ago. . . . These food crops are already growing on millions of acres all around the world" (Teitel and Wilson: 1–2).

Similar sentiments were expressed in *Genetically Engineered Food* by Ronnie Cummins, national director of the Organic Consumers Association, and Ben Lilliston, a health and environment writer and communications coordinator for the Institute for Agriculture and Trade Policy in Minneapolis: "Genetic engineering . . . is a revolutionary new technology still in the early experimental stages of development. It enables molecular biologists to permanently alter the essential characteristics or genetic codes of living organisms. This technology has the awesome power to break down fundamental genetic barriers—not only between species but between humans, animals, and plants. . . . For the first time in history, the scientists and corporations using this technology have become, in effect, the architects, builders, and 'owners' of life" (Cummins and Lilliston: 17).

Introducing the genes of one type of food into another, thereby changing the genetic structure of an organism, gives the second plant or animal beneficial characteristics, such as resistance to disease, improved nutritional value, and better growth. These modifications enable foods to grow faster, stronger, or bigger, all while using far less pesticide. There are now tomatoes that last longer and corn that is resistant to pests. "The acreage devoted to herbicide-resistant crops has been expanding because planting them reduces the need to plow more ground, decreases the amount of herbicidal chemicals needed, produces higher yields, and can deliver a higher grade of grain and other products" (Marwick: 188–190). In 2001, an article in *American Scientist* noted that transgenic or genetically modified crops "can be developed for pest resistance, improved yield, tolerance to biotic and abiotic stresses, use of marginalized land, improved nutritional content, and the production of vaccines and pharmaceuticals" (Follett: 76). A 2000 story in *Popular Science* said, "Genes from flounders can help ordinary plants like tomatoes and strawberries fight the cold. Researchers are also inserting bacterial genes into corn and soybean plants to better protect them from insects or render them immune to certain herbicides" (McInnis and Sinha: 66).

Cross-breeding has been around for a long time. "Virtually all common fruits and vegetables look and taste the way they do because of hybridization" (Gower: 256–262). However, biotechnology has added a whole new dimension to selective breeding. "This process allows for the transfer of only one or a few desirable genes, thereby permitting scientists to develop crops with specific beneficial traits and those without undesirable traits. Current technology permits scientists to alter one plant characteristic at a time, thereby not spending years trying to develop the best tasting and hardiest plants" (International Food Information Council Web site). For example, Craig Nessler, professor and head of the Department of Plant Pathology, Physiology, and Weed Science at Virginia Tech University, inserted genes from rats into lettuce seeds. This produced leafy greens with much higher amounts of vitamin C. "Rats, it turns out, carry a gene that allows their bodies to manufacture vitamin C, which is why the little four-legged fiends never develop scurvy on long sea voyages" (Gower: 256–262). Years ago, such science would have been unthinkable.

In *The Ecological Risks of Engineered Crops*, Jane Rissler and Margaret Mellon further explain the differences between traditional breeding and genetic engineering. "To give a simple example, a traditional breeder interested in producing a yellow tomato must find the yellow trait in a plant that will breed with the tomato by natural mechanisms. The only plants that can breed with tomatoes are closely related ones. Unrelated plants like oak trees or cantaloupes could not breed with tomatoes, and thus could not contribute new genes. A genetic engineer, on the other hand, can consider any organism—even a butterfly or a daffodil—as a source of the yellow trait. If the gene that determines yellow color has been identified and isolated, it can be directly transferred into tomato plants" (Rissler and Mellon: 9–10).

The International Food Information Council maintains that because GMOs reduce the amounts of pesticide used by farmers, they are healthier for the environment. "Insect protected crops allow for less potential exposure of farmers and groundwater to chemical residues, while providing farmers with season-long control. Also by reducing the need for pest control, time, effort and resources spent on the land are less, thereby preserving the topsoil" (International Food Information Council Web site).

It is almost impossible for the average consumer to know whether there are GMOs in his or her food. Playing on consumers' fear of the unknown, a few innovative marketers include "No GMOs" notations on their labels. However, the vast majority of products do not indicate whether they are comprised of any genetically altered ingredients. "Legal authority for food labeling rests with the Food and Drug Administration. Foods derived from biotechnology currently must be labeled only if they differ significantly from their conventional counterparts—for example, if their nutritional content or potential to cause allergic reactions is altered" (U.S. Department of Agriculture Web site).

SUPPORTERS AND OPPONENTS OF GMOS

Should consumers feel comfortable eating genetically altered food? The controversy surrounding GMOs, or Frankenfoods, as they are called by those who oppose them, is filled with heated discussion. In general, the federal government, big business, and many researchers and numerous well-respected publications maintain that genetically altered food is perfectly safe. They contend that GMOs offer the potential to feed healthier food to far larger numbers of people. That is of particular significance, they say, when considering the vast amounts of food needed to feed the populations of developing countries. A 2000 article in *Environment* noted that about 15% of the world's population—about 800 million people—consume less than 2,000 calories per day. They are always hungry and live in a state of chronic malnourishment. Large numbers of these people are women and children. "More than 180 million children under five years of age are underweight, that is, they are more than two standard deviations below the standard weight for their age. This represents one-third of the under-fives in the developing countries." These groups are growing at a staggering rate. "By the year 2020, there will be about an extra 1.5 billion mouths to feed. If the proportion of the population of the developing countries deprived of an adequate diet remains the same, the number undernourished 20 years from now could be well over one billion" (Conway: 8–18).

Not everyone agrees. Sizeable numbers of equally esteemed researchers and consumer and environmental groups worry about a variety of factors. "Concerns include ethical issues related to potential long-term health effects of eating bioengineered foods, labeling, and potential environmental risks" (U.S. Food and Drug Administration Web site). In Europe, particularly Great Britain, large numbers of people have supported a ban of GMOs. Grocery stores are refusing to carry foods containing GMOs. Other countries are following Britain's lead. A long article in the *American Behavioral Scientist* reported that "a recent observation in a bulletin for U.K. agricultural lawyers noted ... that many farmers refuse to field test GM [genetically modified] crops because of their fear of both anti-GM activists and potential liability to neighbors for damage. Moreover, concern about risk of lawsuits and decline in land value has made rural land managers hesitant to authorize tenants to grow GM crops." Within the European Community, there is enormous apprehension. "Consumers worry about the impact of any health risks that might eventually be discovered, especially if whole national populations have ingested GM food. Health effects, moreover, may stem from risk related to questions that scientists have not yet asked rather than those questions for which reassuring answers have been found" (Grossman and Endres: 378–434).

In *High-Tech Harvest*, Elizabeth L. Marshall, a science writer, notes that the most serious GMO controversy has centered on food labeling. Usually, opponents of GMOs favor labeling. They want to know which foods have been changed and believe that shoppers, when presented with such information on the label, would shy away from them. "But some supporters want labels too. They believe that labels would help pave the way to consumer acceptance" (Marshall: 9).

GMO HISTORY

Genetic engineering food research began in the 1980s. In 1990, the enzyme chymosin was the first genetically engineered food to receive the approval of the FDA. More than half of the hard cheese currently sold in the United States is made with chymosin produced by genetically engineered fungi. The rest is made with chymosin obtained from rennet, an enzyme from the stomachs of slaughtered calves. "Although cheesemakers can use chymosin from either source, the chymosin made from genetically engineered bacteria is easier to obtain and more pure" (Marshall: 10).

Two years later, in 1992, the FDA approved the first genetically engineered whole food—the Calgene Flavr Savr tomato, which became available for sale in 1994. Because of a change to a single gene, the Calgene Flavr Savr tomato ripened without getting soft. However, the Flavr Savr tomato encountered a number of problems, such as an inability to tolerate shipping. "Contrary to Calgene's expectations, the tomatoes were often so soft and bruised that they could not be sold as fresh produce, and most of the . . . varieties did not have acceptable yields or disease resistance in tomato-growing regions" (Anderson: 44–45). The Flavr Savr marketing campaign was unsuccessful. The tomatoes received a good deal of negative press, and consumers refused to buy them. "Calgene even tried marketing the tomatoes as a gourmet product under the friendly sounding 'MacGregor's' brand name, but despite their presence in thousands of U.S. grocery stores, consumers did not want to pay more for genetically engineered tomatoes." In 1996, the Flavr Savr tomato was removed from the market. Teitel and Wilson noted that "the Flavr Savr grew well in the laboratory but encountered serious obstacles in the field" (Teitel and Wilson: 21).

Nevertheless, genetic engineering moved forward. By 1996, genetically engineered seeds for corn and soybeans were available, followed by seeds for potatoes, squash, tomatoes, and rapeseed. "Each type of seed offers a characteristic that natural seeds did not. Some protect the plants against insects or disease, while others delay ripening or protect the plants from chemicals used to kill weeds" (Marshall : 47).

REGULATION OF GMOS

It is important to realize that genetic engineering is a tool that may be used in a variety of ways to make many different food products. That is why, Marshall contends, the FDA decided in 1992 that genetically engineered foods would be reviewed "based on their individual safety and nutrition, rather than on the methods used to produce them." The FDA deemed them "as safe as foods developed through other agricultural technologies" (Marshall: 20–21).

As a result, the FDA regulates GMOs as it does any other food. If a new product contains food items that are already considered safe, the manufacturer does not need to obtain special permission to sell the item. "In other words, a transgenic [another word for genetically engineered] catfish containing a trout gene would be considered safe to eat because it is already well-known that trout is harmless to humans. . . . The only time the law requires testing of a new food is when it contains an additive that is not known and, therefore, not generally regarded as safe" (Marshall: 77–78).

In 1992, the FDA determined that there would be exceptions to this rule. If a new food contained ingredients that were likely to trigger allergic reactions in allergic individuals or if the manufacturing process dramatically altered the nutritional content, a label would be required. Unfortunately, this is not as clear-cut as it may initially appear to be. Foods are constantly combined together to form new foods. Should everything be labeled? The government and sizeable numbers of people within the food industry say that such labeling would be confusing and expensive. In *Pandora's Picnic Basket*, Alan McHughen, a senior research scientist at the University of Saskatchewan, Canada, wrote that "in North America, regulators and companies agree that mandatory labels should be reserved for those products carrying a documented health risk or substantial change in nutritional composition. If the GM products are 'substantially equivalent' to conventional counterparts, the companies argue, the GM label would be misleading" (McHughen: 203). Nonetheless, many consumer groups consider labeling to be an absolute necessity. EarthSave International explains that genetic engineering "introduces new proteins into the human and animal food chains. This means that human beings are now consuming products that have never before been considered foodstuffs. There is concern that these new proteins could potentially cause toxic or allergic reactions or other health effects. Unfortunately, there is no easy way to predict the allergenic potential . . . since allergic reactions typically occur only after the individual consuming the food is sensitized by initial exposure to the allergen" (EarthSave International Web site).

It is true that the government has mandated the labeling of other products such as foods that are processed and those containing sulfites. Labels must note the source of hydrolyzed proteins, and they are required to state if a food—other than a spice—has been irradiated. Cigarette labels have a warning from the surgeon general. "These legal requirements are in place because large numbers of citizens want such information, and a specific fraction needs it. An identifiable fraction of consumers actually needs information about genetic modifications—for example, regarding allergenicity . . . and almost all consumers want it" (Council for Responsible Genetics Web site).

Lawrence Kushi, an epidemiologist at Columbia University, notes that it is simply untrue to say that genetically modified food is no different from the conventional equivalents. He maintains that labeling such foods would give consumers the information they want while allowing scientists to examine whether they have any negative impacts on human health or the environment (Gower: 256–262).

ARGUMENTS IN FAVOR OF GMOS

Some people contend that the negative publicity that consumer groups generate about GMOs is most harmful to the world's most vulnerable people—the poor. They say that unlike residents of wealthier countries, large segments of the population of developing countries worry about dying from malnutrition and starvation. By using GMOs, farmers in developing countries may harvest more crops with less pesticide. Playing on this theme, frequently appearing television and magazine ads have featured rice that has been genetically altered with a daffodil gene. As a result of that modification, the rice contains beta-carotene, which the body converts into vitamin A. The ads claim that by eating this form of "Golden Rice," countless numbers of people in poorer countries will be spared blindness.

According to the Rockefeller Foundation, about 400 million people may be in danger of vitamin A deficiency. Of these, 100 to 200 million are children. Mammals do not manufacture vitamin A, so it must be obtained through the diet. People who eat lots of fruits and vegetables and animal products obtain adequate amounts. Millions of people are not as fortunate. "1.0 to 2.5 million deaths per year of preschool children—up to 30% of total deaths in that age group—could potentially be averted by bringing vitamin A deficiency under control worldwide. . . . Combined with expanded vitamin A supplementation programs—which will continue to be important—Golden Rice is expected to make a major contribution to improving the health of millions of the world's poorest children" (Rockefeller Foundation Web site).

Commenting on a March 2001 advertisement for Golden Rice that appeared in the *New York Times*, Michael Pollan, author of *The Botany of Desire* and a contributing writer to the *New York Times Magazine*, noted, "Watching the pitch, you can almost feel the moral ground shifting under your feet. For the unspoken challenge here is that if we don't get over our queasiness about eating genetically modified food, kids in the third world will go blind." But Pollan asserts that there is far more to the Golden Rice issue than is initially evident. For example, in order to meet the minimum daily requirement for vitamin A, it would be necessary for an average 11-year-old to eat 15 pounds of cooked Golden Rice. Moreover, in order to convert beta-carotene into vitamin A, fat and protein must be present, and these are lacking in the diet of malnourished children. Pollan also wonders whether Asians will accept rice that is golden in color. It is already well known that brown rice is healthier than white rice, yet Asians consistently prefer white rice. Apparently, at some point, Confucius "extolled the pure whiteness of rice as the ideal backdrop for green vegetables" (Pollan: Section 6, page 15, column 3). Pollan further questions the ethics of an industry that is using the suffering of children to sell its food.

In "Vitamin A Deficiency Disorders: Origins of the Problem and Approaches to Its Control," Alfred Sommer writes that there are some "hurdles" to be overcome before Golden Rice may have an impact on society.

"The strains must be able to grow under the varied conditions in countries with vitamin A deficient populations. The yield and the cost must be attractive to the farmer (or benefit from public sector subsidization). The organoleptic [sensory] qualities of the rice must be acceptable to the target population (women and children). The beta-carotene needs to be bioavailable, the degree dependent on its concentration in the rice, the matrices to which it is bound, the effect of traditional cooking methods and the amount consumed" (Rockefeller Foundation Web site). Sommer warns that Golden Rice will never be a complete solution to the problem of vitamin A deficiency. "Many deficient populations do not consume rice, and even within traditional rice-consuming countries, some high-risk groups will not be able to afford it" (Rockefeller Foundation Web site).

Regardless, it is impossible to deny that the population of the world is growing at a sometimes mind-boggling rate. Presently, the world has about 5 billion people. By the year 2050, that figure will double to 10 billion. Large numbers of these people will live in the developing world, where hunger is rampant. The International Food Information Council states that "by increasing a crop's ability to withstand environmental factors, growers will be able to farm in parts of the world currently unsuitable for crop production. Along with additional food, this could provide the economies of developing nations with much-needed jobs and greater productivity" (International Food Information Council Web site).

Feeding so many people takes a staggering toll on the environment. "Erosion can claim precious topsoil, farm chemicals sometimes reach streams, rivers and ground water supplies, and livestock can deplete grazing lands. Wetlands and other sensitive habitats sometimes get plowed under for use as farmlands. And, in the world's tropical forests where an estimated 90 percent of the world's species exist, poor farmers clear trees in order to provide food and a living for their families." The International Food Information Council believes that GMOs may play a pivotal role in mitigating this burden. Crops that have been genetically modified are often more resistant to disease and require a reduced level of insect control. Therefore, fewer acres need to be planted to reap the same amount of food (International Food Information Council Web site).

One of the key players in the effort to increase the production of rice in Asia has been the Rockefeller Foundation. The foundation believes that GMOs will enable Asian farmers to obtain more rice from the same amount of land. "By the year 2005, the Foundation's hope is to increase rice production in Asia by 20 percent through the use of biotechnology without degrading the environment or reducing farm incomes." The Rockefeller Foundation has also been conducting similar work in Africa. Former President Jimmy Carter, who has become well known for his humanitarian works, has observed that "responsible biotechnology is not the enemy; starvation is. Without adequate food supplies at affordable prices, we cannot expect world health or peace" (International Food Information Council Web site).

EarthSave International disagrees with the notion that genetic engineering may play an important role in feeding the world's growing population. "World hunger is not a problem of technology or insufficient production, but primarily one of unequal distribution and economic inequality. As farmers lose their land and move to the cities, they also lose their food-independence and begin to rely on money, often in dramatically short supply for many in the third world, in order to buy food that they formerly grew themselves" (EarthSave International Web site). In *The Ecological Risks of Engineered Crops*, Jane Rissler and Margaret Mellon agree. "Even if research is done on the right crops and result in increased agricultural productivity, increased production is only one factor in the complicated equation of world hunger. Poverty, trade policies, subsidies, soil erosion, and water shortages are also important causes of hunger. Increases in productivity obtained through genetic engineering will have mixed effects if not developed with due regard to the other important aspects of the hunger problem" (Rissler and Mellon: 20).

In *The Future of Food*, Brian J. Ford, an English scientist, writer, and television host, says that a number of everyday farm animals and crops—such as pigs, cattle, wheat, oats, barley, and rye—are the result of human intervention. "Traditional farmers have been producing new animals and plants by cross-breeding for ten thousand years." While genetic engineering "offers a more radical way of manipulating characteristics," it is fast becoming a part of daily life. "Genetic modification is inevitable. Like electric power, road transport, or computers, it is a facet of the future and the public will gain little by campaigning to ban this potentially rewarding technology. Properly applied, it could offer us so much" (Ford: 64–65).

All the same, Ford does not believe that the public should simply accept whatever the bioengineering companies do. Rather, he calls for a careful monitoring of the industry and the introduction of safeguards. "This is a huge new industry, and it will have pronounced effects on us all. . . . We will need to control it" (Ford: 66). Ford suggests the following controls:

- Approval for new experiments should always be sought from a regulatory authority well versed in the subject.
- None of the members of such a committee should be in a position to benefit commercially from approval.
- No genes conferring problematical properties (e.g., antibiotic resistance) shall be used, whether as markers or otherwise, outside enclosed laboratories.

- Agents capable of transfer to wild plants, like pollen-carrying genes conferring resistance, shall not be liberated into the environment.
- The public shall be consulted about the siting and the benefits of experiments.
- All GMO products should be properly labeled and the source declared.
- Records of possible unwanted side effects should be meticulously maintained. All such events should be investigated by an organization unconnected with the source of the product. (Ford: 78)

ARGUMENTS AGAINST GMOS

The controversy shows no sign of diminishing. GMO opponents present some compelling arguments. The Organic Consumers Association contends that genetic engineering deconstructs basic, fundamental genetic barriers between species. "By combining the genes of dissimilar and unrelated species, permanently altering their genetic codes, novel organisms are created that will pass the genetic changes onto their offspring through heredity. . . . Animal genes and even human genes are being inserted into plants or animals creating unimagined transgenic life" (Organic Consumers Association Web site). Completely new organisms will be created. The association believes that these have the potential to compromise human health and well-being, animal welfare, and the environment. The following are a few examples of ways in which this might occur:

- Genetically engineered organisms can reproduce, migrate, and mutate. If they escape or are released from the laboratory, they could wreak environmental havoc.
- Gene splicing can have unpredictable and dangerous results.
- Genetic engineering of crops and food-producing animals can produce toxic and allergic reactions in humans.
- Safety testing and regulation of genetically engineered organisms are inadequate or lacking.
- Patenting genes they discover and living organisms they create will enable a small corporate elite to own and control the genetic heritage of the planet. (Organic Consumers Association Web site)

The Organic Consumers Association Web site features an ABC News poll on American attitudes toward GMOs. The poll found that only about one-third of the Americans surveyed view GMOs as safe to eat. A little more than half found them unsafe for human consumption. Women, who tend to do the family shopping, were even more against GMOs than men. While 40% of men think that GMOs are unsafe, 62% of women feel that way. A striking percentage of those surveyed—93%—want the federal government to require food labels to indicate the presence of GMOs. Fifty-seven percent said that they were less likely to purchase food that contains GMOs. There are even age differences. "People under 45 are about 10 points more likely than their elders to think genetically modified foods are safe to eat. But a majority of young adults still calls genetically modified foods unsafe" (Organic Consumers Association Web site).

In *Brave New Seeds*, Robert Ali Brac de la Perrière, an international consultant, and Franck Seuret, a journalist, contend that throughout the world, GMOs will weaken the role of small-scale farmers who lack the wherewithal to pay higher prices for genetically modified seeds and lack the expertise that more technically oriented farming demands. Increasingly, large farms will absorb the smaller ones. Further, farmers are losing control over their products. "With transgenic plants, the freedom of agricultural practice and liberty of choice is reduced as the farmer works with a patented product which is subject to very specific conditions of use. For example, contracts for the use of a transgenic soya variety that is resistant to the herbicide RoundUp forbids, amongst other things, the cultivation of other varieties, the use of herbicides other than those allowed by Monsanto and the exchange of seeds with neighbours" (Brac de la Perrière and Seuret: 16).

An article entitled "The Ecological Impacts of Agricultural Biotechnology" by Miguel A. Altieri, which appears on the BioScience Productions Web site, stated that the use of genetically modified herbicide- and insect-resistant crops has limitations. According to Altieri, who teaches agroecology in the Department of Environmental Science, Policy, and Management at the University of California at Berkeley, the most serious problem with resistant crops is that they "steer efforts away from crop diversification and help to maintain cropping systems dominated by one or two annual species." Crop diversification reduces the amount of herbicide and synthetic nitrogen fertilizer that may be needed, improves the quality of soil and water, controls insect-pest and pathogen populations, increases crop yield, and reduces yield variance. Insect-resistant crops may have unintended victims and disrupt other forms of pest control. Also, toxins from these products may remain in the soil for extended periods of time and reduce the level of soil fertility (BioScience Productions Web site).

As if this were not sufficiently problematic, there is the issue of "terminator" seeds, genetically altered plants that are programmed to kill their own seeds. Unlike most plants, these do not regenerate. "After the seeds are planted and the crop matures, the [seed-killing] toxin is produced, killing the new seeds the plants carry" (Kluger: 44). In the previously noted *Genetically Engineered Food*, Martin Teitel and Kimberly A. Wilson say that terminator seeds end the long-held practice of saving seeds for future plantings. "Farmers who use terminator seeds will be forced to buy new seeds for every planting, ending an age-old tradition of seed saving and creating a perpetual cycle of dependence on big seed companies" (Teitel and Wilson: 30). In *Brave New Seeds*, Brac de la Perrière and Seuret observe that terminator seeds "achieved their supreme goal—enslaving their clients" (Brac de la Perrière and Seuret: 26). There is an even more alarming possibility. "Some doomsday scenarios suggest pollen from Terminator plants could drift with the wind like a toxic cloud, cross with ordinary crops or wild plants, and spread from species to species until flora all around the world had been suddenly and irreversibly sterilized" (Kluger: 44). That is probably a huge exaggeration. Gene drift does not occur that easily. A large number of crops pollinate themselves. As for those that do not, border fields may be established to contain genes.

This product was first developed by the U.S. Department of Agriculture and Delta and Pine Land, a Mississippi seed company. Taxpayers funded this effort. Later, it was purchased by Monsanto, a massive biotechnology conglomerate. In 1999, as more reports about terminator seeds were published, there was a huge outpouring of public sentiment against the seeds. Responding to mounting pressure, Monsanto withdrew the terminator seeds, but it is possible that this decision could be reversed.

In "Genetically Modified Foods: Are They a Risk to Human/Animal Health?," Arpad Pusztai, a biochemist who has written about 300 primary peer-reviewed papers as well as several books, concluded that there is a lack of hard data on the effect GMOs may have on humans and animals. Generally, when testing products, the industry has compared a GM food to a non-GM food. "When they are not significantly different the two are regarded as 'substantially equivalent,' and therefore the GM food crop is regarded as safe as its conventional counterpart." Pusztai said that "substantial equivalence is an unscientific concept that has never been properly defined and there are no legally binding rules on how to establish it." Additionally, there are currently no reliable methods to test new genetically engineered crops for food allergies. "It is at present impossible to definitely establish whether a new GM crop is allergenic or not before its release into the human/animal food/feed chain" (BioScience Productions Web site).

CONCLUSION

People who are worried about the safety of GMOs want to reduce their intake of foods in which they may be found. There are no complete guarantees, but there are ways to reduce the risk. Alan McHughen offers some suggestions in his previously noted *Pandora's Picnic Basket*: Organic foods and individual food items are less likely to be genetically modified. A listing of approved genetically modified foods can help one avoid genetically modified fruits and vegetables, which may include tomatoes, potatoes, squash, radishes, and Hawaiian papayas. Meat is usually not genetically modified, but animal feed often is. Ingredients derived from soya or maize are often suspect and can be hidden in many processed foods. In general, convenience foods, snack foods, and highly processed foods are likely to contain genetically modified ingredients (McHughen: 240–241).

Though the controversy shows no sign of diminishing, the market for genetically engineered crops continues to grow. In 1995, global sales were projected at $75 million. Five years later, that had reached about $3 billion. By 2005, the figure is expected to climb to $8 billion. But, future research may change the public's opinion of genetically modified foods.

TOPICS FOR DISCUSSION

1. Before reading this chapter, had you ever heard of genetically modified organisms? Now that you know more about them, would you want to eat them? Why or why not?

2. Do you believe that there is a significant difference between food that is grown using the traditional methods and food that is genetically modified? Why or why not?

3. Should genetically modified foods be labeled? Why or why not?

4. How did you respond when you read that genes from rats were inserted into lettuce seeds? Do you believe that such modifications should be permitted? Why or why not?

5. What role do you think genetically modified foods are able to play in feeding the millions of hungry people in the world? What are some of the limitations?

REFERENCES AND RESOURCES

Books

Anderson, Luke. *Genetic Engineering, Food, and Our Environment*. White River Junction, Vermont: Chelsea Green Publishing Company, 1999.

Brac de la Perrière, Robert Ali, and Franck Seuret. *Brave New Seeds*. New York: Zed Books, 2000.

Cummins, Ronnie, and Ben Lilliston. *Genetically Engineered Food*. New York: Marlowe and Company, 2000.

Ford, Brian J. *The Future of Food*. New York: Thames and Hudson, 2000.

Lappé, Marc, and Britt Bailey. *Against the Grain*. Monroe, Maine: Common Courage Press: 1998.

Marshall, Elizabeth. *High-Tech Harvest*. Danbury, Connecticut: Franklin Watts, 1999.

McHughen, Alan. *Pandora's Picnic Basket*. New York: Oxford University Press, 2000.

Rissler, Jane, and Margaret Mellon. *The Ecological Risks of Engineered Crops*. Cambridge, Massachusetts: MIT Press, 1996.

Teitel, Martin, and Kimberly A. Wilson. *Genetically Engineered Food*. Rochester, Vermont: Park Street Press, 1999.

Magazines, Journals, and Newspapers

Ando, Amy W., and Madhu Khanna. "Environmental Costs and Benefits of Genetically Modified Crops." *American Behavioral Scientist*, November 2000, 44(3): 435–463.

Conway, Gordon. "Food for All in the 21st Century." *Environment*, January–February 2000, 42(1): 8–18.

Crossette, Barbara. "Move to Curb Biotech Crops Ignores Poor, U.N. Finds." *New York Times*, July 8, 2001: Section 1, page 4, column 1.

Follett, Peter A. "GM: Mark of Excellence?" *American Scientist*, January 2001, 89(1): 76.

Gower, Timothy. "Should You Fear the New Foods?" *Better Homes and Gardens*, November 2000, 78(11): 256–262.

Grossman, Margaret Rosso, and A. Bryan Endres. "Regulation of Genetically Modified Organisms in the European Union." *American Behavioral Scientist*, November 2000, 44(3): 378–434.

Hegarty, P. Vincent. "Covering Issues in Biotechnology and Genetically Modified Organisms (GMO's)." *Quill*, April 2000, 88(3): 25.

Kluger, Jeffrey. "The Suicide Seeds: Terminator Genes Could Mean Big Biotech Bucks—But Big Trouble Too, As a Grass-Roots Protest Breaks Out on the Net." *Time*, February 1, 1999, 153(4): 44.

Kohl, Danny. "GM Food—Another View." *Nation*, April 16, 2001, 272(15): 7.

Marwick, Charles. "Genetically Modified Crops Feed Ongoing Controversy." *JAMA: The Journal of the American Medical Association*, January 12, 2000, 283(2): 188–190.

Maynard, Cindy. "Biotech at the Table." *Current Health 2*, November 2000, 27(3): 22.

McInnis, Doug, and Gunjan Sinha. "Genes, They're What's for Dinner." *Popular Science*, April 2000, 256(4) 64–68.

Parle, Elizabeth. "GM Crops: More Food, or Thought?" *Chemical Market Reporter*, March 20, 2000, 257(12): FR 10, FR 12.

Pollack, Andrew. "E.P.A. Rejects Use of a Gene-Altered Corn in Human Food." *New York Times,* July 28, 2001: Section C, page 4, column 3.

Pollan, Michael. "The Way We Live Now: The Great Yellow Hype." *New York Times,* March 4, 2001: Section 6, page 15, column 3.

Sardar, Ziauddin. "Facts and Friction." *New Statesman,* November 1, 1999, 128 (4460): 42.

Shelton, Deborah L. "Frankenfoods." *Essence,* July 2000, 31(3): 78.

Stipp, David. "The Voice of Reason in the Global Food Fight: Rockefeller Foundation Chief Gordon Conway Has Emerged as the One Thought Leader Neither Side Can Ignore in the High-Stakes Biofoods War—and the Best Hope for an Outcome All Six Billion of Us Can Live With." *Fortune,* February 21, 2000, 141(4): 164+.

Thayer, Warren. "Pardon, Is That a Fish Gene in Your Frozen Veggies?" *Frozen Food Age,* March 2000, 48(4): 34–36.

Organizations to Contact

BioScience Productions, Inc.
423-4486
1401 Casey Key Road
Nokomis, FL 34275
Phone: 941-423-8636
http://www.actionbioscience.org/ (July 29, 2001)

Council for Biotechnology Information
P.O. Box 34380
Washington, DC 20043-0308
Phone: 202-467-6565
http://www.whybiotech.com/ (August 14, 2001)

The Council for Responsible Genetics
5 Upland Road, Suite 3
Cambridge, MA 02140
Phone: 617-868-0870
http://www.gene-watch.org/ (September 2, 2001)

EarthSave International
1509 Seabright Avenue, Suite B1
Santa Cruz, CA 95062
Phone: 831-423-0293
http://www.earthsave.org/ (August 5, 2001)

International Food Information Council
1100 Connecticut Avenue NW, Suite 430
Washington, DC 20036
Phone: 202-296-6540
http://www.ific.org/ (August 8, 2001)

National Food Processors Association
1350 I Street NW, Suite 300
Washington, DC 20005
Phone: 202-639-5900
http://www.nfpa-food.org/ (August 8, 2001)

Organic Consumers Association
6101 Cliff Estate Road
Little Marais, MN 55614
Phone: 218-226-4164
http://www.purefood.org/ (August 14, 2001)

The Rockefeller Foundation
420 Fifth Ave.
New York, NY 10018-2702
Phone: 212-869-8500
http://www.rockfound.org/ (September 2, 2001)

Union of Concerned Scientists
2 Brattle Square
Cambridge, MA 02238
Phone: 617-547-5552
http://www.ucsusa.org/ (August 14, 2001)

United States Department of Agriculture
14th and Independence Ave. SW
Washington, DC 20250
Phone: 202-720-2791
http://www.usda.gov/ (August 3, 2001)

United States Food and Drug Administration
5600 Fishers Lane
Rockville, MD 20857
Phone: 1-888-INFO-FDA (1-888-463-6332)
http://www.fda.gov/ (August 6, 2001)

Index

Acheson, David W.K., 106–7
additives
  adverse reactions to, 4
  approval process, 3–4
  benefits of, 2, 5–6
  color, 3, 4
  concerns about, 6, 17, 20–21
  defined, 1–3
  history of, 2–3
  margin of safety on, 5
Additives (Nottridge), 3
advanced meat recovery (AMR), 90
Adverse Reaction Monitoring System
    (ARMS), 4, 8
aging process, 171, 177–78, 207
AIDS, 155, 174, 179
Ajinomoto Company, 7
Akst, Daniel, 38–39
alfalfa sprouts, 105
All-Bran, 119
allergens, 108, 137–38
alpha lipoic acid, 178–79
Alpha Lipoic Acid Breakthrough, The
    (Berkson), 179
Alpha Lipoic Acid (Sosin and Jacobs),
    178–79
Altieri, Miguel A., 242
Alzheimer's disease
  and ginkgo, 183
  linked with aspartame, 16, 18

linked with MSG, 7, 10
not linked with MSG, 9
and vitamin E, 174
*American Dietetic Association's Complete
    Food and Nutrition Guide, The*
    (Duyff), 225–26
American Heart Association, 102–4,
    128
American Meat Institute Foundation,
    59
amyotropic lateral sclerosis, 195
Anderson, Terence, Dr., 156–57
anemia, 52–53, 110, 184
animal feed, 55
animal rights, 43, 45, 47–48, 54–60
antibiotics, 46
  contamination of milk with, 70–71,
    72, 73, 74
  and organic foods, 193
  resistance to, 74
antioxidants
  aid cancer growth, 175–76
  fight cholesterol, 178–79
  foods high in, 174, 177–78, 180–81,
    183, 184
  function of, 172
  in Okinawan diet, 227
  recommendations for, 184–85
Apple, Rima D., 147, 158–59
Applebaum, Rhona S., 85–86

apples, 178
Arby's, 166
arteriosclerosis, 173
arthritis, 171, 181–82, 206
arthritis, rheumatoid, 49, 109, 113, 181–82
aspartame, 14–18
  adverse reactions to, 15, 17–18
  safety of, 14–16
Aspartame (NutraSweet*): Is It Safe? (Roberts), 17–18
asthma, 4, 8–9, 174, 195
Atkins, Robert C., 205
Atkins Diet, 205–6
Atoms for Peace program, 27
attention deficit hyperactivity disorder (ADHD), 6
autoimmune disorders, 111. *See also* AIDS
Avery, Dennis T., 199
A Week in the Zone (Sears), 207

baby food
  MSG in, 7
  pesticides in, 196–97
bacteria, radiation resistant, 37
Balingasa, Nancy and Eduardo, 2, 4–5
bananas, 113, 222
Bartimeus, Paula, 195
beef
  European consumption of, 88
  ground, 26
  nutritional content of, 45
  U.S. consumption of, 91
Being a Vegan (Weiss), 55
Being Vegan (Stepaniak), 141
Berkely, California, 197
Berkson, Burt, 179
beta-carotene, 112, 113, 183–84
bioflavonoids, and leukemia, 153
birth defects, 18, 46
Blackburn, Henry, 19
Blaylock, Russell L., 7
Block, Keith, 49–50
Block Medical Center, 49–50
blood clots, 114
blood types, 221
blueberries, 177–78, 185

Body Code, The (Cooper and Lance), 224–25
Body Code (diet), 224–25
body-mass index (BMI), 215
Boston Market, 164
bovine somatotropin. *See* hormone treatments for animals
bovine spongiform encephalopathy (BSE). *See* mad cow disease
Brac de la Perrière, Robert Ali, 242, 243
brain
  and aspartame, 16
  damage to, 9
  tumors in, 18
Braly, James, 112
Brave New Seeds (Brac de la Perrière and Seuret), 242, 243
bread, white, 3
Breast Cancer Prevention Program, The (Epstein, Steinman, LeVert), 68–69, 72–73
bribery, 83–84
broccoli, 112, 184, 185
Brody, Jane, 52, 82, 153–54
Brostoff, Jonathan, 108–9
Brownell, Kelly, 163
brown rice, 112–13
bST/rBGH. *See* hormone treatments for animals
bulk-food bins and cross-contamination, 139
Burger King, 134
Burros, Marian, 129

calcium
  foods high in, 112, 113
  in high-protein diets, 210–11
  inadequate intake of, 125
  problems with megadoses, 154
  in the vegetarian diet, 51–52, 53
Campbell, P. Samuel, 155
campylobacter (bacteria), 25–26
cancer
  effect of diet on, 19, 46, 49–50, 104, 119, 206
  foods useful against, 113–14, 178

About the Authors

MYRNA CHANDLER GOLDSTEIN is an independent scholar and the coauthor, with Mark Goldstein, of *Controversies in the Practice of Medicine* (Greenwood, 2001) and *Boys into Men* (Greenwood, 2000).

MARK A. GOLDSTEIN, M.D., an adolescent medicine specialist, is chief of Pediatrics and Student Health Services at the Massachusetts Institute of Technology and assistant clinical professor of pediatrics at the Harvard Medical School. He is coauthor, with Myrna Chandler Goldstein, of *Controversies in the Practice of Medicine* (Greenwood, 2001) and *Boys into Men* (Greenwood, 2000).

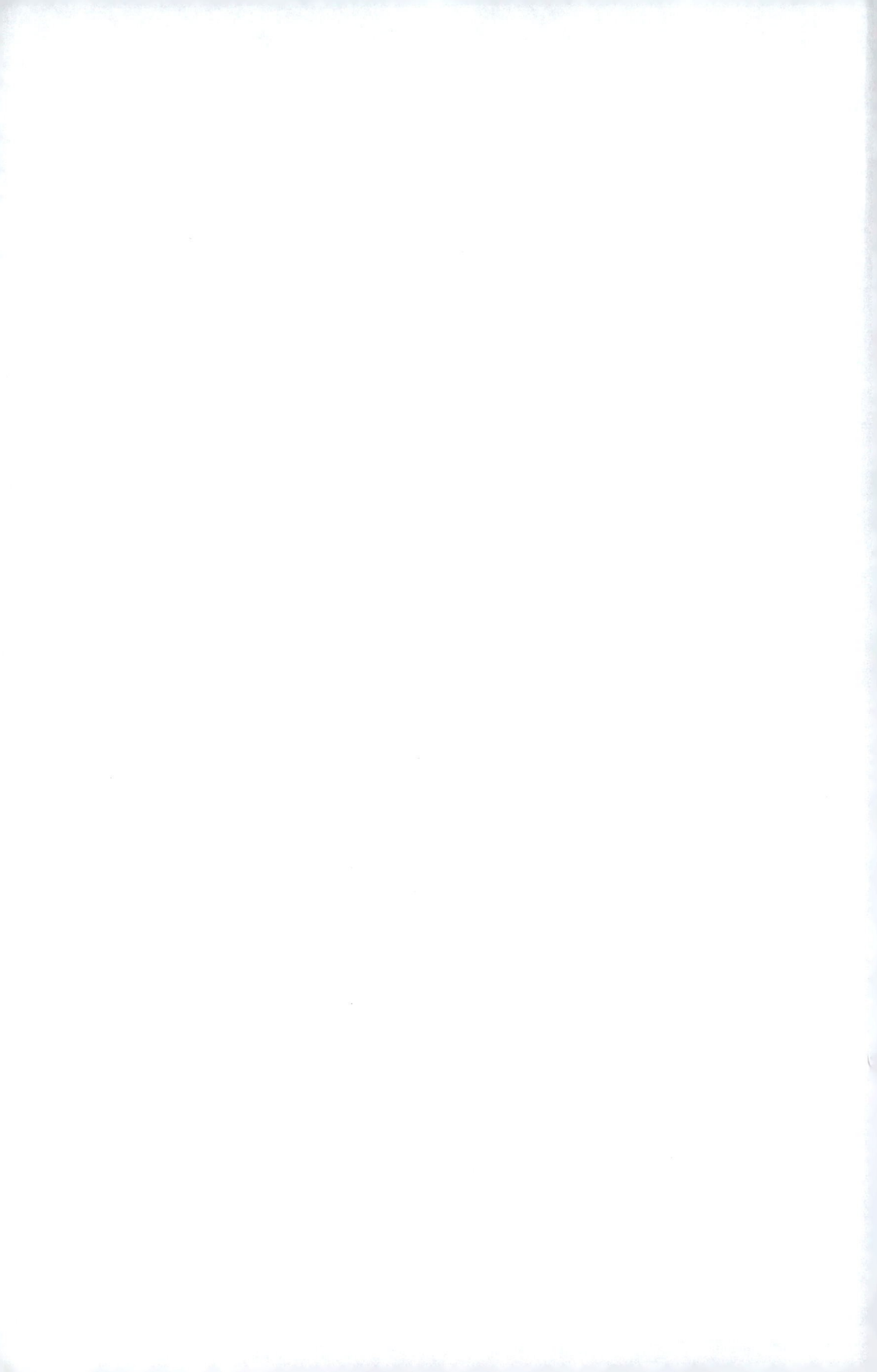

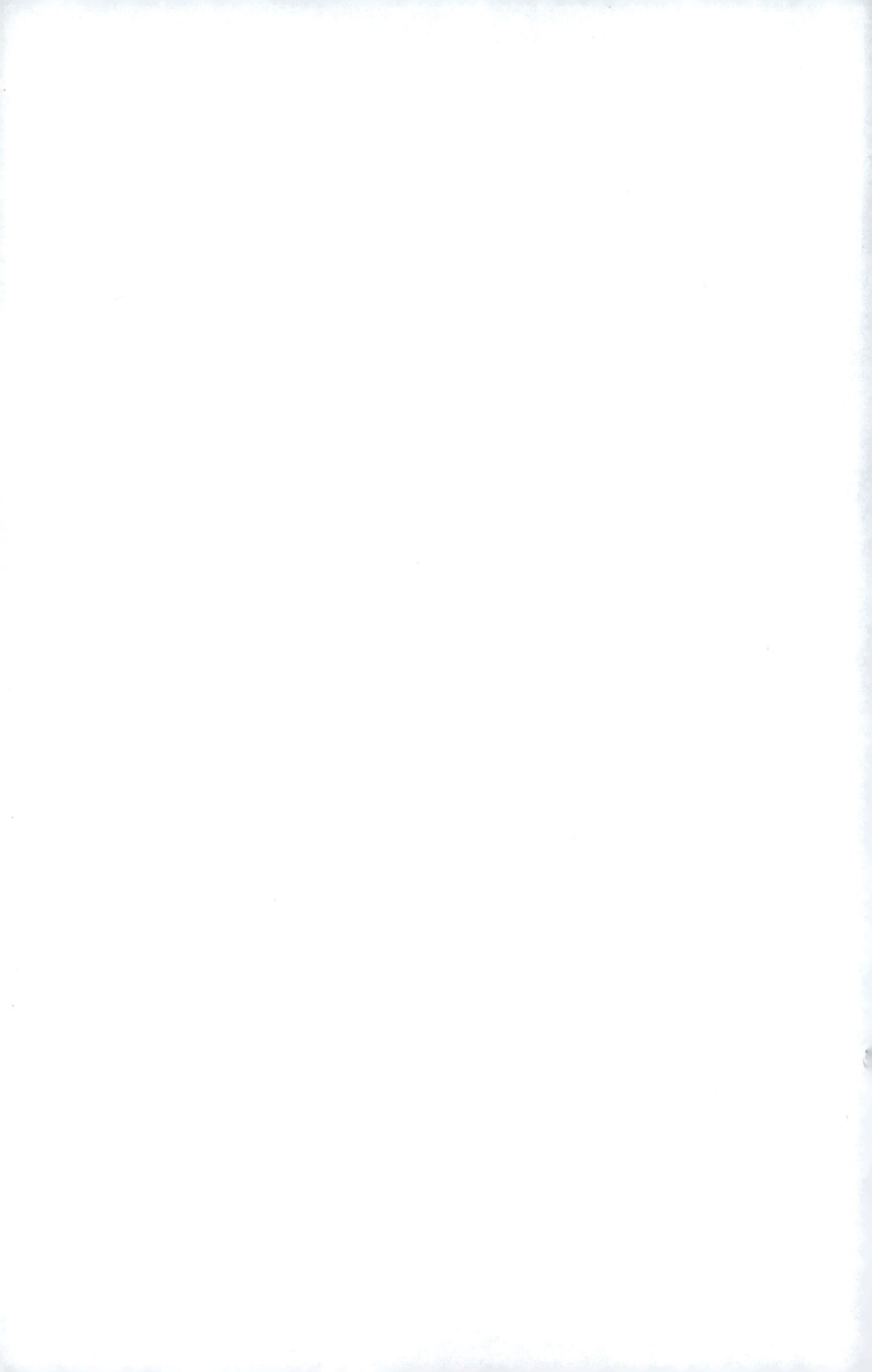